THEOLOGICAL BIOETHICS

Moral Traditions series

JAMES F. KEENAN, S.J., *series editor*

American Protestant Ethics and the Legacy of H. Richard Niebuhr
William Werpehowski

Aquinas and Empowerment: Classical Ethics for Ordinary Lives
G. Simon Harak, S.J., Editor

Aquinas, Feminism, and the Common Good
Susanne M. DeCrane

The Banality of Good and Evil: Moral Lessons from the Shoah and Jewish Tradition
David R. Blumenthal

Bridging the Sacred and the Secular: Selected Writings of John Courtney Murray
J. Leon Hooper, S.J., Editor

A Call to Fidelity: On the Moral Theology of Charles E. Curran
James J. Walter, Timothy E. O'Connell, and Thomas A. Shannon, Editors

The Catholic Moral Tradition Today: A Synthesis
Charles E. Curran

Catholic Social Teaching, 1891–Present: A Historical, Theological, and Ethical Analysis
Charles E. Curran

The Christian Case for Virtue Ethics
Joseph J. Kotva, Jr.

The Context of Casuistry
James F. Keenen, S.J., and Thomas A. Shannon, Editors

Democracy on Purpose: Justice and the Reality of God
Franklin I. Gamwell

The Ethics of Aquinas
Stephen J. Pope

Ethics and Economics of Assisted Reproduction: The Cost of Longing
Maura A. Ryan

The Evolution of Altruism and the Ordering of Love
Stephen J. Pope

The Fellowship of Life: Virtue Ethics and Orthodox Christianity
Joseph Woodill

Feminist Ethics and Natural Law: The End of the Anathemas
Cristina L. H. Traina

The Global Face of Public Faith: Politics, Human Rights, and Christian Ethics
David Hollenbach, S.J.

The Ground Beneath the Cross: The Theology of Ignacio Ellacuría
Kevin F. Burke, S.J.

Heroes, Saints, and Ordinary Morality
Andrew Michael Flescher

Introduction to Jewish and Catholic Bioethics: A Comparative Analysis
Aaron L. Mackler

Jewish and Catholic Bioethics: An Ecumenical Dialogue
Edmund D. Pellegrino and Alan I. Faden, Editors

John Paul II and the Legacy of Dignitatis Humanae
Hermínio Rico

Josef Fuchs on Natural Law
Mark Graham

Love, Human and Divine: The Heart of Christian Ethics
Edward Collins Vacek, S.J.

Medicine and the Ethics of Care
Diana Fritz Cates and Paul Lauritzen, Editors

The Moral Theology of Pope John Paul II
Charles E. Curran

The Origins of Moral Theology in the United States: Three Different Approaches
Charles E. Curran

Shaping the Moral Life: An Approach to Moral Theology
Klaus Demmer
James F. Keenan, S.J., Editor

Who Count as Persons? Human Identity and the Ethics of Killing
John F. Kavanaugh, S.J.

THEOLOGICAL BIOETHICS

Participation, Justice, and Change

LISA SOWLE CAHILL

GEORGETOWN UNIVERSITY PRESS
Washington, D.C.

Georgetown University Press, Washington, D.C.

Printed in the United States of America

10 9 8 7 6 5 4 3 2 2005

This book is printed on acid-free paper meeting the requirements of the American National Standard for Permanence in Paper for Printed Library Materials.

As of January 1, 2007, 13-digit ISBN numbers will replace the current 10-digit system. Hardcover: 978-1-58901-074-1; paperback: 978-1-58901-075-8.

Library of Congress Cataloging-in-Publication Data

Cahill, Lisa Sowle.
Theological bioethics : participation, justice, and change / Lisa Sowle Cahill.
p. cm.—(Moral traditions series)
Includes bibliographical references and index.
ISBN 1-58901-074-4 (alk. paper)—ISBN 1-58901-075-2 (pbk. : alk. paper)
1. Medical ethics—Religious aspects—Christianity. 2. Religion—Social aspects. 3. Religion and politics. 4. Theology. I. Title. II. Series.
R725.56.C34 2005
174′.957—dc22 2005010167

To my sister,

Maryann Sowle, R.N.,

who has raised six children, foster-mothered many more, serves as a cardiac intensive care nurse at George Washington University Hospital, keeps our dad company, and still finds time to ride her Harley.

CONTENTS

INTRODUCTION

THIS WORK AIMS to take theological bioethics beyond the parameters that usually define its role in public discourse today. Secular bioethicists and policymakers seem anxious to keep explicitly religious views off the table and assume that religion leads in a socially conservative direction, obstructing scientific advancement and going against the tide of enlightened social policy. Many theologians react either by accusing most theological bioethicists of having been co-opted by the minimalist morality of the policymakers or by giving up entirely on the prospect that theological engagement in the public sphere will have any significant social results.

Religious *activists,* especially from the political right, fight for their causes with grassroots organizing, political tactics, and overtly religious values and rhetoric. But this is much less true of *academic* theologians and scholars, especially those on the left. Theologians informed by the common good tradition of Catholic social teaching are among those who most consistently try to present justice concerns as integral to bioethics. Yet Catholic advocates for health care justice seem to keep getting sidelined by public debates that reduce Catholic moral commitments to the protection of embryos and fetuses, as embodied especially in the perceived priorities of the pro-life movement. This situation has been exacerbated by the choice of many Catholic bishops in recent years to throw their support behind the rights of the unborn more publicly than behind health care reform.

I propose that Christian theological bioethics should make justice in access to health care resources its first priority. This priority includes justice in global access to the goods essential to health. While justice for the poor and the reform of health care systems to make them more inclusive might be associated with progressive or even liberal politics, I am convinced that these goals are mandated by the New Testament depiction of Jesus' healing ministry to society's outcasts, a portrayal to which all Christians subscribe. According to the Catholic theologian Edward Schillebeeckx, "On the basis of Jesus' message, parables, and his praxis of the reign of God, we see how the biblical concept of God is essentially bound up with a praxis of persons who liberate their fellow human beings, just as Jesus did before us."[1] This work of liberation is not just a secondary pastoral application of revealed doctrine. "No, the option for the poor is *a datum of revelation*." The incarnation is "an identification of God in Jesus with the poor, oppressed, and finally executed innocent individual, for whom Jesus stands as a model."[2]

Jim Wallis—a Protestant social ethicist and editor of *Sojourners*, an ecumenical and countercultural social justice magazine—not only agrees that the biblical portrayal of Jesus demands work for justice but believes that the so-called left and right wings of the Christian churches need not be so far apart on this issue. "Religion and moral values don't fall neatly into right and left political categories." In fact, "poverty, and a serious commitment to address it at home and globally, could become part of a new common ground because the conservative and liberal sides care about it."[3] Christians on the right and the left could come together in a new politics that is progressive on the goal of economic justice.[4]

The language of the common good, inclusion, distributive justice, and solidarity can be valuable in helping theology to raise the profile of justice in public discourse.[5] Explicitly religious narratives and symbols can also have a public role in widening the moral imaginations of people from diverse traditions and faiths. Most importantly, however, theological bioethics is not just about talk. It is about action. The "truth" and viability of the vision of Christian theological bioethics is warranted not just by cogent theory or argument but by the emergence of transformative practices that join with other movements in global civil society to encourage human solidarity, empower "the poor," and motivate the powerful to change.

This work will first develop a proposal for the engagement of theology in public bioethics, then apply this proposal in the following areas: aging, decline, and dying; health care access reform; AIDS; "beginning of life" technologies; and human genetics and biotechnology. The primary thrust of the argument will be that bioethics in the twenty-first century must in every case be social ethics, not just as theory but as engagement. This is particularly true in light of globalization. However, even when the focus is what has traditionally been called "individual" moral decision making, it is now recognized that the knowledge, options, and judgments of individuals have always been highly context dependent. Thus individual bioethical decisions cannot be and never have been separated from social ethics. This has become evident, for instance, from work on casuistry, virtue, the social location of knowledge, and the growing contributions of philosophers and theologians from the developing world to bioethics.

A new item on the agenda of both theology and public bioethics is examining critically the connections among individual decisions and social practices, with the aim of showing how practices that favor the privileged and enable their free choices and access to resources carry a negative impact for global health patterns and the resources and choices of the poor. This phenomenon has been amply addressed by varieties of Christian bioethics informed by liberation theology and by Catholic social teaching. Building on this analysis, something more is now demanded.

Constructively, this book will argue that theological bioethics must go beyond decrying injustice, beyond taking a "prophetic" stance against social practices that commercialize human beings, the human body and its processes, or important human relationships. It must even move beyond painting a vision of a more egalitarian and solidaristic future. Theological bioethics must critically reflect on, make normative judgments about, theoretically account for, and ultimately take part in a global social network of mobilization for change. Schillebeeckx calls theology "the self-consciousness of Christian praxis" and links theology to Christian practices by means of an obligation to examine those practices critically, as well as to voice theologically what "is implied in the new activities and patterns of behavior of the believing community." In fact, "theology is valueless, whether it is progressive or conservative, as soon as it loses contact with the empirical basis of the praxis of believers."[6]

Robert Schreiter writes of four interreligious "global theological flows" in which Christianity participates: theologies of liberation, of feminism, of ecology, and of human rights.[7] To these can be added bioethics. Religious discourses contribute to joined "antisystemic" action, though they are not uniform because they originate in specific cultural contexts. Yet religions share a drive toward coherence, prophetic resistance to exploitation, and a transcendent framework for evaluating human projects. Although religious symbols can be co-opted by violent and exclusionary social interests, religion still remains a potent political force that can help to form social virtues of solidarity, commitment, and hope.

Theological bioethics can and should take account of grassroots movements, and their midlevel and transnational counterparts, in its normative delineations of the common good and of social organizations that support it. Christian theological bioethics must help make the case that different ways of doing things are both morally desirable and possible. Not resting content with seeking the moral high ground, forming countercultural communities "apart" from society, or inveighing against national and international policy setters, theological bioethics must renew efforts toward involvement in social and political processes. It must recognize, put down roots in, and energetically promote widespread, multileveled, and participatory efforts to change the status quo.

One distinctive implication of this line of argument is that theologians can and should be involved in *public discourse,* sometimes even by introducing explicitly religious symbols and narratives. Another is a working assumption that many *common moral values* regarding life and health can be defended across cultures, despite the particularity of moral practices and perspectives. Further, patterns of *social sin* need to be targeted adamantly by theological analysis and action in bioethics. The approach proposed here will be critical of disproportionate social valuing of individual choice and of scientific progress, skeptical about whether technological "advancements" are truly beneficent, politically engaged on behalf of a "preferential option for the poor"[8] and of gender equity, and confident about the possibility and potential of concerted action for change.

Activism and theory are interdependent, and this has implications for the way bioethics should be conceived theoretically today. Theological bioethics must incorporate the fact of mobilization around health care issues into bioethical theory and into a reconceptualization of the "field" of bioethics and its "public voice." Catholic social teaching, with its commitments to the dignity of persons, common good, and subsidiarity, offers one helpful resource for theorizing and advocating a normative, activist, and transformationist Christian bioethical stance. For example, subsidiarity implies both the relative autonomy of local organizations and the responsibility of government to reign in or modify "subsidiary" action that is detrimental to the common good. In the globalization era, what has changed is the idea that a global "public authority" can ensure this balance internationally. Therefore subsidiarity has to be reconceived so that the vertical dynamic of influence expands to include horizontal and much more pluralistic exercises of authority and efficacy, characterized by collaboration and power sharing. The emphasis in this work will be on Christian, especially Catholic, theology, but ecumenical and interreligious connections and resources will certainly be valued. A critical renegotiation of Catholic social tradition is essential to correct the bias toward placing power, responsibility, and authority at the top of a social pyramid, rather than recognizing and endorsing the power of popular social movements and of emerging forms of global civil society, such as nongovernmental organizations (NGOs) and activist networks.

An outline of subsequent chapters will provide an introduction to the way essential theses of this work will be displayed and defended in relation to the history of contemporary bioethics and to essential topics in the field. Chapters 1 and 2 offer an interpretative history of the field of theological bioethics, along with a proposal regarding the practical role of theological bioethics in changing social relationships and institutions. This overview will allow the reader to see in advance how the more theoretical considerations in the first chapters are important for and will eventually be connected to the specific bioethical issues addressed in the final five chapters. The trajectory of the book is not only to analyze problems like physician-assisted suicide, abortion, commercialized reproduction, lack of access to health care, and AIDS, but to make the case that theological bioethics can alleviate the social conditions that create these problems.

A complaint frequently heard about the current state of Christian bioethics is that theology has become marginal to the whole enterprise and that the distinctive impact of the theological contribution has been miserably reduced as a result. Early theological participants in the formation of bioethics, some argue, had credibility precisely because of their clear identification with faith communities (e.g., Paul Ramsey, Richard McCormick, James Gustafson). Because later theologians have downplayed religious roots and identity in their efforts to be heard in "secular" clinical settings and policy forums, it is said, they have paid the ironic price of increasing irrelevance. While some recommend a return to a more distinctive community witness against cultural trends, others try to reinvigorate community commitment to what is still ultimately an engagement with legislators and policymakers on their own terms. Yet neither of these alternatives fully appreciates the potential of religious communities to engage with others for the common good, while voicing rather than repressing their own identities.

Chapter 1, "Theologians and Bioethics: Some History and a Proposal," asserts that what is needed is a new synthesis of Christian bioethics that takes into account the contextuality and historicity of moral knowledge; the reality and changing manifestations of social sin; the emerging social infrastructures and superstructures entailed by the globalization of communications, travel, finance, and science; and the practical and theoretical opportunities that now exist for theological bioethics to make an impact on all these realities. Christian theological bioethics can and must compete with other equally "thick" and more dominant cultural narratives of liberal individualism, scientific progress, and the market.

Theology and theological bioethics do not proceed in the abstract, however "over the heads" of the persons and groups whose lives they affect. Theological bioethics is a form of participatory discourse, offering a vision, a voice, and action that can carry into the sphere of democratic activism, both locally and globally. Participatory bioethics is partly embedded in and partly a reflection on action for social change. It links normative theory with the practical conditions that allow change to occur. A new, more self-conscious and critical participatory theological bioethics is crucial both for health care reform in North America and for health care justice worldwide.

Chapter 2, "Participatory Theological Bioethics in Action," illustrates more specifically why participatory bioethics is possible and necessary and what it looks like in practice. Evidence and examples are drawn from Christian social ethics, history, sociology, theories of democratic politics, and the record of religious lobbying and community organizing around issues of labor, housing, and health care. Parallel concepts or precedents to "participatory theological bioethics," joining forces with other moral traditions and organizations, can be found in the Protestant language of "middle axioms" and the Catholic language of "subsidiarity" and "contributive justice." Historical and sociological descriptions of the development of the twentieth-century Western (especially U.S.) ethos of "participatory democracy" are brought into conversation with political science literature on consensus-building "deliberative democracy" and on the emergence of new forms of decentralized global governance. These resources reveal many contexts and opportunities in which participatory theological bioethics can flourish.

Contrary to the hypothesis that modern societies inevitably become secularized, religious participation and activism are alive and well in the United States and have been in the past invested in both conservative and liberal causes, including protests against the Vietnam War, in support of civil rights, and about end-of-life medical care, school prayer, abortion, and gay rights. Yet, in recent years at least, conservative groups have been much more willing to use overt appeals to ultimate values and worldviews, enabling greater success at grassroots conversion to their goals. More expansive normative discourse, including the judicious use of religious stories and symbols, would enhance political participation by "progressive" theological bioethics that aims at social justice, defined as inclusive participation in the common good.

At the global level, participatory bioethics must seek out opportunities for democratic participation in the quickly changing and decentralized world order, and it must find ways to explicitly name and claim its own ultimate values, while engaging practically and productively with other faith traditions that are doing the same. Jewish and Muslim scholars join Christians in cautiously optimistic evaluation of the prospects for identifying common concerns and aims and formulating cooperative forms of participation that can change social conditions for the better in matters of health and elsewhere.

The main thrust of chapter 3, "Decline and Dying: Cultural and Theological Interpretations," is to show how bioethical concerns, especially in Catholic moral theology, have moved from a focus on individual decision making to a social analysis of the conditions under which life and health are sustained cross-culturally. Aging and the decline of abilities are universal phenomena that cultures accommodate differently. It is important to take a broader look at how aging, decline, and dying are experienced and interpreted in modern Western cultures, in comparison with others. Independence, dependence, and interdependence are all part of the human condition and must be balanced in view of personal and spiritual values and relationships. Those who advocate physician-assisted suicide and those who advocate keeping patients indefinitely on artificial nutrition and hydration both reflect an overly technological and overly individualistic approach to decline and death. The elderly live more fulfilling lives when they are integrated into their communities and continue to participate to the degree to which they are able; the same is true of the chronically or terminally ill. In the same vein, discussions of "death and dying" are no longer concerned primarily with which specific interventions should or should not be permitted for which patient.

Efforts of the Catholic Health Association to enhance community care for the elderly, including housing, and the "friendship" with the elderly that is part of the mission of the international lay community of Sant'Egidio exemplify participatory theological bioethics as it creates innovative social practices of support for the elderly and others in physical decline.

This chapter prepares the way for the next two chapters on defining proportionate and disproportionate means of medical care and on health care access, both nationally and internationally. Economics is an important factor in determining that some people are subjected to excessive technologies in serious illness and in the dying process, while others suffer exclusion from the health care system.

The foundation of chapter 4, "Decline and Dying: Principles of Analysis and Practices of Solidarity," is the distinction between ordinary and extraordinary means of life support. This distinction, used in combination with the principle of double effect, functioned traditionally as a way primarily to assist individual patients and their caregivers to ascertain the moral limits of the obligation to preserve life. However, even within this traditional usage, the sociality of the person was implied by the proviso that economic considerations and burdens to families could be taken into account in determining whether a means of life support was morally mandatory or not.

The thesis of this chapter is that social and relational considerations help constitute the "objective" morality of health care decisions made in the face of severe illness and death and that "individual" and "society" are interdependent rather than competing objects of moral concern. However, a corollary of this thesis is that, to the extent that real social circumstances can present agents with no good solutions to dilemmas, "objective" morality can require decisions that are far from ideal. Decisions about sustaining life in situations of scarce resources, for example, often reflect tragic and sinful circumstances that place agents in unbearable yet inescapable conflict situations.

The necessity to define moral truth and goodness against a horizon of forced choices requires a moral theory with room for paradoxical moral truthfulness and the exercise of what might be called "adverse virtue." This requirement is especially evident when even the best medical resources are powerless to make the suffering of the dying person tolerable or when resources are not available to sustain a life that otherwise could go on. Participatory bioethics, taking action to limit if not eliminate such situations, will be illustrated by the hospice movement and by international efforts to provide community-based services for those dying of AIDS.

Traditional analyses of death and dying acknowledge, at least implicitly, that decisions about health care take place in the context of relationships, social interdependence, and social obligations. However, bioethics through the middle of the twentieth century, both in Catholic moral theology and in North American culture and medical practice generally, still concentrated attention on individual decisions and guarantees of "autonomy."

These same decades saw the rapid development of biomedical technology in cultural contexts (such as in North America) where basic health care was assumed to be available to most. In the United States, high-tech end-of-life care became almost routine for those who had access to such care at all. The 1990s produced efforts at health care reform, stemming from the realization that many Americans lack health insurance, that expensive types of technological medicine create a disproportionate drain on the health care system, and that these types of medicine often fail to serve either the wishes or the welfare of the patients to whom they are applied.

Chapter 5, "National and International Health Access Reform," offers a critical overview of the maldistribution of health care resources in the United States and of recent attempts at reform. The larger and more important issue, however, is access to health care worldwide. Beyond decrying the injustice of health inequities, this chapter links them to other patterns of social access (education, gender, market economics). More importantly, it begins to address grassroots and transnational activism for change in these patterns. Heightened awareness of and action for global means to combat diseases of the poor, such as AIDS, tuberculosis, and malaria, while hardly triumphant in the struggle against exclusionary patterns of health care, have had and are having enough impact in the global order to give Christian social bioethics authority and hope. Particular attention is given to the impact of AIDS on women and the poor, to the interconnected global causes of AIDS, and to local and transnational efforts to ameliorate the consequences of AIDS and to halt its spread.

Chapter 6, "Reproduction and Early Life," takes the focus off inflamed and highly divisive debates about the "personal" status of early human life, ostensibly in a life or death contest with the "autonomy" and "needs" of adults, especially women. Instead, this chapter emphasizes social practices and a social ethos that do or do not support birth, life, health, women, and families. Unintentionally, both pro-choice and pro-life advocates can play into a cultural atmosphere in which women's autonomous choice equates to the burden of sole responsibility for enduring or resolving problematic situations surrounding pregnancy, birth, and infertility. The same individualistic and freedom-centered social ethos legitimates the liberty of scientists and researchers to promote technological "solutions" to infertility, claiming the right to use or create embryos for research and to develop and market biomedical interventions based on stem cell and cloning research.

It can hardly be denied that the entire realm and history of social control over reproduction, and of reproductive ethics, shows the need to value respect for the dignity, freedom, and self-determination of all persons, even granting that personal freedom is always conditioned by social contexts and responsibilities. Feminist bioethics has its origins in advocacy for legitimate reproductive freedom and rights for women. Significantly, however, Catholic feminist theologians and ethicists seek equality for women in the areas of sex, marriage, parenthood, and family, without making "abortion rights" the centerpiece of their cause to the same extent that has been the case in the pro-choice movement.

In recent work on reproductive issues, feminist theologians (Protestant as well as Catholic) have turned their attention to the social contexts and practices that approve and permit the use of reproductive technologies and research on embryos. Not limiting their vision to the encroachment of a market and consumer ethos on the sphere of reproductive activity in the "developed" world, they take up the cause of women in less privileged contexts. Here, the most fundamental battle is for the rights of women to bear children—with prenatal, maternal, and child care—and to raise both boy and girl children with adequate nutrition, clean water, and education. Christian feminist social bioethics today is moving forward to place reproductive morality and social practices surrounding early human life in a global context, in which the needs of the poor are establishing a different and urgent new agenda for social empowerment.

The development of the modern science of genetics and the twentieth century's multinational quest to decode human DNA arrived on the world scene during the rapid globalization of the economic and communications sectors of human societies. While communications technologies enabled the Human Genome Project to succeed, economic globalization on a market model is multiplying exponentially the opportunities that exist now and in the future to exploit genetic knowledge for profit. On the one hand, gene-based research and discoveries hold out promise for miraculous new ways to treat disease and even to enhance "normal" human functioning. On the other, they also threaten to exacerbate worldwide disparities in health, longevity, and social advantage.

It is not enough to look at gene-based interventions "in their own right," as if their morality could be determined apart from the social relations they enable. Another part of the moral scenario is the sizeable profits to be gained by biotech investment. The distinctive contribution of theology should be to challenge the for-profit global marketing of research and biotechnology to wealthy consumers. It can do so sometimes in explicitly religious terms, sometimes in terms with interreligious valence, and sometimes in terms with humanistic or philosophical appeal. Moreover, religious traditions and theology have been and are increasingly effective in sponsoring activism for practical change in the ways genetic knowledge is obtained and implemented. Specific applications of genetics that will be considered are stem cell research and genetic enhancement. Chapter 7, "Biotechnology, Genes, and Justice," criticizes both in light of the inequitable distribution of resources that results in investment in these technologies, rather than in addressing the basic health care needs of the developing world, by both genomic and traditional means.

Religious coalitions responding to genetically modified food, in collaboration with other social agents and networks, can provide a case study or role model for future engagement on issues of human genetics. Agricultural biotechnology began in the 1980s; Monsanto developed the first transgenic plants in 1983. A controversial ethical issue is the distribution of genetically modified foods, plants, and seeds in the developing world. On the one hand, it is argued that hardier or vitamin-enriched crops might improve the nutrition and health of poor peoples. On the other hand, seeds that are sold in developing nations often include a "terminator gene"—forcing buyers to repeatedly purchase patented products from U.S. suppliers, rather than having access to a reliable local supply. Moreover, industrialized farming with "improved" seeds is forcing many subsistence farmers into poverty and off their land. Another worry is that European markets bar modified crops. Hence, developing countries may be excluded from trade relationships if they permit the spread of genetically modified organisms (GMOs).

Religious groups and churches, including Roman Catholic officials in the United States, the Philippines, Brazil, and Africa, have spoken out against genetically modified crops and the threat they constitute to food security and economic justice. GMOs are not "intrinsically evil," as some of the more strident voices claim, but in the present world order their use and distribution presents serious social justice offenses. The work of ecumenical organizations will be cited to exemplify the possibility of religious and theological advocacy for justice and a "preferential option for the poor" in a context of market-motivated genetics research and development.

"Final Reflections" concludes the discussion by observing that theological bioethics must own its distinctively religious vision and voice without retreating from the public sphere. Instead it must redefine the public sphere as a social arena in which multiple value traditions and their representatives join together in shaping the social relations and institutions in which all participate. Theological bioethics is not just about distinctive narratives or arguments; it is about creating and sustaining the kinds of practices that embody those narratives. It is also about reenvisioning theology's own horizon of meaning in light of practices in which religious traditions and theologies join with other communities of meaning and value. The key contribution of participatory theological bioethics is to instantiate as well as advocate practices of health care justice, and in so doing nourish hope that change for the better is possible.

CHAPTER

1

THEOLOGIANS AND BIOETHICS

Some History and a Proposal

THE CONTEMPORARY DISCIPLINE of bioethics arose as part of efforts in the 1960s and 1970s specifically to change social practices in medicine and research. One key agenda item was experimentation that exploited vulnerable populations, especially by subjecting them, without their consent, to research projects that were harmful. The names Tuskegee and Willowbrook symbolize the failure of U.S. researchers to meet the moral requirements of the Nuremburg code.[1] Another was the need to find a way to deal with the use and allocation decisions necessitated by new technologies. The Seattle dialysis lottery, heart transplants, and the removal of Karen Ann Quinlan from a respirator made worldwide news and raised public consciousness of the ethical quandaries modern medicine rapidly introduced.[2]

Theological luminaries such as Paul Ramsey, Richard McCormick, and James Gustafson were visible figures in the shaping of the new bioethics. As a result of their efforts, in cooperation with philosophers, medical doctors, and researchers, the practice of biomedicine in the United States shifted directions. It moved decisively toward respect for patient autonomy and informed consent and toward the formation of public policies, laws, and judicial precedents to govern aspects of practice such as research on human subjects and decisions about life-sustaining treatment.

Two of the most prominent early voices, Ramsey (a Methodist) and McCormick (a Roman Catholic), were often in good-natured conflict with one another. Other important players were Joseph Fletcher (an Episcopalian and a situation ethicist) and James Gustafson (a Reformed theologian who increasingly attended to the importance of the natural and human sciences for Christian bioethics). Karen Lebacqz (a Congregationalist) has been a key thinker both in feminist bioethics and in policy discussions. Jewish voices include Fred Rosner, Immanuel Jakobovitz, Elliott Dorff, and David Bleich. Though more names could be mentioned,[3] these clearly illustrate the engagement of theologians in bioethics debates throughout the 1980s.

Topics of central concern included abortion, reproductive technologies, genetic engineering, human experimentation, termination of treatment, direct mercy killing, and the allocation of scarce medical resources. Theologians joined in debates about how medicine and research are institutionalized in U.S. society and about law and public policy. Theologians such as Ramsey, Gustafson, McCormick, and Lebacqz not only served on important policy bodies like the National Commission on the Protection of Human Subjects (1974) and the President's Commission (1979), but were major players in formation of the field of bioethics—helping to establish centers such as The Institute of Religion at the Texas Medical Center in Houston (1954); the Institute of Society, Ethics, and the Life Sciences, later to become the Hastings Center, in New York State (1961); the Kennedy Institute of Bioethics at Georgetown University (1971); and the Park Ridge Center in Chicago (1985). The first edition of the *Encyclopedia of Bioethics,* whose very existence and title lent substance to the new field, was filled with entries by theologians and articles written from religious perspectives.[4] Theologians have continued to hold membership on national commissions, such as the National Bioethics Advisory Commission (NBAC; under President William Clinton) and the President's Council on Bioethics (PCB), formed by George W. Bush in 2001, initially to advise him on stem cell policy.[5]

Richard McCormick provides an especially good example of multifaceted involvement, as he was a commentator on Catholic Church teaching as it affected not only individuals but the policies of numerous Catholic health facilities. In fact, one of his books on theological bioethics is styled as a revised set of guidelines for Catholic health care.[6] He also commented frequently on court cases, especially regarding end-of-life decisions.[7] McCormick's work illustrates the opportunity that theologians have to affect social practices by means of the infrastructure and networks of civil society, such as religious bodies, health care institutions, and professional organizations and norms, as well as by influencing the processes of legislative change and judicial precedent.

"Theology" is essentially a process of reflection on religious experience, in which the systematic coherence of religious narratives and symbols is clarified and their practical ramifications developed. Theological ethics is the explication and defense of the personal moral and the social behavior required or idealized by a religious tradition. Theologians were particularly well-equipped to advance bioethics at its inception because religious communities had cultivated long-standing traditions of reflection on life, death, and suffering and had given more guidance on the specifics of moral conduct than had moral philosophy at that time.[8] Thomas Shannon notes that theologians entered the early bioethics debates so effectively because they—in contrast to most philosophers of the day—were prepared to take on issues of practical decision making.[9] They sometimes, but not always, used religious language and stories in the process.

The early theological bioethicists used religious language, imagery, and teaching to advance discourse within their faith traditions. In public settings they sometimes sought expressions that were more philosophical, but occasionally used religious imagery to destabilize cultural assumptions and suggest a different context for considering biomedical choices. Even explicitly theological language and religious symbols or stories (such as creation in the image of God, the story of the Fall, the healings performed by Jesus, the parable of the Good Samaritan, the ideal of covenant community) can evoke patterns of individual existence and social life that are similarly shared, abhorred, or admired in nonreligious associations. Examples are the universal human vulnerability to illness and need for health; the inevitability of death and the preciousness of life; the reality of social exploitation and the ideal of social cooperation and respect; and the reality of violent ideologies, contrasted with religious and moral traditions of other-concern and altruism.

Theologians participated then and do now in many circles of expression and influence, including teaching, academic and popular publishing, media commentary, conferences (theological and interdisciplinary, national and international), and membership on the bodies and committees that produce the "official" positions and teachings of religious traditions and denominations. Theology is mediated to the public in a variety of ways, including the representative positions of institutional religious bodies; pastors, teachers, and congregations; religiously sponsored educational systems; activist organizations and movements; and representation on public commissions. The bioethicist and audience or constituency are interdependent.

While some thinkers are influenced by their settings to be more concerned about the integrity of their shaping traditions and values, and to resist what they perceive as threatening cultural trends, others are more concerned about adequacy to contemporary experience and challenges and welcome innovative practices. A biblical image or theological concept such as Creation may be invoked to rule out certain biomedical acts or practices as "playing God"; that same image can also underwrite human freedom as part of what it means to be cocreator with God.[10] The uses of images depend in part on the practices and communities in which they are embedded and the practices and policies they are meant to encourage or discourage.

Religious imagery and theological language can be harnessed either to "conservative" or "progressive" social and political agendas, and this is true of theological bioethics. The proposal to be developed in this book, especially in chapter 2, affirms the importance and the effectiveness of the political participation of religious communities and theologies in shaping bioethical practices and policies. However, I do not see all types of religious advocacy as morally equal or equally representative of the ideals of the Christian biblical and theological traditions. Biblically and theologically grounded norms of justice, as the inclusion of all in the common good with a preferential option for the poor, should energize and renew a theological ethics of inclusion, participation, equality, and empowerment, especially for the least well-off.[11]

Theological Bioethics in the Public Forum

From the end of the 1970s until the last decade of the century, bioethics enjoyed great cultural credibility. But theological participation in public debates had to contend with the objection that such debate ought to occur on "neutral" ground and to ward off the idea that theological interventions are attempts to impose religious dogma on those of differing convictions. Such complaints can be rebutted fairly easily if theologians are willing to agree that positions inspired by religious commitment have to be "translated" into moral terms that can be accepted by all in order to have public viability. In other words, they have to sink or swim on the basis of their appeal to secular thinkers and philosophers. According to Daniel Callahan, founder, with Willard Gaylin, of the Hastings Center, most theological bioethicists enjoyed success because they adopted an "interesting and helpful" approach to biomedical dilemmas, rather than railing against the establishment.[12] They "were quite willing to talk in a fully secular way." In fact, bioethics may even have become popular because it was able "to push religion aside."[13]

Making themselves heard in pluralistic debates, often touching on public policy, some theological bioethicists began to operate like moral philosophers, ceding power to a "thin" and "secular" discourse that limits its moral claims to minimal requirements of procedural justice—or so goes a common critique.[14] This became more and more true in the 1980s, as more aspiring bioethicists, even those pursuing theological degrees, were educated specifically for this new field of endeavor and assumed roles in clinical settings. Moreover, many seemed to pay more attention to crises and dilemmas than they did to their theological or even philosophical foundations. Consequently, specifically as theologians, they became marginalized in a field that came increasingly to rely on the kind of moral principles that could plausibly be claimed to be universal, rational, and "secular" and that sought the kind of decision-making and policy resolutions that could be squared with U.S. legal traditions and command public support.[15]

The sociologist John H. Evans offers an interpretation of theological bioethics that resembles the previous description. Focusing especially on genetic science, he laments the ascendancy of an approach to bioethics centered on the four "secular" principles of autonomy, beneficence, nonmaleficence, and justice.[16] Evans employs a distinction between "thick" and "thin" theories of the good that ultimately goes back to John Rawls.[17] Rawls distinguished between "thin" and "fuller" theories of the good in order to get people to come to the table of public decision making and agree that certain primary goods should be secured for all in a just society. He maintained that social inequalities are just only insofar as they work to secure these primary goods for society's least-favored members.[18] Evans's complaint is that the consequent "thinning" of public debate has "eviscerated" the discourse needed to make important decisions about whether human genetic engineering is compatible with worthy societal ends, because discussion of those ends is ruled out of bounds in the first place.

In his view, the policy discourse on genetic engineering in the United States is both exemplified and shaped by *Splicing Life,* a report of a presidential advisory commission on genetic engineering (President's Commission for the Study of Ethical Problems in Medicine and Biomedical and Behavioral Research, 1983). The commission entertained the concerns of theologians and religious leaders about the aims of genetic engineering and its ultimate effects on human life and on societies. Yet the final report termed the theological concerns "vague" and focused on more concrete problems (e.g., creating animal-human hybrids) that the theological objections could not definitively resolve. Thus the concerns that the creation of new life forms oversteps the boundaries of prudence and humility, or that the poor are being left behind in the development of genetic technologies, are left out of the final reckoning of the ethics and legality of genetic engineering.[19] Evans maintains that more recent debates over cloning have served to consolidate the formal rationality of "bioethics" and to further eliminate "thick" traditions and perspectives on the larger ends of biomedicine from public debate. Instead, autonomy has become an unexamined end in itself, and few if any limits have been imposed by law or regulation on the adventures of science.[20]

As a result of theologians' infatuation with public influence, it would seem, they capitulated to a procedural bioethics that reduced all substantive moral values to autonomy and informed consent. Some even see theological bioethics as having "sold out" to the gatekeepers of thin, abstract bioethics debate. As a result, theology lost its power to identify, expose, and challenge social problems stemming from the misuse of medicine and technology. For example, while theological bioethicists have joined the cause of individual autonomy, health care dollars are increasingly directed away from underserved populations; scientists and investors proceed with threats to "human dignity," such as stem cell research and human cloning, anticipating profit-making benefits for the wealthy.

While it is true that many liberal and progressive theologians have backed away from public religious arguments, it is not true that the discourse they have joined is neutral. In fact, it is governed by the values of individualism, science, technology, the market, and profits. By not engaging these other value traditions from the standpoint of their own distinctive commitment to justice and the common good, theologians fail to make any great impact on cultural norms.

The challenge to theology is to recover its religiously distinctive prophetic voice and enter into policy debates as an energetic adversary of the liberal consensus. Theologians ought to stick to their own convictions, remain unapologetically theological in orientation, while still seeking common cause and building a common language with all who are similarly committed to health care justice.

Theological bioethicists, including those backing progressive social causes, must reassert their religious identity while not giving up moral credibility and social impact. Theologians searching for a new model of thinking bioethically should recall postmodernism's insight that even abstract and supposedly universal principles always come to be articulated out of particular and historical communities of practice and discernment. Every political value system or agenda has a past, a context, and a set of investments, whether it be liberal democracy, the scientific research imperative, free market economics, communitarianism, or socialism.

On the one hand, contextuality may limit the applicability range of values and principles. But on the other hand, the practical context is what gives the principles "legs." Context-generated moral insights and proposals can gain a public hearing if they can prove themselves relevant and useful in the various contexts that together make up the common good of interest to the public in question. "Particularistic" references to the originating context need not be abandoned, though they should be introduced with respect for interlocutors and their differences. Conversation partners from other contexts may find these illuminating in light of shared values and commitments and especially in light of the immediate practical contexts of problem solving and decision making that bring the different traditions together around a common need or goal.

Jeffrey Stout has recommended to theologians a style of "immanent criticism" that "claims no privileged vantage point above the fray."[21] This type of social criticism can still manage to unite "people with diverging conceptions of the good to identify the same moral problems and collaborate in common concern," working within "specific social practices and institutions."[22] Sometimes shared problems and the need for mutually agreeable resolutions can lead people toward consensus about the good life and just social relationships, even when their theoretical or conceptual frameworks do not seem to converge. Theological claims, arguments, and conclusions in bioethics are not primarily intellectual products to be deployed scientifically. They are tradition-based and contextual strategies for uniting and concretizing a number of concerns and goals having to do with biomedical trends and behavior patterns. Theories of bioethics have to be understood in relation to the social worlds of their origin; likewise, their public influence depends on the social responses they can generate. The field of such responses is not limited to legislation and public commissions; it extends to nearly every corner of civil society.

Theological Bioethics: Public and Socially Engaged

A premise of this book is that "theological bioethics" is not so nerveless and enervated an enterprise as some of its critics make out, nor is it as marginal to current biomedical practice and policy as some imply. The real conflict is not between "thin" and "thick" moral languages and views of the good, but between competing "thick" worldviews and visions of ultimacy, complete with concepts of sin and salvation, good and evil, saints and sinners, liturgies and moral practices. Several theologians on a spectrum seek a middle path between a seemingly "secular" voice for bioethics that essentially capitulates to the liberal market ethos of modern Western democracies and a richer, more nuanced discourse that coheres with communal religious identities but seems to become less compelling in the public sphere.[23] The impact and potential of theological bioethics can only be seen and appreciated if one's vision is broadened beyond the realms of academia and high-level government regulation. Although these are the spheres in which early bioethics made its name, today they do little to deter the profit-driven race for biotech innovation. The reality of theological bioethics certainly includes scholarship and policy, but its roots and much of its potential influence lie in broader and deeper networks that can exert pressure on research science, health care policy, and biotech investment.

Evans's ideal, for which he believes the prospects to be bleak, is for citizens to listen to professional debates about genetic engineering, take their concerns back to their "thick" communities of belief and value, and then bring the "demands" of their group regarding ends "to the public's elected officials."[24] Evans cites the burgeoning "participatory democracy" literature to bolster his case.[25] In my view, Evans is on the right track in suggesting that greater public participation in bioethical debates would more fully engage the members of religious traditions and other groups whose perspectives do not find a comfortable home in the discourse of "professional" bioethics. I also affirm his interest in maintaining a vital connection between faith communities and public policy. For national commissions, for example, to be truly democratic and representative, they would need to enact much more aggressive and broad-reaching mechanisms to engage the publics they supposedly address or represent. Rather than providing "expert" answers, they should be setting agendas for further public debate and acquiring legitimacy by connecting with "broad, ground-level forms of moral discourse" and "the practical contexts of moral decision-making faced by most Americans."[26] These contexts will often or even usually involve religious experiences, values, practices, and theological explanations. But broad consultation and public legitimacy are very unevenly represented in national commissions to date.

Hence it is striking that Evans and other critics of the secularization of bioethics keep their gaze so firmly fixed on governmental bodies such as public commissions, regulatory agencies, and legislatures. Not only are the decisions and policies of such bodies the ultimate target of influence, but they are also expected to play a major role in the reinvigoration of the discourses that they are claimed to have suppressed. No wonder Evans's expectation of change is modest. And Evans is not alone; in fact, he represents the general assumptions of most of the literature on theology, bioethics, and policy.[27]

In an interesting discussion of John Evans's book, several theologians express varying levels of displeasure and dismay at his analysis of their "public" marginalization. Nevertheless, they fall into line behind the "thin" and "thick" distinctions with which Evans frames his characterization of the public and "religious" spheres and proceeds to argue that theologians are not taken seriously in the former.[28] On closer inspection, though, the description given by some of the theologians of what their work actually does militates against an easy distinction between "thin" public and "thick" religious discourse. It also tacitly links public and religious-theological discourse to practical settings and interests that are complex and interactive.

This is especially true of the interventions of Gilbert Meilaender and James Childress, both of whom have served on presidential and governmental policy bodies (in Childress's case, quite a number).[29] Meilaender seems to accept the "story line" Evans has plotted, in which advisory commissions have moved from substantive to formal rationality. Yet Evans and Meilaender both agree that advisory commissions were created in the first place "as a device to keep science free of regulation" by funneling ethical concerns through professional bioethicists who would keep their sights narrowly set on a few basic principles and not raise any radical questions about "scientific" objectives.[30] This description of the practical activities of bioethics commissions—their membership, their language, and their ritual hearings—should be enough to at least raise the suspicion that their public discourse is not as "thin" as one might suppose.

Indeed, Jeffrey Stout characterizes most such commissions as "the modern, bureaucratic equivalent of feudal councils, with professionals in place of noblemen."[31] A few further questions from Stout bring home the fact that theologians can become involved in languages, symbolic occasions, and social practices that are quite "thick," if not "theological," when they take on the role of bioethicist for "governments, courts, hospitals, universities, and the press. 'What sort of expertise or authority is one claiming to have when one accepts these roles? Who is supposed to defer to the ethicist's findings and for what reasons? What sort of society are we becoming complicit in when we encourage our fellow citizens to defer to our alleged expertise?' "[32] Stout seems fairly convinced of the pernicious effect of bioethical expertise on the theologian, as it works toward the submergence of the exercise of theological ethics in the practices and languages of foreign institutions.

This does not have to be the case. A theological bioethicist may enter the practice and the "thick" multilayered discourse of the hospital, the court, or the government commission. Still, as a theologian, he or she can and should remember to exercise the critical functions of the worldview, symbols, and distinctive practices that he or she brings to each setting and not become overwhelmed by the dominant (and "thick") discourse that typically controls there. Theological bioethics will represent and lift up for attention and endorsement a variety of alternative discourses and practices concerning health and biomedicine that have an impact on the same areas of life that policymakers envision in a more top-down manner.

James Childress warns Evans and others not to underplay the role and effect that theology has had in shaping "the public culture," presumably beyond or below the "thin" air of policy advisory bodies.[33] Moreover, he believes that theologians have been influential even in the latter, pointing as evidence to the theologian members of these bodies and to testimony given by theologians. However, the issue for theological bioethics is the dominant language of the "practice" of advisory commissions—rights, autonomy, and cost-benefit ratios stated in terms of demonstrable harm or risk. This practice-embedded language can govern debates about reproduction, health care, and research in a way that drowns out talk about who has access, who will benefit, and who will profit from any given option or innovation, as well as about practical ways to change the status quo without waiting for formal policy adjustments. The language and practices of modern science, market economics, and liberal individualism are generally unreceptive to consideration of distributive justice and a "preferential option for the poor."

Evans's view that (liberal) theologians are not taken seriously on public commissions is really a way of saying that the practices represented by the commissions and their members have by and large been able to edge out practical and verbal challenges from the theologians invited to participate, especially if they threaten scientific privilege, profits, or the freedom of those who already have control of the resources. One reason some politically conservative varieties of bioethics (e.g., against abortion and stem cell research) have enjoyed more political success in recent years is that they have been abetted by effective grassroots organizing and networking among organizations. But another reason is that they pose little serious challenge to neoliberal economic policies, to the idea that health care should go to those who can pay for it, or even to the idea that any research that can make a profit should be allowed. For instance, even "conservative" policies about *federal* funding of stem cell research in no way limit the freedom of *private* corporations to create, buy, use, or destroy embryos. (Stem cell research will be treated in more detail in chapters 6 and 7.)

Participatory Theological Bioethics: A Proposal

We have seen that, while theologians such as James Gustafson, Paul Ramsey, and Richard McCormick were active and influential in the emergence of bioethics as a field, their counterparts in the next generation of scholars have sometimes struggled to gain a voice in the public sphere. Theological bioethicists have been criticized for having yielded the floor of public debate to a thin, secular, philosophical discourse that excludes and demeans theology and that is incapable of a truly prophetic or transforming contribution to health care, health policy, or research ethics.

On the other hand, the election of George W. Bush as U.S. president in 2000 (and for a second term in 2004) brought into power a leader who is an avowed evangelical Christian and who specifically invoked divine guidance and religious imagery in pursuing his domestic and international policies. His administration is generally viewed as being under the influence of the bioethical concerns and values of the so-called religious right.[34] Bush's reelection showed that many in the American mainstream were at least open to religious influences on the public life of the country. Bush supporters sought to appoint Supreme Court justices who favored modification or reversal of the permissive abortion policy established by *Roe v. Wade,* sought to severely limit federal funding of embryonic stem cell research, and sought to define marriage legally and constitutionally as a union between a man and a woman, with a concomitant curtailment of protections and benefits for same-sex unions. The Bush administration did not seek to extend universal health care coverage to all members of U.S. society or to raise its level of support for the fight against worldwide "diseases of the poor" to the levels achieved by other wealthy societies.[35] The

Bush campaigns and reelection show that religious denominations and theologians can have a public voice. But not all varieties of theological bioethics are equal either in effectiveness or in moral values and outcomes.

Effectiveness requires both the deployment of a vocabulary and imagery with broad cultural appeal and the cultivation of grassroots practices and communities that display and reinforce that imagery. For instance, early in the 2004 election season, evangelical political organizers were already appearing in local congregations in Oregon, Michigan, Montana, Arkansas, and Ohio to collect signatures for state ballot measures against their signature issue, gay marriage.[36] Progressive activists, who were much more interested than the religious right in health care reform, typically tried to advance this and other goals through the national media, national figures, and publications aimed at a college-educated public. In so doing, they failed to engage religious values and theological interpretations to the degree necessary to advance this goal culturally and win votes. According to Jim Wallis, the 2004 campaign showed that the politically conservative "moral values" agenda virtually excluded the issue of poverty, to which the Bible devotes thousands of verses. On the other hand, "Democrats seem uncomfortable with the language of faith and values, preferring in recent decades the secular approach of restricting such matters to the private sphere." He asks, "Where would we be if Martin Luther King Jr. had kept his faith to himself?"[37]

As the next chapter discusses, progressive causes have been advanced successfully under religious and theological auspices in the past, and positive examples can be found today, especially in the realm of Catholic health care institutions, advocacy, and moral theology. However, such measures are underrecognized and underutilized in the preponderance of theological scholarship in bioethics. Theological bioethics should strengthen already existing practices "on the ground" and broaden and deepen the vocabulary of solidarity and care of neighbor, both religiously and by appeal to shared political traditions.

I propose an alternative understanding of public theological bioethics, as *participatory*. Participatory theological bioethics operates simultaneously in many spheres of discourse and activity, from which it is possible to affect the social relationships and institutions that govern health care. Participatory theological bioethics can be either conservative or progressive, right or left, pro-life or pro-choice, market oriented or social-welfare oriented, or some combination of any of these. In my view, the promotion of progressive causes in bioethics through grassroots organizing, participation in the networks of civil society, and the partnering of explicitly religious and faith-based organizations with counterparts from other religious or nonreligious counterparts has been underappreciated.

What Is "the Public Sphere"?

It is a mistake to think that the "public sphere" is a sphere of argument and debate rather than action and that, when public debate does occur, it has legitimacy only when participants engage one another in respectful yet emotionally detached rational argument, offering warrants that are "secular," pragmatic, and nonparticularistic, and, where possible, empirically sustained. The public sphere so defined is inhabited largely by experts and elites. By lamenting their exclusion from this sphere, theologians tacitly validate its authority and importance in defining health care ethics and in constituting the "public" arena above all others in which it is crucial to be heard.

The notion of the public sphere must be reenvisaged to include action as well as argument and to include integral reference to the contexts and interests of those communicating within it. A definition of the public sphere by Charles Taylor serves as a useful point of departure, because it both embodies standard assumptions about the legitimacy of public debates and implies the need for a different approach.

> What do I mean by a *public sphere*? I want to describe it as a common space in which the members of society are deemed to meet through a variety of media: print, electronic, and also face-to-face encounters; to discuss matters of common interest; and thus to be able to form a common mind about these.[38]

Taylor goes on to specify that the common space of discussion that makes up the public sphere is "nonlocal" or "metatopical"; that it is "extrapolitical" or "not an exercise of power"; and that it is "secular" or having do to with "profane," historical time rather than a transcendent realm.[39]

Like many others, Taylor tends to envision the arena of public exchanges as a metaphorical "space," above and beyond the realities of ordinary life and beyond the particular interests and relationships that have created the identities of the conversation partners. But, in fact, parties to public debate continue to participate in the practices and purposes of their lives, including "local" and "transcendent" ones, even as they interact with others about the meaning and goals of practices and interests they share in common. This is indeed implied by Taylor's references to necessary "media" of communication to bridge locations, as well as by the fact that "matters of common interest" engage those who join in the conversation. Matters of common interest exist and come into focus if and when the debaters share practical concerns—when they come together in certain communities, identities, practices, interests, goals, or fears, even as they retain differences in others.

The factor left out in Taylor's definition, then, is that the common meeting space of society's members is filled not only by "discoursing" individuals in the abstract but also by the intersecting groups to which they belong—families, neighborhoods, churches, ethnic groups, age cohorts, political parties, citizens groups, sports teams, schools, professions, types or sites of employment, and more. No individual enters in disconnection from the communities of belonging and worldview formation that are constitutive for his or her particularity and agency. Moreover, it is precisely converging communities and identities that bring people together around "public" concerns. Mediating between individuals and the public sphere and lending coherence to social agency are institutions. Institutions are patterns of social relationship that give normative definition to practices, structure experience, and shape individual character and commitments. Practices and institutions make up the infrastructure of society and are a necessary component of the public sphere.[40]

While the common space evoked by Taylor may be "metatopical" in that it is not limited to participants in any one place, the identities of participants and their concrete conditions of participation bring a variety of physical and social locations into the mix. The public sphere is never outside of or immune to the dialectics of power. Although the common space may not be identified with any one manifestation of institutionalized political power or government, the participants in discourse will have differentials of influence along a number of different axes—income, education, race, gender, age, profession—and so will the practices and institutions in which they participate. The public sphere is a space in which power is exercised and mediated, resulting both in conflict and in shifting equilibria. Although the public sphere may not be the one in which transcendent meaning is most directly addressed, the individuals and groups coming into it will often if not always integrate their actions and expressions with a grounding view of the human condition that refers to ultimate origins or purposes.[41]

The narrow, liberal understanding of what makes up public discourse deters theologians and others from appreciating the integral relation of public ethical debates to practices and institutions. Ethical arguments and their ability to persuade are rooted in and rely on such practices, not just on intellectual cogency and verbal rhetoric. In fact, the debate over whether religious discourse should be "allowed" into the public sphere is virtually beside the point, given that religious persons, groups, and institutions have always interacted on myriad levels with other actors, dialectically constituting the playing field on which cultural interactions about uses and abuses of modern biomedical science take place. All these agents contribute to a common discourse, and potentially to the development of consensuses, by acting individually and collectively, as well as by speaking in public. More socially conservative bioethics grasps the political potential of activism and works hard to reinforce, heighten, and extend the kind of specifically religious identity that provides thick opposition to abortion and the destruction of embryos. Socially progressive theological bioethicists, on the other hand, who see the "secular political sphere" as the important sphere of influence, tend to overlook the potentially expansive appeal of religious symbols and especially to neglect the opportunities for cooperative action and collective power that civil society provides.

The real issue is which tradition has priority, precedence, and presumed authority within the patterns of social exchange about ethics and ethical behavior. The three main contenders in twenty-first-century postindustrial societies are science, economics, and liberalism. Theological bioethics should and can confront these thick traditions with persuasive counter-strategies, symbolic systems, and narratives, as well as with ethical "reasons." The challenge before theologians is not to cast aside a thin discourse for a richer one, but to dislodge the thick discourses that are so widely entrenched that their constituting narratives and practices are no longer directly observed.

Although socially conservative bioethics rightly fights the instrumentalization and commercialization of innocent or vulnerable life (even in its earliest and last stages), merely defending the rights of embryos, fetuses, the handicapped, or the comatose does not do enough to counteract the individualism of health care in this country or, increasingly, worldwide. It also does not offer a strong enough and broad enough challenge to a general "medicalization" and "technologization" of human life and human problems, advanced by the worship of modern science or of the profits it brings.

"Thick" Traditions: Science, Economics, Liberalism

The quasi-religious overtones of scientific ideals and the quest for scientific knowledge have been identified before. Carolyn Merchant was one of the first to search out the religious motivations behind Francis Bacon's drive to restore "man's" dominion over nature for the sake of the human race, and so to redeem humanity from the consequences of the Fall.[42] Geneticists have described the genome as "the 'Bible,' the 'Book of Man,' and the 'Holy Grail,'" viewing it as a "sacred text" with great explanatory power and even as "the secular equivalent of the human soul."[43] Opponents of genetic engineering are thus cast as the enemies of human self-transcendence. Andrew Lustig notes that in debates about cloning, ostensibly non-religious and explicitly religious arguments for and against cloning can function in analogous ways, placing aesthetic and moral concerns against a backdrop of ultimate meaning.[44] Lustig's main point is to show that religious objections to cloning can converge with secular concerns, helping to build consensus. I want also to stress that "secular" justifications of cloning and other genetic techniques often rely on the same kind of framework of transcendence that backs religious arguments but that is labeled unacceptable if put forward in explicitly religious or theological terms.

Science is not the only symbol system of ultimacy, morality, and meaning competing to define the cultural role of the new genetics. Ronald Cole-Turner astutely noted a decade ago that genetic engineering "involves nations, corporations, individual researchers, investors, and consumers" and thus "cannot be said to serve the interests of humanity" as such, as is so often claimed.[45] Cole-Turner's concern is that it would be naïve for theologians to accept the eschatology of genetics, in which the new knowledge serves the future of humanity as a species. But his observation also exhibits why neither beneficence nor the quest for scientific knowledge fully accounts for the direction, claims, and power of the new genomics. New discoveries and patented techniques for cloning, genetic testing, and pharmacogenomics promise prestige for researchers and profits for biotech corporations, pharmaceutical companies, and even research universities. The mystique of science is reinforced and perhaps even co-opted by the ideology of market capitalism as the driving force of liberal democracy's global expansion.

Biotechnology is big business, and industry advocates present it as having a moral role in shaping humanity's future. According to the Biotechnology Industry Organization's (BIO) website, BIO is the "largest trade organization to serve and represent the emerging biotechnology industry in the United States and around the globe." As envisioned by this self-defined "leading voice for the biotechnology industry," "biotechnology's future is bright." BIO's website assures visitors that its "leadership and service-oriented guidance have helped advance the industry and bring the benefits of biotechnology to the people of the world."[46] BIO's projects in 2003 (the fiftieth anniversary of the discovery of DNA) included an ad campaign to guarantee that pharmaceutical companies would be paid for drugs for the elderly under Medicare, to support President George W. Bush's assertion that genetically modified foods can help end hunger in the third world (not displace subsistence farming and create dependency on corporate seed manufacturers, as critics claim), and to celebrate the "modern era of molecular biology" in which the initiative and creativity of scientists have led to the industry's profitable yet humanitarian endeavors. In a publicity statement, BIO president Carl B. Feldbaum celebrates the sacred traditions, search for ultimate meaning, salvific potential, humanistic ethic, and saints of genetic science:

> No doubt in another 50 years we will look back in wonder at just how much suffering will have been alleviated through a chain of events that began in the early 1950s with a couple of scientists looking for "the secret of life" in X-ray diffraction photos and ball-and-stick chemical models.[47]

Unfortunately, according to Dan Eramian, BIO's vice president for communications, "some in the religious community," including "fundamentalists" and "radical anti-abortionists" are trying to "obstruct attempts to further embryo cloning and stem cell research in the United States." Interference would undermine the lead such research has already achieved, thanks to a government that "pumps millions of dollars into basic research." That would mean disaster for the country's biotechnology industry, because the "largest pharmaceutical companies . . . have continued to partner with biotechnology companies to develop new drugs based on this [stem cell] science." Eramian calls for "dialogue" with religious representatives as part of a program to "manage controversy" and permit research, development, marketing, and sales to go forward.[48] The implication is that, while religious objections to BIO's investment agenda are obstructionist and irrational, BIO's advocacy for research dollars is unbiased and backed by sound data.

In a functionalist view at least, this is not a competition between religion and a "secular," "scientific," or "business" worldview, but a contest between missionary agendas. It has been argued that the most powerful explanation of the world is science; the most attractive value system, consumerism; the largest religious denomination, "our" economic system; the theology in service of that religion, the discipline of economics; and the god whom all serve, the market.[49] Traditional religions have been deplorably unable to offer "a meaningful challenge to the aggressive proselytizing of market capitalism, which has already become the most successful religion of all time, winning more converts more quickly than any previous belief system or value-system in human history."[50] The appeal of this new religion lies in its promise of salvation from human unhappiness through commodities, a promise that can never be fulfilled even for the few who enjoy the ability to purchase almost unlimited quantities.

Theological critics likewise have unveiled the "religion of the market" in ways that are instructive for bioethics. The vitality of this religion depends on several myths, nicely laid out in a critique of globalization by Cynthia Moe-Lobeda.[51] First, growth benefits all. The way to growth is through free trade and investment, which in turn lead to greater economic well-being for everyone. The fallacies within the myth are that economic activity translates into social and cultural health; that economic growth brings general welfare, regardless of income distribution; and that the environment and future generations can sustain the costs of current growth. Second, freedom means the right to own and dispose of private property. This notion of freedom disregards the impact of market freedom on the limits posed to human freedom by deprivation of basic necessities for those who cannot find a reliable livelihood, compete in the market, or accumulate property. It also disregards the fact that, especially in a globalized economy, most market exchanges are not "voluntary." Most important, freedom as market freedom dismisses or represses other notions of freedom, including the freedom to participate in a community that includes the common good of all.

Third, the religion of the market depends on the myth that human beings are essentially autonomous agents, who find ultimate fulfillment in acting individually or by contract to maximize self-interest, with "self-interest" defined in terms of acquisition and consumption. Like the previous myth, this one eliminates aspects of life in community and in solidarity with others that most religious and cultural traditions have defined as fundamental. It "dehumanizes" the human and subjects the less competitive to the more competitive and dominating persons, groups, and economies. Fourth, and most dangerously for the fate of theological bioethics, is the myth that market expansion and the growth of transnational corporations (including the major pharmaceutical companies) is inevitable and "evolutionary, a contemporary form of manifest destiny, a step in modernity's march of progress."[52] On the contrary, the market economy can be resisted and changed, both locally and internationally, as can a rapidly globalizing biotech industry.

Along with the "religions" of science and market capitalism, the traditions, symbols, and practices of liberal individualism provide a framework of meaning and transcendence that deserve a challenge from theology. Liberal philosophy and politics are even more deeply entrenched in the U.S. cultural ethos than science and the market and much more explicitly linked to claims of "ultimacy." Liberalism provides a rationale for the ways in which the science and economics of health care and research are institutionalized and discussed. Liberalism, "the political theory of modernity," begins from the proposition that persons have different conceptions of the good life that cannot be reconciled without violence. They therefore must be accommodated within a rational legal system that favors none and allows all to flourish. Hence, a key liberal value is "tolerance." Classical liberalism upholds a political order that aims to ameliorate the human condition "by the peaceful competition of different traditions." According to defenders of liberalism, "the classical liberal advocacy of the free market is, in effect, only an application in the sphere of economic life of the conviction that human society is likely to do best when men are left free to enact their plans of life unconstrained except by the rule of law."[53] Liberalism, in other words, is not in reality "neutral," "pluralistic," or even "tolerant." Its core value—individual freedom—is a foundational dogma that is highly intolerant of any limits imposed for the sake of marginal persons or the common good.

Liberalism is strangely oblivious, for a theory of political economy, of the effects that differences in economic and social class will have on basic material and social goods and hence on the ability of citizens to "enact their life plans." Thus liberalism as a philosophy and political theory has been attacked from almost too many directions to enumerate: Marxist, feminist, liberationist, and more. Its continuing hold on the North American imagination and culture is partly explained by our founding myths of independence and partly by the strength of the economic interests with which liberalism is symbiotic. Yet the irreversible reign of liberal autonomy within the market, within science, and within health care is another myth that can be uncovered. The narratives, moralities, liturgies, and institutions created by the religion of liberal democratic capitalism can be challenged and perhaps reformed.

Each of these cultural traditions owes its strength partly to an important value it advances: the power of science to illumine the world we live in and avoid some of its dangers, the usefulness of efficient production to maximize quantity and circulation of goods, and the recognition of the intrinsic value of every individual person as well as the importance of respecting differences. However, all of these values can be and are distorted by social, political, and economic systems that give only some people access to their promised benefits or rights, then permit the privileged few to have unbalanced power over the well-being of those who are excluded.

Because of their positive value, all of these traditions have been adapted to some extent and in a variety of ways by bioethicists. Among them, liberalism has seemed the most favorable to bioethicists seeking to modify health care and biotechnology in order to reflect the needs of those who are excluded from present systems. Liberalism seems to offer a theory that coincides with basic cultural values (in the United States at least) that allows for the interaction of different parties in a spirit of mutual respect and that is premised on equality. Some philosophical theories of bioethics adapt the liberal principles of John Rawls in a way that affirms the basic good of health care as a good in which all members of society have a right to participate.[54] From a common good point of view, such theories are welcome challenges to a culturally widespread attitude that individuals and families need be morally concerned only about their own access. However, even modified liberalism in health care ethics tends to accept the status quo of modern medical technology and to limit its critical analysis of market-based health care to "our own" society.

For example, an important book on new innovations in genetics uses a Rawlsian framework to urge that health care is a basic primary good that should be provided to all, insofar as it is a prerequisite of normal human functioning.[55] However, when the analysis reaches the point of recognizing that newly developed techniques for modifying genes will almost certainly be used by wealthy consumers to their own advantage, the book's authors incredibly propose that some day gene modifications will be available to all as part of a "basic package" of health care.[56] The weakness of this suggestion lies in the fact that it is advanced more or less within the same cultural parameters that have created exclusive health care institutions and is directed theoretically to philosophers involved in or analyzing national policy discourse in "a liberal society." There is little or no practical incentive for those now benefiting from the system to change the access patterns; those lacking access have little power to make sure their needs are represented. Under these circumstances, health care resources will certainly continue to be allocated according to market advantage, while the "liberal" values of free choice and tolerance sidetrack any serious critique of the ways the choices of some constrain the biomedical realities of others.

Another work, by theologian Richard Miller, proposes that liberalism can serve as a useful "political theory," if not as a "comprehensive" one. Liberalism as a political tool permits theologians to join with others in provisionally setting aside "metaphysical claims" and "particular religious and philosophical doctrines."[57] They can then participate in a consensus about basic principles of fairness, including access to some primary goods. But the question is whether political liberalism actually leads to significant social changes that match these theoretical principles of justice. Although I affirm Miller's desire for consensus on basic goods, I question whether "thin" and "neutral" theorizing[58] can accomplish much change in institutions whose injustice feeds off the liberal groundbed of individual autonomy.

Miller's specific focus is the care of grievously ill and suffering children receiving treatment in an intensive care unit (ICU) in the United States. He sensitively and poignantly renders case studies and offers compassionate and persuasive moral analyses, given the parameters of critical care in major medical facilities. He modifies liberal autonomy to the extent that family privacy must be subject to the limiting criterion of the welfare of the child.[59] Miller also examines pressures on families to participate in drug trials for which pharmaceutical companies have a financial incentive, which suggests a larger problem of the interaction of medicine and business.[60] However, liberalism invoked as a "political theory" does not ultimately lead to more radical questions about why the many agonized children and families described are subjected to "aggressive" treatment rather than provided with hospice, about what happens to children and families without health insurance, or about why medical centers in North America institutionalize pediatric "intensive care" to excess, while millions of children perish worldwide from preventable diseases.

A much more direct, specific, and critical confrontation with liberal political philosophies, and the practices with which they are symbiotic, is necessary to achieve any real progress toward health care justice. Science, the market, and liberalism all underwrite their cultural status with ideologies of reasonableness and beneficence that conceal the harm and injustice perpetrated by their exaggerated and imperialistic forms, especially in terms of global health inequities. What is needed is a critique that creates or connects with alternative, subversive, or transformative practices, practices that go beyond academia and "official" policymakers.

Public Theological Bioethics

Theological bioethics is, then, not embedded in a free-standing religious "silo" from which it must struggle to be heard in a post-Christian, postreligious, "modern," and "secular" policy world, where the natural sciences and economics have claim to a more "objective," "inclusive," "persuasive," and publicly "appropriate" language. Science, economics, theology, and "liberal democratic" political norms all depend on analogous worldviews that define human nature, human meaning, human goods and goals, and the good society.[61] All invoke symbols of ultimacy that capture the imagination, convert desires, direct practical reason, and motivate action. Perhaps even more important, these worldviews and symbols do more than inspire action consequently; they are themselves nourished and shaped by action continuously. Practices, institutions, moral orientations, and symbolic expressions are co-originate and interdependent.

Several years ago, Roger Shinn wrote that the formation of public policies on genetics necessarily represents an interaction of human values and faiths, scientific information and concepts, and political activity. Religious communities are part of the body politic, advocating their political convictions within the political process. They are especially committed to exposing ideological biases and to speak for "the oppressed and those too often despised by elites." The convictions of theologians seek and often find "wide resonance" in a pluralistic society, especially regarding the value of community and of freedom and the concern for justice.[62] Biomedicine, ethics, policy, religion, and theology engage one another in the public sphere in many more and deeper ways than the display of rational, verbal argumentation by individual spokespersons. Practices, institutions, and issue-oriented activism also make up the dialectical common space where bioethics is negotiated as theory, policy, and implementation.

For example, within bioethics, rights language comes from Western political and constitutional traditions, cost-benefit language comes from market economics, the research imperative comes from enlightenment science, and the call for scientific knowledge to be used for human benefit and the relief of suffering owes much to modern evolutionary views of society as well as modern democracy. The "preferential option for the poor" comes from religious traditions, is reflected in philosophical traditions about equal respect and solidarity, can be backed up by democratic politics, and has some roots in Karl Marx's critique of industrial capitalism and others in scripture.

Even religiously indebted images such as "care for the poor" or "we are all children of God" can stimulate the imaginations of those from diverse traditions so that common ground can be amplified. To the degree that any one image, story, moral principle, or concrete moral analysis can appeal to a variety of associational values and commitments, it can have a chance to influence public life by raising the profile of one pattern of associational behavior over another. For instance, when reformers call for universal access to health care over the present U.S. market-based system, they are appealing to fellow citizens to prioritize solidaristic experiences of social life over capitalism and class, and they can use many rhetorical and symbolic incentives to do this. Theological voices should not be ruled out of court simply because they emerge from traditions that are not completely shared by all other participants in civil society.

Five Modes of Discourse

Since the 1960s, virtually all bioethics has been dialectical in its stance toward society and public debate, rather than strictly autonomous or separationist or totally assimilated to and continuous with nonreligious worldviews and language. But theology moves into public bioethics in a variety of modes and languages. Theology's influence arises in large part from its ability to interface effectively with social problems (here, in biomedicine) that have been identified as important across a broad swath of society. James M. Gustafson has identified four varieties of moral discourse in which theology engages: ethical, policy, prophetic, and narrative.[63] I propose a fifth be added: participatory discourse. Although these are intertwined and have all been represented by theologians since the 1960s, the accent falls on different forms of discourse at different times and for different purposes.

First, the definitions. The aim of *ethical discourse* "is to decide how one ought to act in particular circumstances"[64] by finding moral justification linked to a basic theory of morality focused around such concepts as rights, duties, obligations, and justice. In a theological theory, these concepts will be interpreted in relation to a concept of God and God's purposes or claims regarding humanity. Ethical discourse also requires and relies on an interpretation of the circumstances of action, for instance, as provided by the natural and social sciences.

Policy discourse is closely related to ethical discourse. It involves decisions about what kinds of general practices, institutions, permissions, and constraints should guide social behavior or the behavior of individual agents within social institutions. Compared to ethical discourse, however, policy discourse is more driven by the need to acknowledge and accommodate to the conflicts and limitations inherent in any particular situation of decision. "The 'ought' questions are answered within possibilities and limitations of what resources exist or can be accumulated or organized."[65] Theology can bring to policy discourse a sense that all human enterprises are relative and marked by finitude and sinfulness. Theology can also further a commitment to prioritize and defend some basic values, such as the value of human life, the dignity of every person, and the obligation to advocate for those who are most vulnerable and those who suffer most. However, in a public policy setting, theologians will usually seek expressions of conviction that can communicate effectively with their interlocutors. Sometimes this includes explicitly religious stories or references; usually it does not.

A third type of discourse follows from the fact that theology, along with other value systems and outlooks, prioritizes certain values over others and attempts to see that these values are embodied in social practices and institutions. This is *prophetic discourse.* "Prophetic discourse is usually more general than ethical discourse and sometimes uses narratives to make prophetic points."[66] Prophetic discourse can also be used in a policy setting, although its aim is less to settle specific questions and more to widen horizons of vision. It takes the form either of indictment or of utopia (a visionary inspiration of human hopes and aspirations). Like the prophets of the Hebrew Bible, theological prophets today often forward a critique of economic systems that exclude the poor from basic goods such as health care. They combat an overly pragmatic and individualist approach to biomedical decision making and insist that not all human problems can be resolved by more technology. Though their utopia is ultimately eschatological, they hold up a vision of a more equitable society characterized by the virtues of solidarity and compassion and of justice inspired by love of God and neighbor. Narratives that might bring home these points include biblical accounts and stories, such as the ancient Israelite mandate to care for the widow and orphan (Isaiah 10:1–2), the Gospel of Matthew's parable of judgment (Matthew 25:31–46), or Luke's story of the Good Samaritan (Luke 10:25–37).

The fourth type of discourse uses such stories not just to make theological and ethical points but to form communities and persons in the virtues necessary to enact the points as ways of life. It is called *narrative discourse.* "Narratives function to sustain the particular moral identity of a religious (or secular) community by rehearsing its history and traditional meanings, as these are portrayed in Scripture and other sources."[67] Narratives shape the ethos of a community and the moral character of participants so that they construe the world and envision appropriate action in ways that are suitable to the narrative. Narrative discourse is dialectical in that it forms agents who interact in multiple communities at once. Narratives do not aim to provide clear answers to moral quandaries. They engage the emotions and the imagination to illuminate what is at stake in a certain kind of moral choice or way of life.

By means of both prophetic and narrative discourse, theology moves beyond the theoretical identification of ideals, principles, rules, and resolutions to problems and conflicts. Through prophesy and narrative, theology helps reorient the worldviews of persons and communities and forms them with the virtues that will dispose them to act on their ethical understandings and conclusions. By recalling and living within the story of Yahweh's liberation of the people from bondage, or the sacrifice of Christ on the cross, a religiously and theologically informed people will become better prepared to take action on behalf of those without health care or dying of AIDS. When confronted with public policy choices about new biotechnology, they will be more inclined to ask who will have access, who will profit, and who is likely to bear any associated risks or harms. Recalling that religious communities coexist with other kinds of associations in patterns of interdependence and that people in society participate in many communities and associations at once, it is key to stress that theology's prophetic and narrative roles are not limited to the internal life of religious communities, strictly defined. Illuminating insights can be generated even for those who do not share the entire worldview and symbol system of the speaker.[68] Prophetic critique and narrative formation can extend to other groups or activities in which theologians associate with people on the basis of more limited unifying factors.

The use of distinctively religious and theological language and symbols in the public bioethical realm is not always appropriate or appropriate in the same way. But neutral language in public and strong theological language in community (or in a communal "witness" against cultural assumptions) are not the only options. Theological language and religious stories and images are sometimes effective in public settings—not to dominate, alienate, or condemn, but to stimulate the emotions and imaginations of discussion partners. If a "public" theological participant suggests a symbol, value, or principle from his or her specific tradition, the suggestion may resonate with aspects of the experiences and traditions of other participants, either distinctive or common, leading to agreement on certain values, bonds, practices, and decisions, even in the public realm. Theology can tip sensibilities in a certain direction, disposing participants to consider a line of argument more favorably. In such cases, the role of theology is both narrative and prophetic, creating both an ethos and a set of practical dispositions to act that can combat the technology-driven refusal of death or the control of health care by market economics. Religious and theological language can foster better understanding of the human condition and more humane, just, and beneficent practices and policies of biomedicine.

The types of ethical, policy, narrative, and prophetic discourse identified by Gustafson are not easily separable, nor are they ever abstracted from ways of life and patterns of action in which their speakers are involved. Attempts to advance moral ideals and standards and to transform behavior and social relationships depend on active, participatory engagement, as well as on speech. Therefore, as I indicated earlier, to Gustafson's four types can be added a fifth: theology as *participatory* discourse. Participatory discourse refers to a mode of theological and ethical speech in which its practical roots and outcomes are intentionally acknowledged. Theological ethics in the participatory mode recognizes that its persuasive value derives only in part from its intellectual coherence. It derives in equal or greater measure from its power to allude to or induce a shared sphere of behavior, oriented by shared concerns and goals, and its power to constitute relations of empathy and interdependence among the "arguers." To name theological-ethical discourse as participatory discourse is to hold up as an explicit goal the creation of connective practices among interlocutors in order that shared social practices may be transformed in light of religiously inspired (though not necessarily tribalistic) visions and values.

Gustafson's four types—ethical, policy, prophetic, and narrative discourse—all refer primarily to language and verbal or textual expressions—concepts, principles, stories, statements, and so on. To name the participatory mode is to direct our attention explicitly to the kinds of joint activities that give rise to these types of language, bringing interlocutors together in a common practical space or enterprise where the language is mutually understood. Participatory practices are, of course, already implied by Gustafson's scheme. For example, those engaged in an "ethical" exchange will share or potentially share a terrain of values and priorities—such as respect for persons, the common good, or the obligation to do no harm—on which debates about specific applications can proceed. They will also share a cultural or scholarly setting in which the field of "ethics" is acknowledged, even if that setting is created cross-culturally, for example, by publications, conferences, and visiting lectureships.

Those engaged in policy discourse share or potentially share common social and legal institutions, precedents, and expectations that enable mutually intelligible argument about "best" policies—such as self-determination, informed consent, proportion of cost to benefit, or the right to profit by one's labor. These will have already been made explicit by a framing tradition of policy, regulation, judicial precedents, and law. Contemporary theological bioethics rightly engages in policy discussions and the requisite social practices (presidential bioethics commissions, lobbying in Washington, D.C., court testimony). But this is only one sphere of social action and influence open to religion and theology. Theological bioethicists too readily concede the playing field to those who define it in "policy discourse" terms, essentially the terms of liberal democratic capitalism. This means that theologians become captives to the practice of policy making as the exclusive way to engage others on bioethical matters and forget about equally or more important avenues of reform.

Theological bioethics as participatory must explicitly link religion and theology to practices and movements in civil society that can have a subversive or revolutionary impact on liberalism, science, and the market. The public and social effects of prophetic and narrative discourse should be integrated with participatory, inclusive practices. Prophetic naming of injustice and the enhancement of narratives of resistance and empowerment can unite persons of a variety of religious and moral faiths. It is especially critical to recognize that real-world coalitions around shared purposes and goals are a means of rooting and furthering theological bioethics as participatory discourse. The theoretical apparatus of theological bioethics must include specific attention to the public impact of participatory practices.

Social distortions and social reform need to be understood in light of a more comprehensive and multifaceted interpretation of knowledge, moral commitment, and action. The next chapter will build on the dialectical character of early theological bioethics and propose that theological bioethics participate more self-consciously in reformist practices today. Participatory theological bioethics connects public discourse and influence to a variety of political movements and institutions of civil society in which religious groups can be effective.

Moving Ahead: Feminist Bioethics

Most theological bioethicists today are dialectical in that they engage with cultural problems and increasingly do so in a global sphere of concern. They are also committed to maintain intact those tenets of the Christian tradition that they perceive to be essential. Many believe that the dialectical relation of theology and culture cuts both ways in the sense that religious traditions must sometimes be corrected on basic issues in light of contemporary experience. But still needed is a theological bioethics that explicitly connects theories and worldviews to cooperative social action, combating systemic social distortions with reformist or revolutionary practices that create or join coalitions in civil society.

In theological bioethics, feminist authors have been ahead of the curve on this issue, as on that of making a preferential option for the poor definitive of the contribution of theology to bioethics. Feminist bioethics, religious and nonreligious, arose in close connection with struggles for women's social equality in the 1960s and 1970s. Because the stereotyping of women's roles as defined by sex and reproduction was the target of the feminist movement, these also were the focus of the earliest ventures in feminist bioethics. From the beginning, debates about the ethics of reproductive medicine, such as birth control, sterilization, abortion, and reproductive technologies, were carried out by feminists with a close eye to their practical significance and in coordination with practical activism to change women's opportunities.

Many of the first feminist bioethicists, representatively theologian Beverly Harrison, adopted a "liberal" defense of women's autonomy, advocating for a right to abortion.[69] Yet Marxist and radical feminists soon posed a challenge to the idea that a liberal model of women's choice would necessarily free women from patriarchal scientific institutions and the pervasive influence of the profit motive. Remarked one bioethicist with theological training, "Perhaps the most confusing message about the new reproductive technologies is that they are a gift to women, because they appear to give so-called infertile women the ability to reproduce. However . . . more and more areas of female living have been colonized by medical intervention, and staked out as medical territory."[70]

Particularly as feminist bioethics grew to include the testimony of Latina and African American women and of women from the "two-thirds world," the significance of biomedical practices for women's concrete reality was focused on issues of socioeconomic and racial-ethnic as well as gender oppression. This focus has become much more central as feminist ethicists confront the challenges of globalization. In the words of Karen Lebacqz, the "first thing" theology brings to public discourse is "justice as a crucial category," assessed in terms of "the plight of the poor" and requiring "a willingness to let go of the landscape as we know it in order to permit justice to be done."[71]

Some general directions for feminist theology and bioethics are captured by Margaret Farley and Barbara Andolsen. In 1985, Farley grounded feminist theology in the experience and well-being of women and lifted up three central themes: human relational patterns, human embodiment, and human interpretation of "nature."[72] Farley insists that patterns of relationship not be hierarchical and oppressive, especially to women; that women can reclaim their bodies as personal subjects active in the world; and that the domination of nature that goes along with domination of women can be overcome in the name of a sacramental view of creation. Important interdependent principles for Farley are autonomy and relationality, equality and mutuality.[73]

Andolsen gives special attention to issues of race and class, observing that, ultimately, feminist theology is concerned about "the well-being of all persons, including men, and about the good of the entire natural world."[74] In accordance with her interest in the intersection of race and class with gender, Andolsen corrects a theory of justice as detached impartiality with an ethic of care sensitive to the particular circumstances and forms of oppression suffered by women and others. Seeking to jar religious sensibilities into a new way of seeing the relation between the divine and the world, she suggests a reinvigorating use of the image of God as mother, both to empower women as patients and health care practitioners and to foster a belief in "the God/dess who will tolerate no excluded ones."[75]

Conclusion

Two important trends must be emphasized. First, the practice of medicine and the provision of health care are in our culture increasingly scientific rather than humanistic enterprises, and they are even more quickly being directed by marketplace values. Participants in biomedicine—whether providers or patients—are finding this situation ever less satisfactory at a personal level, and many are raising questions about the kind of society that is sponsoring these shifts, in turn to be re-created by them. Because they deal in the elemental human experiences of birth, life, death, and suffering, the biomedical arts provide an opening for larger questions of meaning and even of transcendence. Religious themes and imagery can be helpful in articulating these concerns and addressing them in an imaginative, provocative, and perhaps ultimately transformative way. Religious symbolism may be grounded in particular communities and their experiences of God and community, but perhaps it can also mediate a sensibility of transcendence and ultimacy that is achingly latent in the ethical conflicts, tragedies, and triumphs that are unavoidable in biomedicine. The immense current interest in the spiritual dimensions of health care exemplifies this trend.[76]

A second, not unrelated, trend is toward investment in the social and even global picture of health care ethics by theologians. In religious perspective, justice in medicine and access to preventive and therapeutic care is increasingly seen not only in terms of autonomy but in communal terms. While philosophical and public policy bioethics in this country is still dominated by considerations of autonomy and informed consent, theological bioethics, even when "translated" into more general, nonreligious categories, tends to prioritize distributive justice and social solidarity over individual rights and liberty. This makes theological bioethics more resistant to the market forces that so often control what research is funded, where it is conducted and on whom, who has access to the benefits, who profits from new knowledge and its implementation, and how health care is organized within a society as a whole. Biblical foundations can be found for such a perspective, especially in the Hebrew prophets and in the teaching and example of Jesus about love of neighbor and serving the poor and vulnerable. Warrants can also be found in religious traditions of practice, where care of the sick has often been institutionalized as a work of devotion and self-offering to the divine and where morality has been communal in nature and definition. In today's world, the community in which the neighbor is served and goods shared is increasingly international and global, and theological bioethics is responding directly to these new global realities.

Chapter 2 will propose an understanding of public theological bioethics as participatory in a multiplicity of social movements and networks—from the local to the global—that can give religion's prophetic critique of injustice some traction in the real world.

CHAPTER
2

PARTICIPATORY THEOLOGICAL BIOETHICS IN ACTION

THE PREVIOUS CHAPTER made the case that theological bioethics can and should shape public policy and social practices by engaging cultural assumptions, traditions, and institutions at both a theoretical and a practical level. It emphasized that theological bioethicists committed to justice as participation in the common good should use a variety of symbols and languages, religious or not, in a provocative and critical, yet dialogical, way.

Earlier theological leaders tended to present theological bioethics as interacting socially in theoretical or discursive terms rather than through practical social interventions, even though they themselves were actually engaged "dialectically" about policies and practices. Although they certainly recognized the reality of social sin, they did not fully nuance and integrate their understandings of how sin operates institutionally with parallel understandings of how Christians in faith communities and as citizens can counteract distorting and oppressive institutions, especially at the international level. Nor did they mount a strong critique of sin as inherent to the ideologies of market entrepreneurship and scientific progress that now globally drive scientific investment and biotechnology.

By conceding that public discourse is *not* tradition generated, worldview oriented, and value driven, some in the next generation of theological bioethics undercut their ability to prophetically criticize the substantive values and social relationships that support the status quo. Theologians should not withdraw from policy settings, lose their critical edge, or be seduced into believing that elite policy bodies necessarily control bioethics practices "on the ground." The challenge for theologians is to use narrative, prophetic, and especially participatory modes of discourse to put social justice—defined as distributive justice and the common good—back on the policy table. This Christian theological commitment to public discourse about justice can also be defended biblically through appeals to the doctrine of Creation and Jesus' socially radical ministry.

A new synthesis of Christian bioethics is needed that takes into account the contextuality and historicity of moral knowledge, the reality and changing manifestations of social sin, and the new social infrastructures and superstructures entailed by the globalization of communications, travel, finance, and science. Emerging networks of action and power at the local, national, and global levels offer novel opportunities for the transformative presence of bioethics.

Models of Participation in Theological Ethics

Parallel concepts or precedents to participatory theological-ethical discourse can be found in the Protestant language of "middle axioms" and the Catholic vocabulary of "casuistry," "subsidiarity," and "contributive justice." The reality of and the need for participatory discourse in bioethics can be further supported by sociological and historical treatments of the emergence in the twentieth century of movements for "participatory democracy," "deliberative democracy," and more democratic forms of "civil society" at the global level.

First, "casuistry" refers to a tradition of moral argument developed throughout the thirteenth to the seventeenth centuries, primarily by Catholic moralists, especially the Jesuits. Stereotypically, it denotes a process of logical deduction from abstract principles to concrete cases and was famously satirized by Blaise Pascal (*Provincial Letters,* 1656) for being not only arid and detached from reality but specious as well. As philosophers and theologians have recently noted, this reputation is ill-deserved.[1] Philosophers Albert Jonsen and Stephen Toulmin arrived at a more appreciative view after working with the National Commission for the Protection of Human Subjects in the mid-1970s. Both scholars noticed that, despite different backgrounds and ways of construing the ultimate ground of morality, the eleven commissioners were often able to reach agreement on particular problems. Jonsen and Toulmin interpret this surprising development in light of Aristotle's view that moral reasoning is practical, calling for experience in relation to particulars and concrete situations more than for rigorous logic. Practical reasoning in ethics, guided by the virtue of prudence, is a matter of exercising good judgment, not of "drawing formal deductions from invariable axioms."[2] Today, a companion concept to casuistry is virtue ethics, an approach elaborated in relation to theology and genetics by James Keenan.[3] To connect virtue to moral argumentation is a way of recognizing that analyses of cases are guided by practical reason, habituated in individuals toward wisdom, and by concrete moral struggle, within a community of discernment that shapes perception and judgment according to shared values and commitments.

The concepts of casuistry and virtue clarify why theology can rarely if ever provide master theories for bioethics policy or definitive resolutions of dilemmas and value conflicts. Rather, theology and religion nurture a social and intellectual milieu in which the social priorities of religious communities can be recognized sympathetically. Social practices and policy outcomes are more likely to reflect respect for all human lives and a "preferential option for the poor" if religious thinkers represent these values while engaging with others in the practical negotiation of solutions to problems.

The principle of subsidiarity was generated within papal social encyclicals, aimed not at theoretical certainty but at political flexibility within a normative framework centered on the common good of society. Developed first by Pius XI in *Quadragesimo Anno* (1931),[4] subsidiarity refers to a reciprocal relationship between higher and lower organizations and their governments, especially in the context of the nation-state. The obligation of governing authorities to intervene when necessary for the common good is given increasing emphasis by John XXIII and later popes, as inequities in global resources begin to occupy papal attention to social issues. According to John XXIII's *Mater et Magistra* (1961), "recent developments of science and technology" make it more crucial than ever that "public authorities" assume the responsibility to "reduce imbalances," whether within one nation or "between different peoples of the world as a whole" (no. 54).

The principle of subsidiarity is a means of responding ad hoc to a variety of challenges of international political life; it evaluates particular political arrangements and their adequacy for diverse social contexts. For example, in the context of human and agricultural genetics, subsidiarity can be used to advance the right of local cultures to control the advent of genetic manipulation and to enjoy whatever benefits it may bring. Yet it also implies that international governmental and nongovernmental organizations should limit the power of international researchers and transnational corporations to remove or patent DNA from local species, plant or human, or to introduce modified species into the local environment.

Despite the fact that the concept of middle axioms is even more ambiguous, it has undergone an intriguing revival. Audrey Chapman, expressing frustration with bioethicists' vague "prophetic" stances, calls for the development of "middle axioms" that could mediate between general convictions and principles and the policy evaluations and political strategies that lead to specific genetics policies.[5] Yet the meaning of the category has been contested almost since its invention by J. H. Oldham in 1937, in a paper prepared for an Oxford ecumenical conference on church and state.[6] For example, Ronald Preston leads off his dictionary article on middle axioms with the phrase "A misleading term."[7]

While it is generally agreed that middle axioms are supposed to negotiate the distance between Christian ideals and social realities, some have understood this to occur by means of deduction from more general to more concrete judgments;[8] others, including Oldham, see middle axioms as indicating more a process of interaction between Christian values and social problems, with the church endorsing positions that seem the best available social alternatives at the time. Middle axioms are "definitions of the type of behaviour required of Christians" in their peculiar settings and are produced not by logical deduction but by interactive efforts to embody Christian values amid the perplexities of life.[9] They assume the need to make common cause and to compromise with others. The notion of middle axioms arose to help Christian ethics contend with the era between world wars, in which the certainty of Christian social teaching had been upset and in which its proponents were acutely aware that the kingdom of God would be impossible to establish on earth, and very difficult to even initiate.

In a parallel context of historical angst, the concept has found favor with liberation theologians, including Charles Villa-Vicencio and Robert Schreiter. According to Villa-Vicencio, middle axioms call for the church to renew society even if the gospel demands more than society can deliver.[10] They are part of a corporate approach to theology, in which social renewal and "mental constructs" work together to give theology not only "a *praxiological* foundation" but a role in "democratic participation."[11] Robert Schreiter connects middle axioms to interdisciplinary collaboration, and particularly to the task of building up civil society and its mediating structures and associations, in both local and global contexts. Religion is a powerful source of such renewal.[12]

In sum, the originally Protestant concept of middle axioms conveys a self-conscious attempt of Christian ethicists to negotiate among Christian values, social realities, local contexts, and global interconnections of societies and faith traditions. In contemporary bioethics, middle axioms should be interpreted neither as part of a deductive process of reasoning nor as tools solely with which to engage the policies of national or higher-level governments. The concept can provide a theoretical niche to the multiple ways in which religious individuals and groups interact with the changing practices and institutions of medicine and health care, seeking opportunistically to make Christian social values more effective.

A similar awareness of the need to broaden the scope of theological engagement, and especially to respect and empower within civil society heretofore silenced groups, is conveyed in the development of Catholic social teaching and its ongoing redefinitions of justice. Rising importance is given in this evolving tradition to concepts of solidarity, participation, and "preferential option for the poor," all within advocacy for global justice, termed, since the 1960s, "the universal common good."[13] Since the time of Aquinas, justice has been categorized as either commutative (relations among individuals in society) or distributive (what society owes to each).[14] The neo-scholastic tradition introduced the category of legal justice to specify what each person owes to society.[15] Since Pius XI's *Quadragesimo anno* (1931), social encyclicals, various bishops' conferences, and other Catholic writings have used the category of "social justice," but never define it precisely. However, it is generally accurate to say that social justice is an integrative concept, bringing together and indicating the interdependence of all the just relations and institutions that make up the common good. Social justice is increasingly defined to consist of or include "contributive justice," what all persons bring to the common good by their active participation.[16]

The contributory dimension of justice is essential to theological bioethics, indicating both the need for a preferential option favoring the voice and participation of the poor and the interdependence of the good of all participants, on which the well-being of the whole depends. At an international conference on transforming unjust structures, theologian Julie Clague delivered a paper on modifying and implementing patent laws so that biotechnology benefits are available to those who need them most.[17] In discussion, she suggested that activism in favor of "global public goods" could be linked to a theory of contributory justice recognizing that, with globalization, the motivations of self-interest and altruism cannot be completely separated. This point might be extended by saying that the contemporary requirement of contributive justice integrates the older principle of subsidiarity with the newer emphases on solidarity and participation by calling attention to the fact that all the associations of civil society are in constant interaction. Decisions made and goods sought in one sphere inevitably reverberate throughout the global network, offering theological bioethics multiple points of entry for wide-ranging transformations. Not only does action in a variety of intersecting spheres allow democratic participation, but also it is necessary so that all contribute to the common good—or contributory justice.

Participatory Democracy

The public role and potential practical impact of theological bioethics can be understood as part of a global trend toward activism for "participatory democracy." This phrase was coined in a manifesto for Students for a Democratic Society (SDS), drafted in 1961 by Tom Hayden for a meeting in Port Huron, Michigan.[18] Participatory democracy became one of the era's most powerful ideas. Egalitarian decision making did not abolish structures, rules, or formal procedures, but it combined these with a deliberative style and an experimental character.[19] Referring originally to the internal organization of leftist social movements, participatory democracy captured the sort of society student activists aspired to create through desegregation, civil rights, and women's liberation. Aimed in part at the U.S. government and its legislation, action for participatory democracy also protested state and local policies, and it united groups across racial, class, and religious lines to challenge the status quo. Though the sought-after reforms were only partially effective, both within 1960s organizations and in the larger culture, they made a lasting impact on the consciousness of the nation regarding political engagement. Perhaps their most significant impact was on the expectation about what commitment and organized action can actually accomplish.

A report of Georgetown University's Woodstock Center on ethical lobbying identifies a systemic problem in U.S. democracy, to which a revival of participatory democracy could reply. Competing today with the impetus toward democratic engagement is "a claimant politics based on the pursuit of self-interest and group advantage rather than a civic politics based on the discovery and enactment of the comprehensive public good."[20] A "market-driven mentality" has excluded other conceptions of political life, with access to funds widely defining political influence. A market model of competition, bargaining, and profit winning defines the new norms of political conduct.[21] Understanding the common good as "the proper goal of public deliberation and action,"[22] the report projects the public sphere as a realm in which citizens and federal and state governments interact with intermediary organizations such as civic groups, public interest groups, nonprofits, and advocates for the poor and disadvantaged.[23] Yet the decline of public confidence in the power of these interactions to change the status quo has resulted in widespread alienation at many levels of the political process. Religion, theology, and religious institutions can contribute by recognizing and enhancing political and civic mobilization, especially around their distinctive values, such as compassion, respect, solidarity, and service.

The tradition of participatory democracy is a latent catalyst for change, one amenable to both religious and theological initiatives. Theological bioethicists who feel stifled in "official" policy debates should turn to this tradition for a more optimistic prospect. One model and resource for participatory democracy movements has been religious fellowship, long exemplified by Quaker pacifism. Religion has also been operative in faith-based organizing, which is less focused on authority figures and less resistant to forging new bases of authority.[24]

Deliberative Democracy

In their depiction of the components of democratic social deliberation about controversial matters of the common good, such as abortion, Amy Gutmann and Dennis Thompson provide a similar framework to that of participatory democracy, one that further clarifies the potential contributions of theology.[25] A key point in their work is that members of democratic communities can deal with disagreement in a mutually respectful way that aims to create greater consensus, even though disagreement will never be eliminated and the consensus will never be complete.[26] Instead, as a practical matter, members seek ways to agree on practices that accommodate the interests and commitments of all parties, without demanding that any abandon their convictions or act entirely with motivations of altruism rather than self-interest.[27] Most of this kind of negotiation occurs somewhere between the micro level of individual action and the macro level of theories of justice, though it moves back and forth between particular decisions and ultimate foundations.[28]

Gutmann and Thompson also suggest that, ideally at least, the ambit of moral accountability for deliberative democracy extends to all who could be affected by an outcome, including those who have been left out of the discussion and those in the international sphere.[29] They acknowledge that truly *democratic* practice requires participation by the formerly excluded, not just their consideration on the part of the elites, especially as those who benefit from advantages are not likely to yield them easily. And changing unequal patterns of advantage may well require impassioned testimonials, even in "public" matters, as has been the case in U.S. history, in the fight against racial exclusion.[30] Moreover, participation in the deliberations of a democratic society requires more than the ability to express ideas and values—it requires certain social and political conditions. Democratic deliberation therefore implies and requires substantive principles and goods, not simply procedures.[31] Gutmann and Thompson call for a principle of "fair distribution" to be applied to "basic opportunity goods," such as health care, education, security, income, and work.[32]

The theory of deliberative democracy illuminates the role of participatory theological bioethics in several ways. First of all, its normative values converge with those of religiously grounded approaches, especially with Christian social ethics and the "common good" tradition explicitly endorsed by Catholicism. Second, Gutmann and Thompson offer a theoretical framework to explicate and defend practical ways in which these values can be advanced in social and political arrangements, without expecting or demanding that "success" be measured in absolute terms. Theological advocacy, connected to the practices of faith traditions, provides such a venue.

Third, the theory explicitly takes into account the important and valid role of substantive value traditions (and their corollary practices) in naming basic goods, seeking empowerment, and shaping consensus. In examples they give, including abortion, civil rights, and surrogate motherhood, some of these bearers of substantive values have been philosophical in orientation, some theological, some political, some legal, some economic, some racial or ethnic, some gender based, and so on. All can profitably encounter and debate one another, granting such principles as reciprocity, mutual respect, transparency, universal accountability, and the recognition of basic obligations to protect the liberty and welfare of others in society.

Finally, the theory of deliberative democracy, like that of participatory theological discourse, does not just reflect abstractly on—but engages and advances—actions, policies, and practices that instantiate its values and goals. Both validate their goals, not just by showing an intellectual cogency and appeal but by making the case that they can make a real difference in society—even if that difference is not comprehensive, irreversible, or complete. But the idea of participatory democracy provides an essential complement to the theory of deliberative democracy in that it highlights the possibility of making progress toward a more "deliberative" society by instigating social change from the bottom up and by explicitly involving worldview claims.

Theology, Bioethics, Action, and Justice

A distinctive contribution of theology, especially but not exclusively Christian biblical theology, can be to challenge exclusionary systems of access to social and material goods under the aegis of "love of neighbor," "self-sacrifice," or "the preferential option for the poor." But this challenge must be embodied and mediated through action initiatives developing and operating in concert with narratives, symbols, arguments, and ideals. Historical and sociological studies of social and political activism by churches provide concrete evidence that religiously sponsored and theologically grounded initiatives for change are possible and realistic.

While theology may have been disenfranchised from the "public sphere" of politics, religious communities are present and active in civil society and also, if to a lesser degree, in social movements that aim to affect the economy and government. The field of theological ethics, and theological bioethics specifically, needs to renew the link between theological reflection and argument, and social action for transformative goals. Action is a source as well as outcome of normative ethics. The defining action of theological bioethics takes place in and by faith traditions as they engage other traditions of belief, identity, and practice regarding "matters of common interest" (Taylor).

Both academia and the media have minimized the role of religion in contemporary American politics, despite the fact that religious activism has been rising since the 1960s. This is partly due to the influence among cultural elites and scholars of "secularization theory," the idea that religion loses value in modern societies because "advancing human reason" makes it unnecessary.[33] This conception may validate the cultural authority of the advocates of secularism, but it does not square with the realities of American society.

Taking a broader view of contemporary U.S. society than typically informs debates about thick and thin bioethics, the case can be made that religious communities are effective shapers of individual and collective identity, that they form and inspire members for political engagement, and that they are already identifying their theological voices as politically participatory. Since the 1960s, immigration has increased dramatically, bringing to America novel and rising levels of religious commitment and diversity. But pluralism, while eroding the older Protestant-Catholic-Jewish mainstream consensus, has not had the simple effect of secularizing the culture. Instead, it has brought the "de-Europeanizing of American Christianity and the intensification of religious identity."[34] The accentuation and cultivation of particular identities within specific faith traditions does not necessarily result either in religious conflict or in the retreat of believers from civic engagement. Instead, religious identities become the *basis on which* society is engaged. Sociologist Stephen Warner observes, "The religious cultural reproduction of the sort that I see promoted in black churches, white evangelical churches, Hispanic/Latino churches, synagogues, and immigrant congregations presupposes at least implicitly what mainline churches proclaim explicitly: that society is worth the church's while." The stress on particular identity can be "a religious form of thinking globally but acting locally."[35]

Private devotions such as prayer and reading scripture, as well as public forms of religious expression such as church attendance, are correlated positively with political involvement.[36] A churchgoer relies on his or her religious communities to help make sense of and provide an orientation for his or her attitudes and behavior. He or she "encounters symbolic political messages as part of the religious socialization process and may well obtain politically relevant cues from discussion and interaction with other congregants." Evidence that such messages have an effect is that political distinctiveness persists among religious groups.[37]

Both culturally conservative and progressive religious groups have been politically active and successful in evoking social change. In the early 2000s, the former seemed more visible and politically effective. But in the 1960s, religious groups protested against the Vietnam War and in favor of civil rights. In the 1970s, the introduction of new medical technologies brought into public view quandaries over whether and how to sustain the life of comatose patients such as Karen Ann Quinlan or severely comprised newborns. Religious groups, especially the Catholic Church, were particularly vocal then and have been since in setting standards regarding ordinary and extraordinary means of life support and in diminishing the impact of the movement for physician-assisted suicide. Whereas earlier cases, such as those of Quinlan, Nancy Cruzan, and Brother Fox, were settled in favor of removing or foregoing treatment, on the basis of a Catholic analysis of the optional nature of "extraordinary means," there has been a surge of recent Catholic pro-life protest against allowing even comatose patients to die, as in the case of Terry Schiavo. In the 1980s and 1990s, school prayer, abortion, education, and gay rights were on the agenda, along with international issues such as the conflict in Central America and the end of apartheid. At the turn of the twenty-first century, bioethical issues such as health care reform, the potential uses of knowledge about the human genetic code, and the morality of embryo and stem cell research came into focus.

On all of these topics, as well as on the war in Iraq and on the legal recognition of "gay marriage" or gay civil unions, religious congregations and their leadership have been opinion shapers, with theologians systematically linking moral and social agendas to the worldviews of the religions. Church membership has been mobilized around these and other issues, even though denominational affiliation does not "predict" individual stances or deliver votes on each and every one. In fact, while voting and involvement with political parties have deteriorated, "organized religion has moved in to fill the void," expressing its goals in terms of both practical initiatives and theological analysis.[38]

Common to religious activism on both the left and right is the perception that the influence of government and the state has become too great and "totalitarian," whether on welfare policy, abortion, or war decisions.[39] Religious groups in general act to reclaim democratic authority over actions and policies that reflect special interests, consolidate elite privileges and biases, or base their assumptions on pragmatic cost-benefit calculations rather than moral principle. They usually reflect communalistic rather than individualistic sensibilities. Hence they can be seen as important catalysts for participatory democracy, embodying a force for practical equality, inclusiveness, reciprocity, and empowerment of socially marginal groups, even though their substantive agendas vary. What these groups have in common can be expressed theologically through doctrines of creation, covenant, love of neighbor, and community, for instance.

In all of these movements and cases, theologians and theological ethics have been invoked to explain and justify the religious traditions' moral and social aims. Theological ethics is exactly the normative discourse that fulfills this role and so enhances activist and socially ameliorative commitments. Theological ethics is constituted in the very process of response to the quandaries generated by religious engagement with social problems.

However, as Stephen Hart claims, progressive religious groups too often take for granted the self-evidence of their normative agendas, thus failing to examine critically and clearly why they are so compelling.[40] A theological and religious agenda must be connected to cultural and social funds of meaning; this connection can only be made through practices that express norms and attract others to them via cooperative projects, as well as by "discourse" that makes norms and values conceptually explicit (a role of theology). In recent years, at least, socially conservative groups have done this more effectively than progressive ones.

Progressive voices can talk about justice and equality for all, without necessarily linking these values to the ultimate beliefs and transcendent frame of reference that give the ideals their real power, and explain why the advocates are so highly committed. The cultivation of empathy and the social virtue of solidarity require expanding the cultural symbol system to accommodate ideals of solidarity and justice. The symbol systems of liberal individualism, scientific progress, and market economics legitimate self-interest under the aegis of protecting democracy and liberty. Conservative groups are much more effective in tying anxieties about domestic economic insecurity, the threat of cultural change, and fear of threats from outside—whether from low-wage labor or terrorists—to a sense of privilege and entitlement, legitimated in terms of patriotism, fidelity to "traditional" values, or loyalty to "the American way of life." Progressive groups and movements, including those with a religious orientation, need to retrieve or invent more effective symbols, discourses, and liturgies that imaginatively present solidarity for the common good as a "traditional American" value, as a social concomitant of biblical themes such as the kingdom of God and love of neighbor, and as a cultural and political possibility in the global era. Progressive groups neglect the power of religious narratives to do this constructive and unifying work.

Hart maintains that progressives and conservatives typically employ two different styles of discourse: "constrained" discourse and "expansive" discourse. The difference between the two works to the disadvantage of progressives, including religious progressives; progressive theological bioethics is a case in point, especially when it is operating in the policy mode. Constrained discourse aims to affect the "public sphere"; it assumes that unified action and a public voice depend on taking a narrow focus on specific, well-defined, and agreed-upon issues, while leaving out of the picture all talk of transcendent values, comprehensive worldviews, overall goals for society, or universal standards. In other words, constrained discourse favors the policy mode and avoids prophetic and narrative language, as well as language about ethical foundations.

Expansive discourse, on the other hand, typically invoked by evangelical Christians, is much more passionate. A bioethical example is the pro-life movement, backed by symbols and concepts such as divine providence, the image of God, the sacredness of life, human dignity, and the protection of innocent life. Expansive discourse constantly asserts judgments about transcendent and utopian values, demonic and even apocalyptic threats, and the need for clear, universal standards of right and wrong. Limited to constrained discourse, progressives in the public sphere tend neither to examine nor to advocate issues of ultimate purpose and meaning. Religiously based progressive politics "often uses modes of discourse that are cautious and constrained to the point of being anemic."[41] Progressives lose sight of the larger challenges they could make to society, instead becoming fixed opportunistically on small, incremental changes.[42]

Hart claims that progressive religious movements and advocacy lose contact with cultural processes and symbols that could help instigate and motivate effective political action. One might argue further that while they have lost touch with the cultural resources for change, they are not only in touch with but held in place by the cultural processes and symbols that help legitimate the status quo (liberal individualism, a market economy, the scientific imperative). This is particularly unfortunate, because although Republicans have had more success in elections in recent years, and although pundits decry the "culture wars," public opinion polls show no general trend toward the right in popular conviction. Grassroots views on most issues have remained more or less stable since the 1970s.[43] Yet progressives have failed to capitalize on this latent cultural consensus in the policy arena. Mainline churches, through official statements; activities of highly placed representatives; and lobbying efforts make it a major focus to knock on the doors of the custodians of the public sphere. Yet they fail to exploit to full effect the potentially powerful base membership that could be working for change through the institutions of civil society and engaging in grassroots political initiatives.

Hart warns that "recovering the capacity to express moral outrage, universal claims of justice, and visions of a better society is essential if progressive political initiatives are to prosper—or deserve to prosper."[44]

Prophetic religion explicitly places human interests against the horizon of the absolute. It declares human enterprises to be dependent, fallible, and frequently malicious. It names the domination and deprivation of the many by the few as *sin*. In the words of Reinhold Niebuhr, "The moral and social dimension of sin is injustice. The ego which falsely makes itself the centre of existence in its pride and will-to-power inevitably subordinates other life to its will and thus does injustice to other life."[45] To name something as sin is also to assert that it can and should be changed. The category of sin and its social extrapolation as injustice are a distinctive contribution of theology. Participatory theological ethics is a solidaristic, active, and empowering response to social sin that conveys the reality and promise of change and that overcomes alienation. Only a more expansive, normatively committed, and substantive discourse, carried into the public sphere by talk and action, can tie in to the deeper cultural and social values that progressive politics needs on its side.

Examples: Religious Lobbying, Faith-Based Organizing, and Academia

In a study of religious lobbying, Daniel Hofrenning concedes that "in terms of conventional wins and losses on specific pieces of legislation, religious lobbyists often—but not always—come up short." Theological ethics and religious activism obviously do not always succeed in mediating their ideals into society as a whole. Nevertheless, they transform politics significantly, because of their consistent calls for moral reform. "With these calls, religious lobbyists register a challenge to the state and offer mediating organizations for citizens to voice their discontent."[46] Clearly participatory, the strategy of religious lobbyists is also both narrative and prophetic in character, offering scathing criticisms of the status quo, based on age-old strands of their religious traditions.[47] This fact alone is an obvious reason why religious groups are viewed with suspicion by the state and by state-sponsored advisory or policy bodies.

Religious lobbyists tend to keep in view a bigger picture than specific pieces of legislation or the gain of a particular client; their goal is to make fundamental changes in the U.S. political system, in particular to reinvigorate the moral dimension of politics. In places such as Poland and the Philippines, religion has been an essential factor in successful resistance to totalitarian governments. Although religions themselves can be totalitarian in outlook and aims, democratic activism on the part of religious groups can effectively challenge unjust and elitist state policies if it emanates from or engages the grassroots, if it works through persuasive social criticism, and if it embodies "alternative" practices that attract cooperation.

To recognize the value of lobbying is not to say that the federal government is the only available conduit for social change. At the opposite end of the spectrum from the Washington lobbyist is the faith-based community organizer, mobilizing local interest to contend with local problems. In his study of congregation-based activism, Stephen Hart displays another side of the impact of religion on politics. He asserts the power of community organizing to link spirituality, theology, and politics; to unite different religious traditions with partially contrasting theological and political stances; and to accomplish change at the neighborhood, city, or state level. Congregation-based community organizing empowers individual leaders. It also creates discourse between religion and "secular" politics, partly by "translating" religious values and theologies, sometimes by invoking them directly in political action, and always by making connections among religions, their theologies, and the values most Americans believe in, such as democracy, human rights, and civil rights.

Supporting the hypothesis that religious participation in politics has increased in the past half-century rather than declined, Hart compares the results of a 1994 and a 2000 survey on congregation-based community organizing programs in the United States. He finds that there were 48 percent more such projects in 2000, with the average number of congregations involved increasing from twenty to twenty-six, for a result of 95 percent more congregations involved nationally in community organizing than in 1994—a total of 133.[48] The movement is ethnically and racially diverse, with member congregations that are predominantly black, Hispanic, Asian, Native American, interracial, and European American.[49] Faith-based organizing takes political objectives seriously and influences debate and outcomes in many cities. Theologically, community-based organizing is influenced by modern Catholic teachings about the economic order, African American Christian social action traditions, liberation theology, the Social Gospel tradition, and the "Christian realism" of Reinhold Niebuhr, which demands a realistic approach to the need to back up moral persuasion with pressure.[50] Theological "policy" bioethics would gain significantly in effectiveness if it could overcome what Hart refers to as "the decoupling of civil society from politics."[51] Religious communities have tremendous resources for civic engagement that could be engaged on behalf of health care justice. In Hart's view, "congregation-based organizing may be the largest coherent contemporary movement for economic justice—either secular or religious—that engages grassroots Americans locally in face-to-face political activity."[52]

Congregation-based community organizing provides a model for a more expansive form of theological bioethics that is ecumenical, ideologically inclusive, and practical. Hart illustrates with the example of Milwaukee Innercity Congregations for Hope (MICAH), which he studied from 1991 to 1993. A focus of MICAH during these years was to improve inner-city housing, preferably by an increase in publicly subsidized rental housing. As the next chapter will illustrate, housing is a crucial health-supporting resource, one that has been prioritized by the Catholic Health Association as a public-action agenda item.

MICAH began by targeting the problem of boarded-up houses—havens for drug dealers and signs of neighborhood deterioration that made banks even more likely to divest from the inner city.[53] The organization included members and supporters as different as the Catholic Archdiocese of Milwaukee, Lutherans, Presbyterians, Quakers, and the Church of God in Christ. (The latter is a historic African American church, whose all-male governing board adopted a resolution in 2004 against gay marriage, but that also hosted Martin Luther King Jr. as a speaker at its Memphis headquarters.) Despite differences on sex and gender issues, for instance, the thirty-five congregations involved in MICAH agree that religion and politics should be linked and that the prophetic message of Judaism and Christianity demands a commitment to improve the well-being of the poor, especially by empowerment of the poor. MICAH cuts across stereotypes of "liberal" and "conservative" but is clearly a stimulus to progressive social change.

MICAH organizers do not hesitate to couch their commitments in references to their own religious beliefs and spirituality. Their trust in God, or gratitude for what God has bestowed on them, form powerful motivations for their commitment to strengthen their communities or to help others. They refer to housing as a divine right, as well as a civil right and a human right.[54] Having been frustrated in a number of other measures, MICAH members finally staged a march on the mayor's house and through this public action won a favorable housing ordinance. The city never did commit significant funds from its general revenues to fulfill this ordinance, but it did obtain outside money, primarily from the federal government, to convert around one hundred abandoned buildings into subsidized housing.[55] Obviously, theologically informed themes such as "preferential option," "common good," "liberation of the oppressed," and "reign of God on Earth" could be invoked to defend or explain MICAH's normative vision of a good society in which the basic need of housing is met for all. Yet theologies of liberation and divinely willed justice are symbiotic with politically motivated cooperative action in civil society.

The theological ethics embodied in MICAH's organizing for fair housing was in the mode of participatory discourse. It accomplished some of its goals, whereas theological "policy" discourse, or even "ethical" discourse, might have been less effective. Participatory discourse, accompanied by prophetic and narrative forms of theological expression and reflection, was able to bring about change at levels that would be "invisible" to interlocutors whose gaze was fixed on the arena of federal legislation or regulation debated in a detached, nonlocal, public sphere.

The work of the Southwest Industrial Areas Foundation (IAF) further confirms the link between religious organizing and political participation.[56] Though not a faith-based organization as such, the IAF gains much of its power from religious leadership and congregations, and the ecumenical cooperation the IAF engenders. Paul Osterman opens his book on the IAF with an account of a convention in Austin, Texas, that exemplifies his view that participatory democracy can resist "politics" as "increasingly a game played by the economic and political elites operating out of Washington."[57] Successful mobilization against economic inequality, the core of the progressive agenda (as well as of theological bioethics), should and does locate alternative ways to exert pressure.

Fifteen hundred people, many of them Spanish speaking, and most of them traveling with church groups, convened in a hotel ballroom in April 2001 for a rousing send-off of prayer and political exhortation, then wended their way through several sessions of workshops. Afterward they repaired to a downtown church for an "accountability session" in which six IAF representatives shared a panel with about a dozen state representatives and senators. Addressing health issues first, including Medicaid eligibility and government insurance for children, the six IAF representatives went down a list of agenda items, demanding that the lawmakers answer yes or no as to their support of each item. Then two thousand people marched to the state capitol to locate (and if necessary outwait) members of the legislature who had not agreed to attend, to whom they posed the same questions. Every workday thereafter for several weeks, IAF delegates returned to "work the legislature."[58]

Organizing and activism in the local community provide windows for success, even when legislatures and policymakers are resistant and slow to produce concrete changes. Seemingly powerless groups can become sites of resistance and advocacy with real impact on the social order. Osterman tells of two women from Mexican immigrant families who joined with city, health, and business leaders to create the free Milagro health clinic. This required securing state funding, overcoming opposition from the local health care establishment that wanted all efforts focused on a research facility, and identifying a nonprofit corporation to manage the clinic.[59]

As a contrasting example of ineffective advocacy for change in health care access, Hart describes an academic paper he once heard delivered on the subject. The author lost out rhetorically to a religious conservative, because she did not invoke a bigger perspective on the sources of human dignity, the importance and limits of freedom, the necessity to honor mutual responsibilities as well as rights, and the priority of basic physical health over the bottom lines of insurance companies.[60] The "expansive" style does not shy away from these questions. Nor would it direct its energy primarily to "official" or academic policy discourse, focused on the formal cogency of abstract principles such as a right to health care. This can be a problem with theological scholarship, even when it assumes a more expansive style.

Consequences for Participatory Theological Bioethics

Theoretical discourse becomes relevant to the practical realm only insofar as it can validate patterns of relationship that match the terms of the verbal explanation or argument. Intellectual or scholarly discourse (including theological and philosophical discourse) challenges the status quo in an area, such as housing or health care, by expressing and reinforcing symbols, concepts, and arguments (the image of God; human dignity; that the common good requires distributive justice) that in effect cause a tension between the status quo in that area and alternative practices and behaviors (basic housing for all, universal access to health care). The alternatives are part of a different worldview or orientation (the reign of God mandates a preferential option for the poor, the nature of moral experience mandates equal respect for all) that challenges the prevalent worldview and the social arrangements that follow from it. The power of alternative discourse increases in proportion to the fact that it is not "merely" intellectual, but a conceptual expression of alternative realities taking shape in practice.

Theological bioethics can engage civil society, invoke transcendent values, and empower the disenfranchised. Yet these actions can be harnessed to very different political objectives, either conservative or progressive. Thus theology and theological bioethics should promote open, sustained, and nuanced debate of substantive values and goals as they are embodied in existing social practices. Theological bioethics must be attentive to and integrated with the various levels of civil society and political action, in the "participatory" theological mode. But broad participation in itself is not the chief political goal of faith-based activism. The ultimate goal of theological bioethics must be the achievement of social arrangements that are more consistent with the core messages of the involved religious traditions about the uses and limits of liberty and the meaning of the common good and social justice.

Dimensions of the core message and, even more so, its political ramifications will be controverted. Hence the need for open, explicit, and public value discussions, as well as active and sometimes high-pressure negotiation of concrete political aims regarding priorities, budgets, and programs. Progressives can only engage persuasively and productively in this process if they become involved at its many levels, putting their values and worldviews in action.

Theological bioethics that favors political change toward equality and inclusive participation in the civic and material goods of society will need to adopt a forthrightly "expansive" and substantive style, as well as an activist dimension. Its task is to communicate its message clearly and on the basis of both religious and humanistic authorities, narratives, and arguments. The message of progressive theological bioethics is that basic human dignity, the imperative to alleviate human suffering, and the ideal of more cooperative local and global societies demand a "preferential option for the poor" in health care. The flip side of this demand is a healthy skepticism about claims that new medical technologies unfailingly serve the human good or that the market economy is an acceptable mediator of access to basic health resources at home and worldwide. Such claims must be tested in light of their transparency, respect for disagreement, relation to the availability of basic "opportunity goods" for all, and positive or negative effect on universal social and political empowerment.

Globalization, Participation, and Interreligious Dialogue

The central social message of Christianity is inclusion of the poor, a message that has always presented a radical and often intolerable challenge to the hierarchies of status on which most societies are built. For most of the centuries in which institutional Christianity has existed, this radical message has been compromised by power relationships in the church itself and in the civil arrangements in "Christian" societies. Although this has not ceased to be true, the modern era has seen in Western democracies, at least to some degree, a coalescence of Christian ideals of individual worth and of inclusive community with political and cultural ideals of democracy, rights, and participation. In such societies, Christianity can and should still challenge tendencies toward individualism and the co-optation of the rhetoric of democracy to serve the interests of more powerful groups and nations. To the extent that religion does promote inclusive participation, it makes the powerful accountable and thus advances the "option for the poor."

This potential is not limited to Christian religion and theology. Indeed, if Christian theological bioethics is to foster global participation for change, and do so in a religiously "expansive" manner, it will have to assume or discover other religious traditions whose symbols of ultimacy yield a similar commitment. In a lecture delivered to the American Academy of Arts and Sciences, the economist Amartya Sen makes the case that religious prioritizing of respect and inclusion is not unique to Christianity.[61] He cites precedents that hark from many religious and cultural traditions, including ancient Greece, Buddhist India, seventh-century Japan, Maoist China, and modern-day South Africa, and Christian practices influenced by African traditional cultures. In the 1590s, Sen observes, "the great Moghal Emperor Akbar . . . was busy arranging organized dialogues between holders of different faiths (including Hindus, Muslims, Christians, Parsees, Jains, Jews, and even—it must be noted—atheists" while "the Inquisitions were still flourishing in Europe."[62]

In an address to theologians, political scientist Richard Falk (who is Jewish) waxes hopeful about "the re-emergence of religion as a world-political force" that is ecumenical and inclusive. For Falk, not only are religious ideals democratic in essence, they also bring optimism and hence greater investment regarding real social change. Religion can help overcome the paralyzing "politics of impossibility" that is the condition as well as the outcome of "political realism" and that feeds into theological resignation to being marginal to any vital political debates, especially about the future shape of globalization.[63]

A Muslim scholar, Abdullahi An-na'im, takes this confidence in the role of religion into the institutions of social life that concretely link members of societies and of global society in practices and institutions. He proposes "a synergistic and interdependent model of the relationship between religion and global civil society."[64] Religion contributes to a "politics of solidarity and alliance formation" in which people are motivated to claim the multiple media of global civil society in their cause of "justice and human dignity."[65] An-na'im agrees that there is no sharp dichotomy between the religious and the secular, or between religion and politics.[66] Religious communities acting and speaking in ways reflective of their specific identities and theologies can extend progressive social practices by working with others for common goals, even if their worldviews, ethical theories, and moral expectations do not conform to one another on every point. Although the clash of fundamentalisms and the neocolonialist powers of "democratic" societies will not easily be erased from the worldwide scene, scholars and practitioners of religion from various continents and experiences (Asia, North America, Africa) are converging in an experience-based idealism that holds up religion as a force for solidarity and change.

Participatory theological discourse can help create community and democracy worldwide and facilitate shared protests against certain consequences of globalization. Religions and theologies are concrete in their cultural settings and practices, yet "they are intelligible to discourses in other cultural and social settings that are experiencing the same failure of global systems and who are raising the same kind of protest." This has already occurred in theologies of liberation, feminism, ecology, and human rights.[67] Theological bioethics as participatory has potential to address and change inequitable conditions of health care access. In fact, this mode of theology may be even more important globally than nationally, in the absence of any single global authority comparable to the federal government of a nation or any unitary sphere that could be designated the locus of public discourse. Participatory action is an essential vehicle of the theological vision and voice of religious communities, and those communities on the whole rank compassion and respect as key and constitutive values. Participatory action regarding health care justice is essential to the substantive expression and effective presence of twenty-first-century theological bioethics.

But Will It Happen? Windows of Opportunity

Students of global governance today invest a decentralized approach to social change with great potential. In the past few decades, "supranational decision making" has expanded, through forms of authority and sanctions that are pluralistic and overlapping. Considerable powers have been transferred from nation-states to intergovernmental organizations such as the European Union and the World Trade Organization. Powers are also shared through interstate agreements or cooperation, such as the G7/G8.[68] In the view of its critics, "this new supranational decision-making power has remained hidden and unaccountable to democratic processes, and exercised largely by specialized government officials and international 'technocrats.'"[69] However, the elitist tendencies of globalization are moderated by the huge number of lower and midlevel centers of control and regulation that provide opportunities for broader participation in governing world social and economic affairs. "Hundreds of organizations now regulate the global dimensions of trade, telecommunications, civil aviation, health, the environment, meteorology, and many other issues."[70] Recent years have seen the emergence of "an informal global system of governance" composed of networks of regulatory bodies, judiciaries, and even legislators in different countries, as well as cabinet-level ministers, financial officials, and even chief executives, who cooperate toward mutually beneficial goals.[71] Fostering an ethos of "positive comity," these officials and their noncoercive alliances "open new institutional horizons for the possibility of global justice."[72]

The danger of elite control is moderated partly by the fact that political legitimacy depends on democracy and transparency and partly by the fact that midlevel and "grassroots" initiatives are mobilizing, organizing, and magnifying their agency through cooperative networks of resistance. For example, the international summits of supranational organizations have spawned parallel summits of groups and coalitions—primarily from the developing world—who perceive themselves to have been excluded from the "official" forum where issues are framed, rules made, policy guidelines developed, and enforcement measures implemented.[73] Parallel summits have grown in strength since protesters disrupted the 1999 World Trade Organization summit in Seattle, Washington. In 2003, a much more organized constituency of dissenters from the developing world managed to sidetrack trade negotiations in Cancun, Mexico. Parallel, and often directly oppositional, summits "challenge the legitimacy of government summits, confront official delegates, give visibility to the emerging global civil society, resist neo-liberal policies, and propose alternative solutions to global problems."[74] They exploit means of mass communication, especially the Internet, to widen and empower their constituencies.

Utilizing similar measures, citizen initiatives are also creating a sizeable "global backlash" to the world economy.[75] A force to counteract corporate-led economic globalization is emerging from a coalition of movements representing the interests of labor, the environment, access to patented drugs, subsistence farmers, and other sectors.[76] At the very least, such forces have managed to displace "the Washington consensus" and force elite power brokers to give some account of their concerns, as was acknowledged in a 2001 article in *Fortune* magazine that portrayed backlash proposals as inimical to business interests.[77]

Richard Falk writes of trends toward "globalization from below" as evidence of a "Grotian moment." As in the time of Hugo Grotius, the seventeenth-century father of international law, ours may be an era of change that permits a new type of international order to emerge, one less focused on governance by nation-states complicit in market norms and one more open to "global public goods."[78] Falk identifies this prospect as a sort of "rooted utopianism," in which the aspiration for a better future appears currently out of reach, but is supported by recent developments toward more participatory ways of resolving conflict and distributing goods.[79]

Participatory Theological Bioethics, Justice, and Global Change

Various religious institutions of global civil society are becoming advocates for health care for the poor, including transnational organizations such as Church World Service, Christian Aid, the evangelical Christian adoption and welfare agency Holt International Children's Services, the evangelical children's agency World Vision, and religious orders such as the Roman Catholic Society of Jesus, Catholic Relief Services, and Caritas International. All of these incorporate aspects essential to a theological-bioethical perspective that can marshal resources from above and below and can take form in multiple practical initiatives under a shared vision and compatible aims. They examine social, economic, scientific, and medical decisions from the perspective of the least well-off. They build strategic alliances at different levels around the world, among different cultures and social contexts, in order to resist forms of oppression (such as excesses of the market and technology) that burden all. They also engender critical attitudes toward the way local communities and families, including those with a religious identity, can themselves perpetuate social injustices that result in health risks and deprivations. In a recent review of challenges to Western bioethics, Maura Ryan sees all of the above as demanded by theological bioethics, but as also amenable to the convictions and aims of philosophers, bioethicists, and activists who are committed to a framework of distributive justice.[80]

Some examples will help validate the social potential of participatory theological bioethics. Although grassroots and local activism may provide a more ready illustration of the potential of theological bioethics to engage society and make practical gains, the mainline Christian congregations have not been entirely absent from this process, and they have taken it into the global sphere. One example is Christian intervention in the behavior of transnational corporations, especially interesting in light of the close and increasing connection of health care and research to corporate funding and marketing. International business interests may seem among the most invulnerable determinants of health care access with which religious advocates for the poor have to contend. Pharmaceutical companies and genomics companies are far more concerned with return on investment and maximizing profit than with addressing the underserved. Yet the Interfaith Center on Corporate Responsibility (ICCR) and the mainline churches have had significant impact through the movement for socially responsible investing. The ICCR is a vehicle for ethically motivated investment choices of the major denominations and for shareholder activism at the annual meetings of major corporations.[81] Such efforts lend global reach to the local or national efforts of faith-based advocacy: for example, access to lifesaving vaccines and medications (e.g., for AIDS, tuberculosis, or malaria) for those in the developing world is highly dependent on the way transnational corporations develop and market products.

Religious activism in favor of socially responsible investment has had an impact on health via campaigns against the marketing of infant formula and of tobacco products and, more recently, against the use of patent rights to charge insupportable prices for AIDS drugs in Africa and elsewhere. In 1975, religious investors began introducing shareholder resolutions against the marketing of infant formula in developing countries. By 1984, Nestlé, a Swiss corporation, agreed to the guidelines created by the World Health Organization (WHO) covering infant formula, thus ending a boycott of Nestlé products in the United States that had been begun in 1977 by the Newman Center at the University of Minnesota. This concession put pressure on other companies to accept the WHO code. Among the factors that between 1975 and 1984 contributed to this outcome were a suit brought by the Sisters of the Precious Blood against Bristol-Myers, and shareholder resolutions at Bristol-Myers and American Home Products meetings by the United Church of Christ, the United Presbyterian Church in the U.S.A., and the United Methodist Church.[82]

In 1981, the ICCR began a campaign against the sale of tobacco products, nationally and abroad, by introducing a shareholder resolution at the annual meeting of Philip Morris. It soon targeted the marketing strategies in the developing world of both Philip Morris and R. J. Reynolds, and in the 1990s extended its efforts to American Brands, Loews, and Kimberly-Clark, then to companies that supported tobacco companies, for example, by carrying tobacco ads in publications. In 1996, the American Medical Association called for divestment from tobacco in its own portfolios, and 3M agreed not to accept billboard advertising from tobacco companies. President Bill Clinton publicly recognized the role of the ICCR in his administration's campaign against tobacco products.[83] Though the efforts against infant formula and tobacco have been the ICCR's most visible endeavors, it has also pressured to keep genetically modified foods off the U.S. market and to arrange more favorable pricing of pharmaceuticals to the poor.[84] ICCR targets elites in that it pressures for change in corporate behavior via top-level decision making. However, it mobilizes resistance to corporate practices by drawing on many other levels and types of social agency. Shareholders, consumers, would-be beneficiaries, victims, colleges and universities, and local activist networks all reinforce one another's efforts for a common cause.

In recent years, Christian organizations have become even more self-consciously global and more explicit about the need for reinforcement of initiatives at many social levels. They are also increasingly committed to partnership with other public and private bodies and with other religious traditions. Just before the fifteenth International AIDS conference in Bangkok in 2004, the British humanitarian organization Christian Aid released the report *God's Children Are Dying of AIDS.* The report calls all the world's religions to cooperate in reducing the stigma of AIDS and in educating young people about HIV transmission. Christian Aid has wide experience working with partner organizations in developing countries to disseminate information about HIV to a wide cross-section of the population. During the Bangkok conference, Christian Aid sponsored a workshop cooperatively with the Asian Muslim Action Network, to be followed by an interfaith meeting of religious leaders to build more effective networks of cooperation.[85] According to Rachel Baggaley, chief of Christian Aid's HIV unit, religious leaders have a crucial role to play in reducing discrimination against those suffering from HIV infection. "There is evidence that good theological reflection can encourage people to change their perceptions of HIV. When God is perceived to be benevolent rather than punitive, this can lead to significant changes in attitudes towards life and health."[86] In fact, one of Christian Aid's partners, Anelera+, has established a support network for HIV-positive faith leaders, who then conduct retreats throughout Africa and become catalysts for change.

Even more remarkably, the efforts of religious leaders, organizations, and theologians have elicited cooperative responses from health care and corporate leaders as the practices, narratives, and values of science, business, and religion mesh in areas of mutual involvement. For example, in March 2003, a conference on biotechnology, ethics, and policy brought together theological and philosophical bioethicists, researchers, clinicians, industry representatives, and policymakers.[87] At the meeting, Catholic, Protestant, Jewish, and Muslim scholars raised social justice concerns about new health technologies, both nationally and internationally.

Una Ryan, CEO of Avant Immuno-therapeutics (Needham, Massachusetts), voiced her company's aim of enhancing access to lifesaving drugs for the world's poor. Avant uses profits from products in the "first world" to subsidize drugs sold more cheaply or developed expressly for "third world" populations. For example, it plans to use sales from vaccines for travelers, food safety, and antibioterrorism to support vaccine sales to developing nations.[88] As the chairperson of the Biotechnology Industry Organization's subcommittee on global health, Ryan may enjoy further significant opportunities to introduce religiously informed values into corporate behavior regarding access to basic health goods. This does not mean that the profit motive will be replaced with altruism, of course, but rather that corporate profit-making behavior can be modified in light of religious and moral critiques, whose appeal may be strengthened by potential positive results for corporate image and morale, the satisfaction that comes with relieving the suffering of others, and an expanding corporate culture of prosocial and globally responsible behavior.

These examples raise the question "What is to count as success in measuring the effectiveness of theologically-informed, faith-based activism on behalf of health access and equality, or of participatory theological bioethics?" The success that theological bioethics and related advocacy can expect will rarely amount to a complete reversal of federal policy or a comprehensive transformation of institutional behavior. Yet theological engagement in the ethical, policy, narrative, prophetic, and politically participatory modes can bring about adjustments in the social-cultural milieu. It can enhance democratic participation and enable critical interaction among traditions and groups about the substantive values and practices that make up the common good. It can introduce real changes in health care and other realms and keep open the possibility of greater public participation in shaping access to health.

Conclusion

Subsequent chapters offer further examples of successful local and international religious-theological action for health equity. These include Catholic health care ministry and its mission to the poor and underserved; the hospice movement as an answer to physician-assisted suicide; religiously sponsored pressures for health care reform, both nationally and internationally; religious networks supporting the availability of AIDS drugs, AIDS education and condoms, care for persons with AIDS, and care for AIDS orphans; adoption as an alternative to expensive, low-success reproductive technologies; and international networks resisting in the name of social justice the implementation of innovations in human and agricultural genetics.

In the end, the idea that theology has disappeared from public bioethics is a fallacy that distracts attention from the competing and equally elaborate symbolic narratives of science, the economic market, and liberal individualism. However, for theological bioethics to reassert and confirm its authority in emerging local and global practices of research and health care distribution, it will be necessary to take the option for the poor beyond rhetorical or abstract conflicts with countervailing social norms. Theological bioethics must become a self-conscious mediator between participatory movements for equity in health care; religious and philosophical worldviews and language; dominant institutions of civil society, state, and market; and policy-setting agencies at the grassroots, local, national, regional, and global levels.

Theological bioethics must self-confidently take shape in broad, inclusive, participatory networks that bear out the conviction that more just practices are not only obligatory but a "possible impossibility" (to reverse the terms of Karl Barth's definition of sin). Religious liberation movements show that theory and practice are interdependent. History confirms not only the doctrine of sin but also the amelioration of the social order through conversion when possible, and forceful intervention when necessary, sometimes "from below." The energy of emerging global practices of equity in health care verifies that theological bioethics prioritizes the criterion of justice in public advocacy and, through vision, voice, and action, can make good on its hope that new possibilities for the common good will emerge.

CHAPTER
3

DECLINE AND DYING

Cultural and Theological Interpretations

FOR THREE DECADES, controversy over legalizing physician-assisted suicide has dominated much of the U.S. bioethical scene regarding end-of-life care and decision making. The movement for physician-assisted suicide has been met by an equal and opposing force: the movement to keep seriously ill patients on life-sustaining technologies as long as possible. On the surface, these two movements appear completely antagonistic. One is humanistic, the other motivated by religiously grounded pro-life concerns; one appeals to freedom and autonomy, the other to moral obligations; one equates meaningful life with self-determination, the other with continued physical survival; one prizes a right to die and to kill, the other a right to life and a duty to preserve it.

At a fundamental level, however, these movements have much in common. First, they assume a context of access to medical resources for dying patients, indeed, quite extensive access. Second, they focus the moral question on the individual patient, whose own particular welfare is the governing concern. Third, they envision the cultural context of illness and dying primarily as medical, and even as highly technological. The legal and moral conflict between these two movements over *how* to use modern science and technology to gain control over death is actually a distraction from a bigger problem: the fact that modern science and technology supply the major moral and hermeneutical framework within which death is considered in modern culture.

A four-year study of end-of-life care in the United States estimated that half of all deaths occur in hospitals, "surrounded by the technologies of medicine, embedded in a highly specialized, sophisticated setting."[1] The seriously ill, the aged, and their families seek out hospitals to stave off death, but often find themselves trapped by a medical momentum that seems immune to their own sense of dignity and need for understanding and companionship. The drive toward physician-assisted suicide is a reflection of both the modern patient's need for control and the modern medical institution's inflexible grip on the most profound human transition. Ironically, the insistence of some on sustaining life by artificial nutrition, as long as possible, and in the most desperate of circumstances, reinscribes technological domination over the experiences of decline and death, rather than referring those experiences back to the more intimate circles of love, friendship, family, and church.

Timothy Quill, a physician who has written extensively on the ethics of palliative care and of hastening death, remarks that "medicine and technology have taken an increasing role in providing meaning and ritual at the end of people's lives. In some circumstances, medicine has almost become a religion, and prolonging life at all cost by using medical technology is its primary objective."[2] Physicians may well feel torn between the types of expertise demanded of them and at a loss to fulfill the roles of both spiritual and medical sage. Those seeking medical help with suicide can also look to the physician and his or her arts to legitimize or ritualize their deaths. Even Timothy Quill, who goes to extraordinary lengths to assure himself and others that his patients choose death at their own initiative, and who sees suicide as a very undesirable last resort, seems unable to evade the expectation that he fulfill a quasi-priestly role in bringing it about. He was put on trial, in a case dismissed by a grand jury, for having given one patient, "Diane," enough barbiturates to end her own life. She did so alone, so as not to expose her physician or family to legal consequences. In retrospect, he feels that Diane's solitude in death "violates every principle of humane care for the dying." Concluding that his own role cannot simply be reduced to that of the medical expert, he vows that his future actions will be different. "As a physician, I make a solemn promise to my dying patients that I will not abandon them no matter where their illness may take them."[3] After all, "caring humanely for the dying and trying to help them find a dignified death is a fundamentally vital role for physicians."[4]

The way Western cultures treat decline and death is symptomatic of three contemporary trends. The first is *individualism,* especially a focus on autonomy and self-determination as essential to personal meaning. The second is the *medicalization of social problems,* such as relations among generations and balancing independence and dependency. The third is the *refusal to accept that life has limits* that science, technology, and money will never remove. This is not to say that modern medicine has not made huge strides in eliminating many forms of human suffering. But medical approaches to aging, decline, illness, and dying need to be better integrated with the personal, social, and spiritual relationships that constitute life's highest meanings. This integration is a task few modern health systems accomplish well, but one that is integral to religions.

Christian theological bioethics should respond to decline and dying not just by analyzing specific medical interventions but by assuming a participatory style. It should foster social practices that represent alternative experiences. These practices would reintegrate the ill and dying with spiritual avenues of transcendence and with communal structures of support. This chapter pursues the connection between the proliferation of medical technology and conflicts over physician-assisted suicide and artificial nutrition and hydration; between liberal individualism and the isolation of the elderly, who also make up the majority of dying patients; and between the marketing of high-tech medical care and the dearth of more adequate resources to resolve the suffering faced by the elderly, the chronically ill, and the dying. However, this chapter also notes that the problem of care for debilitated members is not unique to modern culture. Hence the special role of religious communities and theological bioethics in enhancing solidarity with the vulnerable and an ethos of care.

A report of the Hastings Center on the "goals of medicine" cautions that the synchronization of medical and social welfare services for the chronically or terminally ill and the elderly is of special importance. Such services should include economic support and social programs; support for family care of the elderly and ill; the provision of coordinated health care, so that a person's physical well-being is overseen as a whole; and the nurturing of spiritual and psychological well-being, hope, and peace, even for those facing death.[5] This vision is hardly representative of the way most persons face old age, illness, or death in the United States. Medicine and bioethics often approach terminal decline and death as unfortunate medical events to be prevented if possible, and medically controlled when they cannot be avoided. Theological bioethics brings a larger spectrum of values to the human realities of decline and death, including the values of equity and justice in access to the resources necessary for a good life and a peaceful death.

The next chapter will discuss euthanasia and the refusal of technological supports for life, in the light of a framework provided by the Roman Catholic tradition, which has for centuries provided guidance about practical decision making in times of illness and danger of death. This is the distinction between ordinary and extraordinary means of life support, which is implemented with the principle of double effect to evaluate end-of-life care. Both these tools of moral judgment developed out of Catholic moral theology but have come to enjoy much broader currency in biomedical ethics. Chapters 3 and 4 together aim to show that participatory theological bioethics is still guiding complex decisions and social practices through a multidimensional presence that encourages believers to embody their commitments practically and to partner with other religious, civic, and governmental institutions and groups in seeking the common good around issues of aging, illness, and health care.

The gist of the theological contribution is an understanding of the common good that stresses personal and spiritual values; the social interdependence and contributions of all persons; solidarity in seeking the material, social, and spiritual well-being of all; and a "preferential option" for vulnerable and marginal members of communities and societies. The hospice movement, some programs of the Catholic Health Association (CHA), and the social action of the Community of Sant'Egidio will illustrate this message. The problem of allocation of health resources will be raised in these chapters and pursued more intensively in chapter 6, on health care access.

Decline and Dying in the United States

Obviously, human beings become ill and die at all phases of their existence, sometimes even before birth. But in modern societies like the United States, the moral, spiritual, and cultural problems of decline and dying coincide to a great degree with the problem of old age. Three-fourths of those who die are elderly. They die mainly in hospitals and, to a lesser extent, in nursing homes.[6] The leading causes of death in economically privileged nations such as the United States are heart disease, cancer, and stroke, all of which disproportionately affect older people.[7] The very fact that modern Westerners react with shock to the terminal illnesses and deaths of children and younger adults is because they are, in their experience, blessedly rare. In Western society, modern medicine has developed means to fight off the infectious diseases that killed the young in earlier ages, enabling life expectancy to rise.

Along with longevity comes the likelihood that life in a state of marked decline will be prolonged for many. Yet the social condition of the elderly has not risen along with their lifespan. The rarity of a youthful death has enabled modern culture to construct death as an extraordinary incursion into the normal scheme of things, as a disaster that befalls the unlucky. Longevity has made moderns less able to accept and alleviate the suffering that trails fatal illness and the universal prospect of our ultimate demise. Often exacerbating this suffering are cultural and economic factors that enhance the vulnerability of the elderly, certain racial and ethnic groups, and women in particular.

The contemporary U.S. approach to illness, aging, and death and our public controversies over physician-assisted suicide and euthanasia have evolved as the result of a convergence of several factors peculiar to our national and cultural history. In the colonial era of the United States, "the seniority principle" conferred protected status on elderly people, even as their competencies in many areas declined. Colonial society was built around religion, politics, family, agriculture, and trade. Power and control were based on landownership and position in the family, both of which the elderly could retain. Position was tied to an age hierarchy, partly because of religiously authorized traditions, but also partly because experience enabled success.[8]

The American Revolution accelerated not only the influence of values of individual achievement, pragmatism, equality, and the free market but also an influx of new, younger immigrants. Relationships based on achievement and contract began to displace the rule of familial and communal hierarchies.[9] In the late nineteenth century, the belief in prosperity through the market was coupled with faith in progress and in science and technology as means of improving human life. Physical infirmity increasingly was used to discredit "the old guard," who were viewed as the custodians of tradition. A science of aging as "decline" displaced eighteenth-century respect for elders, and an ethos of efficiency helped promote the value of physical and mental acuity and independence.[10]

In American culture these trends combined to create a paradoxical situation for the elderly and for all who suffer physical and mental diminishment. An ethos of the market and of individual choice and entrepreneurship makes those who cannot contribute productively to society, or who require assistance in the basic skills and tasks of life, seem a burden to themselves and others. Yet only an appeal to the basic cultural values of autonomy and independence has the power to make renewed respect for such persons possible and compelling. The notion that the way to resolve unwanted dependency is through the autonomous exercise of a right to die or even to be killed has enormous cultural appeal. The legalization of euthanasia to resolve the problems brought about by decline and impending death actually confirms that to be extremely ill or debilitated is to have extremely low social status and value. In such a state, individuals would rather choose to be dead, a choice whose premise of low self-worth is validated by those who compassionately defend it.

Keeping comatose patients alive indefinitely by artificial nutrition and hydration may seem like the opposite of physician-assisted suicide, but the two practices have something in common. Both cooperate in the basic social ethos that focuses on the individual rather than his or her relationships, reduces the dying to objects of medical intervention, and normalizes techno-scientific control over human meaning. A difference of course is that the right-to-suicide movement absolutizes the individual's control and autonomy, while the backlash artificial feeding movement absolutizes the value of the individual's biological life. Each exaggerates what the other neglects. Yet they have in common an excessive focus on what they consider to be individual patient rights. The nature and quality of a person's relationships, his or her participation in and impact on the common good, and a critical examination of the market forces behind hi-tech institutionalization of the demented, comatose, or dying all need to be part of a more complete and humane approach to biomedicine. We will return to an analysis of physician-assisted suicide and artificial nutrition and hydration after considering the cultural contexts of illness and decline, which typically take place in old age. Because loss of previous abilities is inevitable for those who survive to old age, cultural, social, and medical responses to aging are an important part of the ways cultures and health care systems approach death.

In modern U.S. culture, approaches to old age are often as individualistic and medicalizing as is the response to death, and just as uncritical of inequities in patterns of access to health care. In 2002, a background paper on aging research, prepared for the President's Commission on Bioethics, identified an investigative thrust beyond the diseases of the elderly (e.g., Parkinson's, Alzheimer's, and cardiovascular disease) and toward significant lengthening of the lifespan and prevention of the general deterioration that accompanies advancing age. Several fronts of research were identified, including free radicals and mitochondrial dysfunction, caloric restriction, genetics of aging, regenerative medicine, and hormone treatments.[11] Ethical questions had to do primarily with the effect of such technologies on the societies and populations who would have the opportunity to use them. Would they be beneficial to these people overall? "How will social and political institutions—like the education system, the retirement system, the healthcare and insurance systems—deal with such changes?" "How could our ability to control the length of life affect our thinking about the breadth and depth of life?" "Should we in general do everything possible to extend life as far as possible? . . . Our advancing technical powers may soon force us to decide."[12] The narrow purview of the ethical concerns expressed here is remarkable, even though only a discussion starter for the commission. Certainly the majority of the world's population would never have access to such interventions and would continue to suffer old age, not only with physical degeneration but in poverty. And even as a policy-guiding body in the United States, the President's Commission appears, at least initially, to be considering aging research of, by, and for the elites.

Circumstances are different and worse for minorities and women than for white men, even in this country, with regard to accessing end-of-life medical treatment. For minorities, the problem is not so much how to use advanced technology, but how to access even basic and lifesaving care. Miguel De La Torre recounts the history of an African American family that was reluctant to remove their elderly father from a respirator, though this is what the doctors had "respectfully" recommended. The family feared the advice was motivated by a desire to transfer the machine to a white person. They felt their worst suspicions were confirmed when, after their father's death, they reentered the unit and saw the respirator being used by another patient. De La Torre reminds us that "we should not be surprised that ethical dilemmas such as the use of euthanasia are approached quite differently by people of color. As society debates the morality of assisted suicide, people of color cannot help but wonder if this could be used as a new opportunity to victimize the marginalized."[13]

Actually, fewer people of color than whites will have occasion to require respirators in old age in the first place. Death is more likely to occur at a young age for minorities than for whites, and to have social in addition to physical causes. For black males, homicide, HIV infection, and unintentional injuries are among the leading causes of death. Hispanic males are more likely to die of unintentional injuries and HIV than of stroke. Suicide is among the ten leading causes of death for American Indian, Alaskan

Native, Asian, or Pacific Islander women. White infants are most likely to die of congenital abnormalities while black infants are more likely to die of complications from short gestation and low birth weight; and when they do have congenital abnormalities, they are more likely than white babies to die from them.[14]

Poverty is at the root of many of the health disparities and higher rates of death experienced by disadvantaged racial and ethnic groups, disparities that have a magnified impact on the elderly. Women within these groups are poorer than men. Poverty signals not only low income but poor housing, poor nutrition, inadequate information about health, lack of access to preventive care, inadequate access to acute care, and fear and distrust of a biased health care system.[15] Poverty rates for older African American couples are three to four times higher than for white couples. For individual blacks, the risk of poverty also increases with age, especially for women.[16] Native Americans have the lowest median income among disadvantaged populations of the elderly.[17] Among all these populations, greater poverty and lesser health status are associated with gender. Retirement incomes for women average only about 55 percent of those of men, and "for older African American or Hispanic women, poverty is the rule rather than the exception."[18] This would hold even more for Native Americans.

Aging and Well-Being across Cultures

It might appear that the solution to the incredible expansion of medical-technical expertise and control, as well as to the disparities resulting from racial and ethnic discrimination, could be found by turning to the wisdom of more communal and less "scientific" societies. Perhaps a stronger ethos of communal reciprocity and of family unity can provide support and dignity for the ill, the elderly, and the dying. Traditional roles prescribing honor to elders, as well as residence in an extended family rather than a nuclear household, could ensure more consistent companionship and care.

This is certainly true up to a point, as studies in Asia and Africa have shown.[19] However, conditions are changing, as traditional societies shift to a market economy and as birthrates decrease.[20] Moreover, highly communal societies can reinforce disparities of social status, especially those based on gender, just as is the case among ethnic populations in the United States.[21] Sociologists offer evidence that even more "primitive," less technologically advanced societies exhibit various types of death-inducing behavior aimed at the elderly and others who have become a burden.[22]

Unfortunately, although the medicalization of decline and death may be peculiar to modern societies, the exclusion and elimination of those who are physically weak is not. While we modern Westerners no doubt have something to learn by looking at cultures different from our own, it is important not to romanticize more communalistic alternatives.

That being said, there are a variety of cultural understandings of the elderly that provide provocative models for a reconsideration of the contexts within which decline and eventual death are approached in the United States and in other modern and postindustrial societies. For example, women who are past their most "productive" childbearing years can sometimes capitalize on the value of their mothering experience to locate new roles in family and society. In Africa and Asia, elders frequently reside with adult children and assume an active role in raising grandchildren and sharing domestic responsibilities. They may also take on such roles for families or individuals to whom they are not related by blood or marriage. Older men sometimes take on roles in the household that they did not when they were more engaged in productive economic and in political activity.[23] Elders are also important transmitters of cultural and religious traditions to grandchildren, especially in cultures under transition or duress.[24]

The epilogue to a volume on Africa explicitly takes issue with a Western concept of aging "that is burdened with connotations of gradual decline" and takes to task the Western medical model of intervention that focuses disproportionately on individuals rather than on communities.[25] The authors propose that in many African cultures aging is an asset, not a liability. The elderly are thought to have access to unseen or "occult" forces that affect daily life, offering power, knowledge, and opportunities. Even the poorest of elders can devote their time to "social contacts, decision-making in village affairs, giving advice in all types of matters and initiating younger generations."[26] Elders who are extremely weak or who do not have children of their own can still be anchored in a caregiving network constituted by both male and female caregivers.[27]

In African American culture, the meaning of aging derives from family, religion, and the experience of slavery. Elements of African heritage are important too, including the power and authority of elderly women, especially in passing on oral traditions. The old are "the wise."[28] They have the duty and prerogative to instruct and correct any children in the community. Older women may take an active role in raising children to whom they are not related, even providing shelter and primary care.[29]

Data from a study of Taiwan, Singapore, Thailand, and the Philippines indicate that, despite rapidly shifting demographic and socioeconomic conditions, "Asian families have worked out a variety of financial and exchange arrangements, and the emotional bonds that sustain them."[30] These arrangements typically involve the elderly and their relatives, especially their children. The elderly report remarkably few serious health problems under these circumstances and are able to undertake daily life activities. They also score well on emotional health.[31]

Stresses do result from factors such as educational and cultural differences between the generations, relocation of younger families to urban areas, decreasing rates of coresidence of elder parents with adult children, and delay of marriage by young people. Some groups among the elderly are, of course, more vulnerable than others. People with no formal education suffer more risks in all areas. Women as a group experience more socioeconomic and health disadvantages than men. Men and women who are not married or who are separated from their spouses also experience above-average risks to health and well-being.[32]

Yet overall the elderly are faring well in the cultures studied. To address the needs of the elderly population, policymakers in Asia are pursuing ways to strengthen the traditional family, as well as to maintain or institute other support mechanisms for the elderly, such as informal support mechanisms and government-sponsored programs. For example, in Singapore, adult children are given incentives to reside with their parents, such as tax rebates and preferential housing choices. Pensions and health care may also be provided by governments. Another strategy is to provide home health care, adult day care, and recreation centers.[33] Senior centers and other health, recreational, educational, and service-oriented opportunities designed specifically for the elderly can help compensate for gaps in family and other social supports and are beginning to emerge in Asia. In the United States, where voluntary organizations have always thrived, focal points in civil society, in combination with state and federal funding, show great promise of being able to create services and social networks for the elderly.[34] Surveys do not bear out the suspicion that concentrating the elderly in activity centers for the aged necessarily exacerbates social isolation or alienation.[35]

Social approaches such as those previously described provide multiple opportunities to place the inevitable process of decline within community relationships that provide positive, valuable roles for the elderly and potentially for those suffering serious illness. It seems safe to agree that the quality of life for the aged, and by extension for those in progressive decline from illness, will be highest when cultures facilitate community and kin roles for them and integrate these roles rather than constructing them on separate planes.[36] Networks within families and communities help those experiencing decline of ability and strength to compensate for their deficits and discover new ways to express the wisdom that can come with experience and even with suffering. While medical and technical assistance and expertise have, of course, a crucial role to play in maintaining health and function, they are not the most powerful sources of human meaning, nor do they provide the most effective means to address the losses that may be associated with illness, decline, and impending death.

In prosperous societies, both men and women live longer and enter their "retirement years" in better health, able to participate in new interests and activities such as community service and "second careers." Nevertheless, decline is an inevitable part of the aging process. The elderly require family and community assistance in order to maximize the potential satisfaction of their remaining years, and to cope with the losses they will face. In the United States, however, multigenerational families rarely live together. Because women survive on average a few years longer than men, there are a disproportionate number of women requiring care. The burdens of care also fall disproportionately on female family members, who themselves are often without the support of an extended family network or the equivalent. They often must cope with conflicts between increased domestic responsibilities and participation in the workplace or other responsibilities.

Caregivers often—even usually—have inadequate access to social and economic supports for themselves and the elderly for whom they care, leading to stress and isolation for both parties. There is an important obligation of society and government to support family care of those in advanced age by ensuring income security, health care, and housing arrangements that facilitate the participation of the elderly in community. The common good demands that the family as primary caregiver for the elderly be supplemented by church, community, and government measures of assistance and solidarity.[37]

These networks are important dimensions of overall health support and should be so viewed by bioethics. In a 1994 joint report on social justice for the elderly, the Hastings Center and a Dutch bioethics institute concluded that health care should be viewed in light of larger public policy concerns and values and that solidarity between the generations should be cultivated as the basis for a just and workable total social approach to their respective needs.[38] Basic recommendations are that old age not be turned into a medical problem; that moral solidarity between the generations become a matter of dialogue and refinement; that priorities for young and old be pursued in an integrated way; that the burden on women of caregiving be alleviated by more sharing in informal care and by governmental programs of support; that the elderly organize politically and collectively, especially to avoid separation of health and welfare programs; and that the public dialogue on the significance of old age be advanced through the media, education, and joint public-private efforts.[39]

Contributions of Participatory Theological Bioethics

Many religious traditions sponsor health-related caregiving facilities and networks. Allen Verhey recalls that "Jesus was not only a healer, not only one who suffered, but also a preacher of 'good news to the poor' (Luke 4:18)." In fact, "Christian hospitality to the sick and care for them" led to the founding of hospitals and eventually to the view that care for the sick poor is a civic responsibility.[40] James Keenan notes that "for two thousand years the church has cared for the weak and the sick" and includes religiously sponsored health care under the corporal works of mercy.[41] Catholic health care in the United States began in the eighteenth century when a delegation of French nuns, the Ursulines, arrived in Louisiana to begin several social programs, including education and care for the poor and sick. Today there are 60 Catholic health systems, 617 hospitals, 3,044 social service centers, 1,117 day and extended day services, and more than 1,500 continuing care ministry facilities. Catholic health ministry also involves 19,484 parishes, 2,988 missions, and 1,069 pastoral centers.[42]

Catholic health care has become more innovative, lay-headed, and community oriented in recent decades. For example, Catholic Health Initiatives, formed in 1996, combines the resources of eleven sponsoring religious congregations committed to an equal partnership with lay health care leaders and providers. The organization creates new models of care that can respond to community needs and collaborate with community groups, agencies, and other health care organizations, especially to assist the underserved and address the social causes of health deficits. Catholic Health Initiatives is comprised of sixty-eight hospitals, forty-four long-term care and assisted and independent living and residential facilities, and six community health services organizations. Located in nineteen states, it serves sixty-eight rural and urban communities with more than 67,000 employees.[43]

Other Christian denominations also sponsor health care. For example, Gundersen Lutheran Health Care System in La Crosse, Wisconsin, is a network including group medical practices, regional community clinics, hospitals, nursing homes, home care, behavioral health services, vision centers, and pharmacies, located throughout western Wisconsin, northeastern Iowa, and southeastern Minnesota.[44] Similarly, health has been an emphasis of the Seventh-Day Adventists since the 1860s when the church began.[45] Smoking and the use of alcohol and other sensory-altering drugs are actively addressed through community programs. The health ministry of the Adventist Church includes a health care delivery system of church-operated clinics and hospitals throughout the world. The Community of Sant'Egidio is a Christian lay organization that also sponsors health-related ministries and programs and is international in scope.[46]

The CHA, representing many different Catholic health care systems and coordinating with the U.S. episcopal leadership, will be treated here as a major example of participatory theological bioethics, uniting religious ideals, ethical analysis, political activism, and health care institutions and practices. Sant'Egidio will exemplify the link participatory theological ethics makes to global justice in health care. Obviously, any of these institutions and networks will have strengths and limits. For example, because the CHA works with a number of different religious orders with different notions of Catholic identity, as well as with the U.S. bishops, it avoids any appearance of direct conflict with official Catholic moral teaching, especially around sensitive issues such as reproduction. Nevertheless, it tries to help member organizations negotiate complicated or conflict-producing situations and disagreements with local bishops, for example, when Catholic organizations partner with non-Catholic health care providers or serve as the only provider in a rural community. The strong suit of the CHA is its emphasis on the social mission of Catholic health care and its political outreach, including inventive ways to contact and partner with health care institutions and professionals, other types of community services, and individuals concerned about health care justice.

Sant'Egidio, on the other hand, prioritizes a commitment to spirituality, community life, and face-to-face relations among members and the people they serve. The organization thus does not have the sort of highly developed bureaucratic infrastructure that might maximize its ability to cooperate internationally with other organizations. In fact, Sant'Egidio is funded largely by the members themselves, who pay their own expenses and raise funds for common works. This ensures the personal investment of members in the works of Sant'Egidio, but it could also skew participation and leadership toward those with more resources. Positively, Sant'Egidio provides an opportunity for laypeople who want to ground social action in a community of prayer and mutual support, while at the same time sustaining family life and professional vocations. These two different ventures, the CHA and Sant'Egidio, will provide two contrasting instances of the potential of participatory theological bioethics.

Catholic Health Association

The CHA is not an official organization of the Roman Catholic Church; it is a professional organization, with voluntary membership in all fifty states, that

> supports and strengthens the Catholic health ministry in the U.S. by uniting members to advance selected strategic ministry issues best addressed together rather than as individual organizations. More than 2,000 Catholic health care sponsors, systems, facilities, health plans, and related organizations comprise the gathering of ministry that is CHA.[47]

A "shared statement of identity" for these ministries mentions Jesus' mission of healing and the gospel values of justice and peace. Their aim is to seek "wellness for all persons and communities" and to give "special attention to our neighbors who are poor, underserved, and most vulnerable."[48] Catholic health organizations aim not just to serve but to "empower" these constituencies and to strengthen the social presence of the ministry "through collaboration, networking, and community-building" with various other entities and groups.[49] They exercise leadership in both health care and "broader societal issues" related to health and well-being.[50] The CHA aims for social transformation, claiming that "Jesus not only healed the sick; he also challenged unjust structures and called for fundamental social change. So too must the contemporary ministry."[51]

The CHA sponsors an "eAdvocacy" link on its home page, informing members of public issues of concern to their health care mission and offering them the opportunity to have a voice and become involved in change. Legislative and policy developments, concerns, and items for engagement are also circulated to members through e-mail. Social justice and access issues, such as Medicare reform, appear frequently among issues identified.

Other issues of note, in July 2004, for example, were a decline in enrollment revenues for the State Children's Health Insurance Program (SCHIP), the retirement of Congressman James Greenwood to serve as the head of the Biotechnology Industry Organization, legislation that would protect health care workers from legal repercussions as a result of investigations of patient safety, and the announcement of a White House conference on aging in 2005.

The CHA website integrates many projects and ministries among its members, in coordination with CHA leadership and in relation to advocacy for social change. Implementation of practices that represent its worldview and members is a key priority and function of the CHA. A project called "Continuing Care Ministries"[52] serves the aged and chronically ill through a spectrum of services, including day care, home health care, senior housing and assisted living, counseling, and case management. The introductory page on the website features statements by the pope, a Robert Wood Johnson Foundation report on race-based disparities in care at the end of life, and resources for planning housing programs.

Communal supports for those in decline are not limited to people for whom death is a near prospect. "Continuing Care Ministries" also includes housing initiatives, especially options for low-income seniors that integrate health and housing services.[53] Sponsored jointly with Catholic Charities USA, these initiatives engage home-, parish-, and community-based services, assistance in living at home, nursing facilities, affordable assisted living facilities, and advocacy opportunities, including letters, reports, and testimony in favor of legislation.

On the occasion of an international conference at Vatican City on "The Church and the Elderly," John Paul II noted that the increasing proportion of the elderly population presents a worldwide challenge to social planning, to economics, and to the relationships among the generations. An important point is that the elderly should be seen as active and participating members of the communities in which they live. "Although often regarded as only the recipients of charitable aid, the elderly must also be called to participate in this work. . . .They too have a valuable contribution to make to life. Thanks to the wealth of experience they have acquired over the years, they can and must be sources of wisdom, witnesses of hope and love."[54] The elderly must be assisted "to live with security and dignity," with their families when possible.[55] The papal remarks connect the outreach of CHA programs with the prophetic and narrative dimensions of the theological worldview. They also make clear the implications of that worldview for justice and the common good.

Twenty-five percent of people eighty-five or older live in nursing homes, 50 percent of those not in institutions need help with daily activities, and most older people have at least one chronic health condition. Some of these are unable to live alone, for example, those with Alzheimer's disease.[56] About 1.5 million elderly receive some federal housing assistance, but of the 5.3 million people in the United States with "worst case" housing needs (i.e., spending more than half their income on shelter), 1.5 million are elderly. In the United States, there are about 3.5 million who are eighty-five or older, a number that will quadruple by 2030 to 14 million.[57] Clearly, not all the elderly will be able to live with families; those that do will need extensive community support, and those who reside outside the family unit will need means to be in connection with family members and with institutions in the community that can offer the elderly meaningful ways to participate in the common good, in proportion to their capacities. In 2000, the Elderly Housing Coalition created a working paper for the U.S. Department of Housing and Urban Development (HUD) that recommended supporting legislation that could lead to "a national health and housing policy agenda" to ensure access for elders in federally subsidized housing to "a continuum of care that provides the support and services they need to continue to live independently in their apartments and community." This should include programs that integrate shelter, support services, health care, and social services to assist elderly residents to remain as independent as possible, whether residing in federally subsidized housing, assisted living facilities, or family homes.[58] Members of the Elderly Housing Coalition included Jewish organizations, two Lutheran and one Catholic organization, and several professional and nonprofit organizations dealing in elderly services.

Beyond advocating for legislative changes, Catholic health care leadership is moving ahead with incremental projects in civil society, in cooperation with other nonprofit organizations, religious groups, and state and federal government to make changes in the ways the elderly, ill, and dying participate in their communities. For example, CHA created an exchange of information among parish-based programs serving the aging and the chronically ill,[59] convened national long-term care providers to address Medicare payment policy, and developed and distributed a letter to Congress to express its concerns.[60] CHA has set several policy priorities to enhance the delivery of long-term care and provides information, informs its members of existing opportunities and benefits, and organizes advocacy on the part of CHA members, as well as coordinating multiple ventures to improve access and care in the immediate environment.

Sant'Egidio

As we have seen already, and as will be developed further in subsequent chapters, a huge challenge for theological bioethics today is globalization. Global trends, especially economic trends, carry weight for the elderly. For example, shifts in corporate investments and employment may affect retirement and pensions, the pricing of pharmaceuticals, and the extent of insurance coverage. Movement of employment opportunities from locale to locale affects prosperity and decline of neighborhoods, place of residence and income of the younger generations, and the influx of immigrants into communities. Transnational trade and financial institutions such as the World Bank, the International Monetary Fund, and the World Trade Organization have "fed into the crisis construction of ageing" with dire predictions about retirement rates and effects on pension funds. They have also pushed trade liberalization and pressured governments to privatize social services, which means that more in the future will be motivated by the need to bring in a profit.[61] It is possible that these trends may be countered by forms of transnational government, such as age discrimination legislation passed by the European Union.[62] However, the impact of global trends on aging, decline, and dying is still relatively unexplored territory for theological bioethics,[63] except in the case of the AIDS crisis.

One effort with wide appeal among young people is the lay community of Sant'Egidio, begun in Rome in 1968 as a student organization dedicated to community living, prayer, and social action.[64] Whereas CHA is an umbrella organization and action network, Sant'Egidio aims to provide a spirituality and way of life for its members. Founded by a high school student in the wake of Vatican II, Sant'Egidio's earliest members aspired to the ideals of the early Christian communities and of Francis of Assisi and began work in the slums of Rome, where they founded a school for children. Sant'Egidio has grown to an ecumenical Christian international organization with forty thousand members in sixty countries, concentrated in Europe. American communities exist in New York and Boston. Among the social projects of Sant'Egidio are friendship with the elderly, one of its oldest; friendship with the mentally disabled and those in prison; work against AIDS in Mozambique and other African countries; peacemaking efforts in Mozambique, Sierra Leone, and Eastern Europe; and efforts to rehabilitate child soldiers. Sant'Egidio has responded to humanitarian emergencies in at least eleven countries and sponsors ecumenical dialogue with Judaism and Islam.

Sant'Egidio first began work with and for the elderly in 1972, when older people were among the first congregants at its prayer services in

Rome. In 1988, Sant'Egidio mounted an organized program to help the elderly stay in their own homes, coordinating family members, doctors, hospitals, and social services.[65] Eventually, a variety of creative ways evolved to strengthen supportive, mutual connections among the elderly and other segments of their local communities, as well as between local needs and city, regional, and national funds and services. Among these, of course, is the Sant'Egidio network itself, a transnational entity sharing a vision of gospel identity, a voice for suffering and oppressed peoples, and practices shared through literature, the Internet, travel and cooperative international projects (e.g., on AIDS and peacemaking), and an annual convocation and spiritual pilgrimage for members in Rome. In May 2000, an international conference for and about the elderly was held in Rome, attended by more than two thousand international Sant'Egidio delegates.

Since 1988, Sant'Egidio has helped more than twelve thousand elderly find appropriate living arrangements. One creative solution has been to house the elderly in family-style communities in apartment buildings of about thirty units. Residents receive consistent support from Sant'Egidio members, who run projects in the building and serve as conduits for social services. In Rome, immigrants who likewise need housing have been placed with the elderly as companions. The Sant'Egidio community has published a resource guide for the elderly and those who serve them, collaboratively produced with the city of Rome, the newspaper *Corriere Della Sera,* and the organization Christian Family.[66] The guide contains information on economic planning and services, medical and health services and practices, social services, charitable organizations, emergency numbers and resources, information on how to get about the city, and information about cultural, leisure, and volunteer opportunities.

Sant'Egidio aims to provide the elderly with the continuing ability to contribute socially and to express solidarity with others. In Italy, more than six hundred persons over sixty-five are involved in "service to those in difficulty." Groups in Italy and elsewhere prepare meals distributed to the homeless; collect food, clothes, medicines for the poor; and hold "charity sales" to raise funds for Sant'Egidio projects. Others write to prisoners and those who are alone.

Sant'Egidio places a high value and emphasis on building personal relationships between members and those they serve. Creating a lifestyle of spirituality, prayer, and "friendship" is key to the identity of Sant'Egidio. At the same time, as an international network, it connects local action to solidarity across cultures and makes use of an international presence to share knowledge, resources, and a common spiritual identity. Making a preferential option for the poor on behalf of the elderly, Sant'Egidio also builds up the participation of the elderly in local and international efforts to serve the common good. This illustrates the importance of subsidiarity in defining solutions to concrete problems, but also the importance of contributive justice, seen in global perspective, for members of every generation. Sant'Egidio exemplifies the potential of religious communities to catalyze cooperative efforts in public and private spheres, to connect such efforts to personal religious identity and commitment, and to create social practices embodying the virtues of solidarity and justice.

The examples of the CHA and Sant'Egidio have placed aging and decline in the context of the cross-cultural need for social supports in the form of family care, community networks, and public policies that support the elderly and the chronically ill. In modern postindustrial societies, these resources are less available than in the traditional societies of Africa and Asia, for instance, even though much more money may be spent on medical technologies. Religious groups and religiously inspired health care organizations can and do move into the breech, not only to provide care but to help create better supportive structures for the aging and others in decline, both locally and internationally. These positive responses have not, however, eliminated dangers to the elderly. In "advanced" and "developing" societies alike, the weak and debilitated often become marginalized from community resources. This fact continues to present a moral and social challenge to which participatory theological bioethics must respond.

Euthanasia across Cultures

The elderly and the ill need stronger structures of solidarity and justice, because they are so often the victims of discrimination and exclusion across cultures. Communalistic patterns of social life provide important insights and models for dealing with decline and dying, but even strongly communal societies are not immune to the idea that the old and weak should be killed or allowed to die. Even in societies in which the medical-technical regime has not displaced familial, communal, and religious sources of meaning, the elderly and chronically ill can still be marginalized and even exterminated. Apparently, conflict and despair over the burdens of old age and degeneration are alive and well virtually everywhere. Theologian William E. May rightly observes that the loss of mental and physical abilities is the accompaniment of old age that cannot be romanticized away and that old age may bring its specific vices as well as virtues. In democratic societies, the older age cohorts even form their own voting blocs and pursue their self-interest as avidly as the younger generations, refusing, for example, to support local school budgets.[67] Controversy over whether the elderly consume more than "their share" of resources, medical or otherwise, is not unique to any one culture.

In more "primitive" societies, the moral ambiguity surrounding "death-hastening behavior" bears a striking resemblance to the ambivalence inherent in U.S. debates over "letting die" and "euthanasia." In an introductory essay to a book on aging, the sociologist Jay Sokolovsky retells a 1928 account by an anthropologist who lived among the people of a tiny South Sea island, the Tiwi. Among the Tiwi, the healthy elderly were accorded respect and support. However, as they grew more decrepit, and especially if they were senile and a burden or embarrassment to their kin and neighbors, elderly women were sometimes subjected by their sons and brothers to a ritual known as "covering up."

> The method was to dig a hole in the ground in some lonely place, put the old woman in the hole and fill it in with earth until only her head was showing. Everybody went away for a day or two and then went back to the hole to discover to their surprise, that the old woman was dead, having been too feeble to raise her arms from the earth. Nobody had "killed" her, her death in Tiwi eyes was a natural one. She had been alive when her relatives last saw her.[68]

Sokolovsky notes that most societies incorporate a variety of ways to treat their elderly. Access of the aged to supports and opportunities decreases in proportion to loss of function.[69] Anthony Glascock coined the term "death-hastening behavior" to refer to "killing, abandoning and forsaking of the elderly."[70] He reports that some type of death-hastening behavior was found in twenty-one of a sample of forty-one societies.[71] Glascock provides four examples from anthropological literature. Among the Chukchee, a reindeer-herding people in northeastern Siberia, few old people die a natural death. When an old person takes ill and becomes a burden to the family and community, he or she asks a near relative to kill him or her. The oldest son or daughter or son-in-law then stabs the elder in the heart with a knife. The horticultural and fishing people of the Lau Islands off southern Fiji abandon the old and feeble in a cave filled with the skeletal remains of other aged members of the community who had been led to a similar fate. The Bororo, a horticultural people in the Amazonian forest of Central Brazil, generally give old people meat or fish after a hunt. However, sometimes the indigent elderly are "forgotten." The Yakat herders of north-central Siberia show little care for decrepit old people who are no longer able to work, providing little food or clothing. Old people are beaten by their own children and are often forced to beg from house to house.[72]

In the twenty-one societies studied in which death-hastening practices exist, direct killing is the most frequently used means, occurring in fourteen societies. The decision is usually made within the family and includes consultation with the elderly individual. In three societies the elderly are beaten to death, in three buried alive, in two stabbed, and in one strangled, with no significant differences based on sex. Old people are "forsaken" in nine societies and "abandoned" in eight. Death-hastening behavior is directed at individuals who are no longer active and productive members of the group, instead straining community and family resources.[73] Probably the most striking difference between these cases and contemporary North American society is that, in the former, the rationale behind the induction of death is overtly and clearly oriented to the community and to what is viewed as overconsumption of scarce resources.

Such instances are a reminder that decline and death are approached in many cultures in the world in a much more communitarian and less rights-based way than in the United States. They are also a reminder that rights language, while often excessive in liberal cultures, arose as a response to clear violations of human dignity and the exclusion from common resources of society's most vulnerable members. Just as rights language can be used to promote self-interest rather than the common good, so an overemphasis on the good of the majority or elites can sacrifice the human dignity of the weak to the interest of the strong.

Euthanasia in the Modern West

In the United States, the primary reason to cause or "permit" death is, at least ostensibly, the welfare of the ill or elderly individual. Although some raise the suspicion that burdens may occasionally be an unacknowledged factor, the bigger question of whether expensive end-of-life care is just in view of the common good is generally avoided in the United States. Instead, practically limitless "care" is given to the very ill and dying who are insured, while 45 million other people of all ages are deprived of access both early and late in life.[74]

In modern, liberal societies, the major focus of public ethics and law is the individual and his or her rights, so it is hardly surprising that the language of rights frames the debate about euthanasia in the United States. The key argument in favor of legalizing medical assistance in causing one's own death is autonomy. The most culturally and legally prevalent form of assistance is "physician-assisted suicide," in which the medical provider is not directly involved in the killing, but provides "medical" means to patients, in the form of prescription drugs. Physician-assisted suicide is claimed as a right by those otherwise facing what they consider to be unendurable suffering or even intolerable loss of control over physical and mental faculties.

From a theological perspective, the concern to maintain self-control throughout the dying process is fairly easy to rebut, at least in some of its more insistent and exaggerated forms. Insofar as autonomy is the main impetus behind the movement for physician-assisted suicide, leading to the voluntary deaths of persons who are still in meaningful relationship with family members, this movement should be and is resisted by most religious communities that value community, covenant, reciprocity, altruism toward those who suffer, and so on. According to the Vatican, "What a sick person needs, besides medical care, is love, the human and supernatural warmth with which the sick person can and ought to be surrounded by all those close to him or her, parents and children, doctors and nurses."[75] Coopting the "rights" language of the movement for euthanasia and suicide, religious critics frequently resort to a similar vocabulary. "No one can make an attempt on the life of an innocent person without opposing God's love for that person, without violating a fundamental right, and therefore without committing a crime of the utmost gravity."[76]

It is possible to make a strong argument that, even when suffering is significant and the effect on relationships grave, better alternatives than the direct causation of death can be found. These alternatives are psychological and spiritual accompaniment of the suffering person; palliative or "comfort" care; sedation, even "terminal sedation"; and the withdrawal of all measures that would unnecessarily prolong life. However, the testimony of those who have worked with such patients or cared for them as family members leaves considerable ambiguity as to whether these measures are always adequate, effective, humane, and genuinely the best expression of the mandate to "love your neighbor as yourself."

Compassion and autonomy have both motivated the cause of those who defend voluntary killing of the very ill, both in the United States, where physician-assisted suicide has been legal since 1997 in the state of Oregon, and in the Netherlands, where euthanasia has been permissible since 1981. The "right to die" movement has been gathering momentum in the United States since the 1970s. The Hemlock Society's *Final Exit,* written by its founder, gives the terminally ill patient instructions for a painless and nonviolent suicide.[77] This book maintains that the patient has control over determining when pain is overwhelming or diminishment too severe. Patients are advised to ask physicians for a prescription for barbiturates, if necessary under the guise of experiencing sleeplessness or pain. The ill person can hoard a lethal dose and consume it at an appointed time, arranging the scenario to permit last farewells to family and friends. Companions are requested to put a plastic bag over the head of the patient, who, if not already dead, is provided a guarantee that the sought-for outcome is attained. Comments Timothy Quill, "Current laws create a paradox by prohibiting physician participation under any circumstances, but allowing explicit information about suicide methods to flow through the impersonal, uncontrolled, and potentially dangerous format of a book."[78]

This "impersonal" format and pragmatic approach help reinforce the ideas that dependent life is meaningless life and that the individual's tolerance for dependency is an adequate barometer for gauging the acceptability of continued survival. The Hemlock Society newsletter published an account by one woman who used the Hemlock method to satisfy the demand for death of her eighty-eight-year-old father. Happily married and active, the father was able to carry out daily activities, but was failing in vision and hearing as well as bored, depressed, and lonely for many friends who had already passed on. After his death, the daughter reflects, "I had always known him as a man in control. The last year of his life, he had truly become a wimpy old man. By his final action, he left life as he lived it—by making his own choices. I hope I have his strength."[79]

Jack Kevorkian, M.D., also known as "Doctor Death," provided "suicide machines" that have administered barbiturates to dozens of patients, not all of them terminally ill. He furnished this service for patients, mostly women, with whom he had no extensive relationship, nor did he explore with them alternatives of care and support. Kevorkian was convicted of second-degree murder in his home state of Michigan, in 2001, after he videotaped himself giving a fatal injection to a fifty-two-year-old man, which was televised on "60 Minutes." Before being sentenced to a ten to twenty-five year jail term, Kevorkian vouched that he had participated in 130 deaths. Again Quill: "We should begin to ask ourselves how the medical profession can be found so lacking that a superficial, bizarre approach to death can appeal strongly to the general public."[80]

Other physicians have admitted acceding to patient requests for aid in dying, including Timothy Quill. When such decisions are left up to individual patients and physicians, moral deliberation about their justifiability is not only limited but understandably biased, and often rash. In a now famous essay in the *Journal of the American Medical Association*, an anonymous doctor recounts how, as an overstressed resident, he was summoned in the night to the bedside of a young woman with ovarian cancer, suffering grievously from deprivation of sleep, food, and oxygen. She says, "Let's get this over with." Without investigating measures to improve her palliative care or engaging her in further conversation about her suffering or needs, he responds with an injection of morphine that brings death within minutes.[81] Quill tells the story of "Diane," a patient whose death he assisted, and for which he was brought to court, though not finally tried. His own decision process was nuanced, consultative, prolonged, and agonizing. The very difficulty of the decision and its aftermath motivate Quill's conviction that social norms for ending life in similar cases should be public and clear.[82]

Social Experiments: Oregon and Holland

In 1994, Oregon voters passed a referendum to legalize physician-assisted suicide. After surmounting legal challenges and gaining support from a second referendum, the Oregon Death with Dignity Act was implemented in 1997.[83] The law specifically prohibits the administration of lethal drugs by a physician, but permits patients to request and receive prescriptions for them. The patient must make two verbal requests, separated by fifteen days, and one written request. The requesting patient must be an adult (eighteen or older) and an Oregon resident. He or she must have a terminal illness and have fewer than six months to live. The prescribing physician and a consulting physician must confirm the prognosis, determine that the request is voluntary, and refer the patient for counseling if psychological impairment is suspected. The physician who prescribes the medications must also inform the patient of alternatives, such as pain control, comfort care, and hospice care.[84]

The experience of the first five years in Oregon suggests that a relatively small percentage of patients choose to request lethal medications and, of those who do, a significant percentage—almost one-third—never go on to take the drugs. In the first five years, there were 42,235 total deaths in the state of Oregon, 198 requests for prescriptions to enable suicide, and 129 persons who actually carried out suicide using the prescriptions.[85]

However, of these persons, only 22 percent gave pain as a reason for their action, while 33 percent feared being a burden to family, and 2 percent mentioned financial constraints. Much more prevalent reasons were loss of autonomy and independence (85 percent), "decreased ability to participate in enjoyed activities" (79 percent), and loss of control over bodily functions (58 percent). The underlying illness of 79 percent was cancer. Their median age was sixty-nine.[86]

It is notable that the legalization of physician-assistance suicide in Oregon was a catalyst for efforts to improve end-of-life care. The law requires a state agency, the Oregon Health Division, to collect data and monitor compliance with the new regulations. This resulted in extensive interviews with physicians who had enabled suicides. However, there is no provision made for an independent assessment and evaluation.[87] The passage of the Death with Dignity Act also prompted the Oregon Health Sciences University's Center for Ethics in Health Care to convene a task force on improvement of care. The task force is a consortium of health professionals, organizations, agencies, and institutions "which seek to promote excellent care of the dying and to address the ethical and clinical issues posed by the enactment of the Death with Dignity Act." Not all members take the same ethical or practical views of physician-assisted suicide. They collaborated in a guidebook to resources on end-of-life care, based on a consensus that requests for suicide often derive from unmet pain needs or depression, that alternatives to suicide must be realistically available, that health professionals who do not want to participate in suicides should not have to do so, and that physician-assisted suicide, when used as a last resort, should be carried out in compliance with the law.[88]

The nonprofit advocacy group Compassion in Dying, describing itself as "a client service organization" and a national leader in "the reform of end-of-life care," includes under its "primary goals" the improvement of pain and symptom management, increase of "patient empowerment and self-determination," and the expansion of choices "to include aid-in-dying for terminally ill, mentally competent adults."[89]

Statistics indicate that the increased attention to end-of-life issues in Oregon has resulted in the lowest rate of in-hospital deaths of the fifty states (31 percent), a higher frequency of advance care planning and "do not resuscitate" orders, and potentially an improvement in pain management. However, in 1997–98, family reports of pain experienced by dying patients remained about the same for those in nursing homes and at home, while pain of those in hospitals was reported to have increased—and the prescription and administration of painkilling drugs to have decreased. In 1999, the Oregon Board of Medical Examiners became the first in the country to discipline a physician for providing inadequate pain care to six patients.[90]

There are problems and questions stemming from the Oregon experiment. Physicians interviewed are recounting events after the fact, based on their own impressions and memories. Physicians who choose not to comply with requests have no specific forum in which to voice their experiences, those of their patients, or other options that may have been discovered. It is also difficult to ascertain exactly what level of expertise and resources regarding palliative care were actually commanded by the physicians who complied with suicide requests, for how long they had worked with the requesting patients or families, and on what basis they arrived at judgments of competency and voluntariness.[91] And, obviously, the prognosis for persons with "terminal illness" is always an estimate.

Critics have also disputed the idea that data support the conclusion that suicides are not prompted by economic considerations. Even for those who have insurance, there are both economic and social burdens that result from the need to receive and provide intensive care. The effect of such factors on decisions to die could be expressed in terms such as loss of autonomy and fear of becoming a burden to family. Kathleen Foley and Herbert Hendon report that the official Oregon data "does not assess the high care needs of patients who requested assisted suicide, nor does it assess the caregiver burden." They claim that there are "significant disparities according to sex, ethnicity, age, and income" with regard to the economic and other burdens of terminal illness.[92] And even when patients have insurance, end-of-life care can create hardships such as loss of family savings, loss of income, and changes in educational plans and employment status.[93]

There are, however, a few things that both critics and advocates of the Oregon law agree on. There is a great need for improved palliative care. Physicians are in the best position to make determinations of terminal disease, to judge the patient's ability to make an informed decision, and to decide what drug dose will bring death most easily—however, physicians are ill-equipped to do so in reality, partly because of the ambiguity of many cases and partly because of their own lack of knowledge. Finally, whether one accepts euthanasia in principle or not, there is general agreement that the United States as a society does not have in place the protections and safeguards that would save the practice from abuse and vulnerable patients from mistakes.[94]

The Netherlands provides a longer-term case study in social acceptance of directly causing the deaths of the terminally ill.[95] There are some significant differences, primarily that Dutch law requires that the patient be in a state of severe suffering, but it does not exclude euthanasia (killing by the physician rather than suicide). In the Netherlands, a 1991 decision retained the status of euthanasia as a criminal offense under the penal code, but established that physicians providing voluntary euthanasia would not be prosecuted, if certain conditions were met. These were that the patient must make a free and informed request; he or she must be in a state of intolerable, unrelievable suffering; the appropriateness of the decision must be confirmed by consulting physicians; and the facts of the case must be reported to the coroner, to allow supervision of instances. However, reports on actual practice through the mid-1990s indicated that, in addition to the approximately 3,600 cases of physician-assisted suicide and euthanasia reported annually, there were also about 1,000 cases of nonvoluntary euthanasia. In most of the latter cases, the patients killed were no longer competent and thus were not able to request or give informed consent to the action. In some cases, these patients were newborns.[96] According to one estimate, physician intervention in actively causing death rose 27 percent from 1991 to 1995, while 40 percent of the cases involved no explicit request from the patient to do so.[97]

In 2001, the Dutch senate passed a new law regulating euthanasia and physician-assisted suicide. According to its provisions, these actions, still criminalized under the penal code, can be exempted explicitly from criminal liability if they meet several conditions. In general, these are the same conditions under which physicians had not been prosecuted in the past. The law concerns only termination of life on request—involuntary euthanasia remains forbidden. A new development, owing to case law, is greater concern that a doctor have an established relationship with his or her patient before agreeing to assist death.[98]

The Dutch health system is accessible to all and provides full coverage for palliative and terminal care. Since 1995, hospice care initiatives have been established in almost every region of the country. A Dutch physician, specialist in palliative care, and director of a hospice reports that levels of nursing care in the Netherlands are sophisticated and that such care is virtually always covered by insurance. Most patients who are afraid, depressed, control-oriented, or suffering "burnout" can be counseled and supported so that their expressed desire for euthanasia is alleviated. Those in physical pain frequently have conditions that have not yet been treated with the best resources; those few in "extreme" pain are given barbiturates for "terminal sedation" as a last resort (to be discussed below).[99]

Doctors in general seem to be more cautious about conceding to euthanasia requests. In 1998, in the Netherlands, legislation established five regional review committees to ensure that doctors exercise due care in making decisions, with patients, about euthanasia. Based on numbers furnished to these committees, reports of euthanasia cases have declined. However, it is not clear whether this represents an actual reduction in the occurrence of physician-assisted suicide or euthanasia.[100]

In 2002, a new Christian Democrat government came into power in the Netherlands, replacing the socialist and liberal coalition that had been preparing initiatives for legislation on nonvoluntary euthanasia, voluntary euthanasia for children, and a right to assisted suicide "for people who are 'tired of life.'" Instead, the government intends to monitor and enforce compliance with existing regulations. Theo Boer, a bioethicist and a professor of Christian ethics at Utrecht University, is skeptical about arguments that the Netherlands is heading down a "slippery slope" toward ever-greater expansion of rationales for legal killing by doctors. He believes that the situation has reached an equilibrium, that many doctors openly express a change of mind about the acceptability of euthanasia, and that palliative care initiatives are abundant and effective.

Nevertheless, he concedes that the right to active euthanasia has become a norm, so that those arguing against it carry the burden of proof; active euthanasia is performed even on patients who are not competent, despite the fact that this is supposedly against the law; and the grounds for euthanasia and assisted suicide have shifted from beneficence (requiring a demonstration of intolerable suffering) to autonomy (based on the choice of the patient, but not actually requiring voluntariness in every case).[101] Others have expressed concern that, because the population of the Netherlands is aging and care may be more difficult to provide in the future, "there will be increasing pressure on those who are sick and frail, chronically ill, or dying to consume less care and fewer societal resources."[102]

Theological-Ethical Analysis

The reason that one is disconcerted by the accounts of "Debbie" and of persons who committed suicide with the help of Kevorkian or the Hemlock Society is that their main characters seem to define "compassion" simply as respect for autonomy regarding time of death. Missing are the reciprocity and contextualization that would better ensure that the choice exercised truly advances the patient's well-being. As a 1988 report of the Hastings Center states, "Autonomy is not some a priori property of persons abstractly conceived. It is an achievement of selves who are socially embedded and physically embodied."[103] A person's true interests—that define his or her good and well-being—do not exist in advance of or apart from his or her illness and its limits. Illness, aging, or the dying process demands an effort to keep the life-transforming power of illness within bounds and to integrate the afflicted person's subjective desires with new objective needs "into a coherent and satisfying life."[104] The problem is not self-determination per se, but an excessively individualistic interpretation of autonomy, which if accepted cannot ground truly compassionate action, but only a detached regard for "choice" that fails to meet the real and evolving needs of the patient.

Michael Mendiola, a theological bioethicist, urges that a full view of the dignity of the person must take into account relational histories and contexts over which control is limited, but in which our freedom finds its concrete possibilities of expression. "Honoring the demands of human dignity means a recognition of, and positive efforts to enhance and nurture these multiple, rich dimensions. Surely choice and self-direction are a necessary aspect of any ethical attending to human dignity: but they are never sufficient."[105] Gerald McKenny observes that "a community of care" is required to meet these needs and that the attempt to control death, whether through technology or euthanasia, is ultimately futile.[106] For Stanley Hauerwas, euthanasia contributes to the erosion of community and can signal abandonment of a person in desperate suffering.[107]

This insight applies to families and other caregivers. "Choice" about caring for a loved one is a meaningless or even harmful concept, unless there are interpersonal, medical, and community resources available to provide support that truly meets the needs of the patient and of the caregivers as well. These resources might include "publicly financed home care services with appropriate quality assurance and licensure mechanisms, respite care programs, so-called adult day care programs, counseling services, educational programs and support groups, and the like."[108] Individual patient welfare can only be comprehended and served within the networks of relationships that are the components of a meaningful life.

Autonomy as the isolated power of self-determination is an illusion, because true freedom is not absence of limits and constraints, but the ability to pursue cherished and important values and goals within the constraints that human life inevitably brings and the opportunities provided within specific relationships and communities.[109] The need for community and social services for the ill, the dying, and all those in decline raises questions about national resources, the need to set priorities within the health care sector, and the need to measure the good of health care against the worth of other social goods that also sustain individuals and communities.[110] Though such issues will emerge more fully in chapter 4, they are quite clearly at stake in the availability of support for the dying and of life-enhancing services and opportunities for the elderly and the ill.

Religious traditions put the human problems of loss, suffering, and death within a framework of transcendent meaning that holds humans to account, yet offers them hope of reconciliation with the powers of the universe and one another.[111] For those facing decline and death, religious experiences and beliefs can provide meaning and purpose, even when the satisfactions and usefulness of life seem to be over. A religious worldview can be a powerful antidote to the tendencies of technology and pragmatism to control the experiences of radical suffering and threatened nonexistence. But for religion to be truly powerful, it must take shape in ways of life, not in abstract "beliefs."

Religious worldviews are mediated and made practical in a variety of ways, which is important for the role of theological bioethics and the impact that theology and theologians can have on cultural struggles with the meaning of death and the care of the ill and aged. Religious value systems and symbols are in turn affected and nuanced as a result of the practices and conversations in which theologians and other religious persons engage. A religious frame of meaning inheres in and fosters communal values and virtues that are coherent with founding narratives such as scriptures; specific communal practices embody and reinforce these values and virtues; individual values, virtues, and practices are formed by and also form communal participation; and theology expresses, reflects on, and enables individual and communal values, virtues, and practices. Meanwhile, religious individuals and even religious communities participate in practices and discourses that are not exclusively religious or are interreligious. Religious identity, expression, and practice thus have an inherently dynamic, open-ended character.

In relation to aging, decline, and death, religious worldviews are mediated and refined in all of the previously mentioned ways. Stanley Hauerwas has been among the most eloquent of theologians to insist that coherence with the Christian scriptures demands specific, very demanding values and virtues, exhibited not just by individuals but by the Christian community as a discipleship community. According to Hauerwas, the character of Christian beliefs can only be understood in relation to the formation of a community formed by those beliefs. Care for the sick is a practice that both reveals and tests the community of the church.[112] The church is "a resource of the habits and practices necessary to sustain the care of those in pain over the long haul," to be present for the ill and the dying, even when we feel helpless to do much to relieve their condition.[113]

Allen Verhey imaginatively projects a horizon of meaning against which the dilemmas of modern medicine are illumined in different shades. While healing was a part of Jesus' ministry, his larger concern was inclusion of the socially marginal in communities of care and service.[114] The inevitability of suffering and demise is given testament in his own death, along with the trust in God that enables the communal virtue of accompaniment of the sick and dying. In a Christian biblical perspective, the meanings of embodied personhood go beyond freedom and dependence to include sociality and the need for community.[115]

Special Christian virtues can be cultivated throughout life that prepare individuals to overcome the threat of meaninglessness, approach death in appreciation of a community of love and care, sustain in the dying person the virtue of solidarity with the community, and even, as Christopher Vogt puts it, attain a "sense that their deaths might be redemptive for themselves or others."[116] Taking the Jesus of Luke's gospel as a model, Vogt commends especially a faithful and hopeful disposition of patience, cultivated over a lifetime in times of adversity and loss, culminating in the acceptance of the dependency and loss of control that inevitably accompany dying. Despite its bias toward the embrace of physical suffering, the *ars moriendi* tradition of lifetime preparation for a good death can provide a useful model for the cultivation of personal Christian virtue today.[117]

Essentially a tradition of personal prayer, piety, and devotional reading, the *ars moriendi* tradition assumed that death was not an isolated event, that persons had regular opportunities to be present at the deathbeds of others, and that the faith community would furnish the tools to meet death well.[118] The intentional cultivation of virtue in view of impending death and the "great transition" is a well-attested Christian tradition; yet it may imply a degree of control over one's dispositions and moral resolve that those actually in the throes of tormenting illness may not experience.

To confront the reality of inexplicable, undeserved, virtually unbearable suffering, Verhey invokes the biblical rhetoric of "lament," found in the book of Job and in the psalms. Neither petitions nor expressions of personal resolve, laments are simply "great cries to God in sickness and in sorrow, in catastrophe and grief, sad songs of complaint," and even of "doubt and fear and anger."[119] Verhey makes the important point that biblical lament is a communal act, one that deserves a bigger place in liturgical prayer,[120] perhaps especially in prayer for and with the sick and dying.

Verhey also sagely observes that, although the Bible furnishes five or six stories of suicide, it never explicitly condemns it.[121] For Verhey, this does not mean that suicide may be acceptable, but rather that it is not best discouraged by prohibitions but by showing that there are better alternatives. Those alternatives become real to suffering persons only if they are mediated by communal practices of care and accompaniment. The avoidance of suicide is not an obligation only of persons in despair, but also—perhaps even more so—of the communities responsible to minister to them. "A 'more excellent way' [than physician-assisted suicide] will include a ministry to the dying as members of families, as friends, as members of communities of faith, and as members of other communities."[122]

Beyond spiritual and liturgical traditions and practices of care for the sick—but in some ways derivative from and dependent on them—religion and theology provide guidance about how to negotiate circumstances of uncertainty about specific choices and also about how to create more comprehensive social practices and institutions that encourage good behavior. Theological ethics tries to integrate individual and institutional moral behavior with Christian values, as well as to speak to and with other communities and institutions guiding the same behavior, such as medicine and law. Roman Catholicism has had an especially long-standing and far-reaching tradition of medical morality, shaping norms for decision making and institutional policies and practices that affect how care is delivered, at least in Catholic health facilities. A discussion in the next chapter of the (originally Catholic) distinction between ordinary and extraordinary means of life support and the principle of double effect will further address the personal and social morality of physician-assisted suicide, of "allowing to die," and of the use of artificial nutrition and hydration. It will also prepare the way for an examination of the social and institutional presence of theological bioethics in advocacy for better distribution and use of health-supporting resources worldwide.

CHAPTER

4

DECLINE AND DYING

Principles of Analysis and Practices of Solidarity

ALONG WITH OTHER religious traditions, Christian teaching has traditionally opposed active causation of death, even for suffering, terminally ill patients. At the same time, death need not be opposed absolutely. The death of a very elderly or ill person may be accepted as appropriate, and measures to prolong life may be refused. While suffering may have a redemptive meaning when intentionally united with the cross of Christ, the mission of caregivers—indeed, of all Christians—is to serve their neighbor by alleviating suffering. Sometimes this means caring for a person, but not preventing death.

This chapter first examines the principle of double effect and the differentiation between ordinary and extraordinary means of prolonging life to see how Christian values, both theologically and philosophically rendered, shape practice. It considers how these analytic frameworks have been used to exclude euthanasia of ill or dying patients, then reviews some counter-arguments. It also looks at the impact of scarcity of resources on such decisions. Then it considers ways in which Christian bioethics—as participatory—has been effective in justifying and making available alternatives to euthanasia. These are the hospice movement, the CHA's advocacy for the chronically ill and dying, and the work of international Christian organizations with AIDS patients.

Catholic Bioethics: Theology in Practice

From at least the seventeenth century onward, the Catholic Church has distinguished between "ordinary" or mandatory means of life support and "extraordinary" or optional means of life support.[1] While good care must include the former, it need not entail the latter. The definitions, however, are somewhat relative to the condition of the individual patient, as well as the cultural and social environment. There is no measure that is "always" ordinary or extraordinary, no matter what the circumstances. Rather, the church permits the refusal of life-extending measures that do not significantly improve the individual patient's physical condition or that are excessively burdensome for him or her to use, as well as the use of methods of pain relief that will ultimately shorten life (e.g., doses of morphine that depress breathing and heartbeat).[2]

The decisive distinction in Catholic moral theology is between direct means of causing death and indirect means. A patient may never be killed directly, even when there are good reasons to welcome death. It is essential to realize that the seemingly abstract reasoning process that produced and applies the principles of Catholic moral theology is actually a form of casuistry that is embedded in social practices and practical concerns. This continues to be the case, given the interdependence of bioethical analysis and the institutional practice of Catholic health care. Catholic health facilities ordinarily express their mission in terms of adherence to Catholic values and moral principles, while ministering to the sick and most especially while devoting special energies to the care of the underserved. Sensitive to the plight of patients and communities under duress, Catholic health care ministry still avoids solutions such as abortion, sterilization, third-party reproductive technologies, and euthanasia, as well as cooperation with non-Catholic partners (other health facilities or social service agencies) that supply these interventions.

In specific ambiguous or conflict cases, however, what constitutes acceptance or avoidance requires interpretation and, often, flexibility. Ostensibly, there are clear moral norms prescribing conduct and practice in these problem areas, norms that are backed theologically with principles such as "the sanctity of life," "made in God's image," or "the one-flesh union of marriage." However, the theological worldview, the moral implications, and the context of application exist in a constant dialectical relationship, in which the meaning of worldview, principles, and practical morality mutually inform and refine one another.

A vehicle for this process in modern Catholic health care is a set of guidelines, the *Ethical and Religious Directives for Catholic Health Facilities.* The development and function of these directives display some of the ways theological bioethics can be interactive with social practice, respond to contexts and problems, and be reformed in the process. The *Directives* emerge from a Christian worldview and are based on Catholic moral theology, but they also set policies for the operation of Catholic health care institutions, and they are revised in light of the experience of these institutions. The *Directives* today represent the teaching of the national bishops' conference but are under almost constant reinterpretation and negotiation by those providing health services under Catholic auspices, in conversation with theological advisors and with members of the episcopacy in various dioceses.

The original version of the *Directives* was developed in 1949 by a group of U.S. and Canadian theologians and health care professionals and published in a Catholic journal aimed primarily at physicians.[3] The CHA (founded in 1915)[4] produced a more succinct Code of Medical Ethics for Catholic Hospitals in 1954, meant to be placed on the walls of surgical suites. In 1956, moral theologian Gerald Kelly, theological advisor to the CHA, led the development of a second, revised edition of the 1949 *Directives*, which was then published by the Catholic Health Association of the United States and Canada.[5] This edition took effect as official policy in each Roman Catholic diocese in the country as each bishop chose to approve it.

Since the 1971 edition, the *Directives* has served as the official policy of the U.S. bishops.[6] Today they remain the standard by which each bishop may approve or discredit any health care institution under his aegis as "Catholic." Therefore, the content of the *Directives* is important to Catholic institutional policy and practice. The specific elements of the *Directives* are defined in practice with individual bishops and in specific settings, in relation to specific problems, especially in relation to serving pluralistic communities when the Catholic facility is virtually the only provider or the only provider to underserved populations. Each new edition of the *Directives* is hammered out by a committee of authors, including moral theologians, who debate the best way to formulate items so as to be coherent with tradition even as they respond to issues and needs of the day.

Moral theologians and bioethicists Gerald Kelly and Richard McCormick constructed major works around the format and content of the *Directives*.[7] In Kelly's case, it was to propound and defend the *Directives*; in McCormick's, it was to propose a revised version that he considered an appropriate development of tradition. Both wrote in response to concrete biomedical and social concerns and in relation to their theological and ethical heritages. The format they chose illustrates their expectation that theological bioethics would be informed by, responsive to, and influence the social practices of medical and health care. In McCormick's case, it was with explicit attention to the larger culture and legal and policy debates over such matters as abortion, euthanasia, and just access to health care.

These were debates that McCormick himself addressed frequently, with theological and ethical precision, in a series of annual essays on moral theology, published for more than a quarter of a century in the scholarly journal *Theological Studies*.[8] McCormick's March "moral notes" were avidly read by an audience of other moral theologians, parish priests, Catholic health care professionals, church officials, and all those interested in the inner "politics" of the Catholic Church. Many of the issues of "medical ethics," in the early days, overlapped with sexual ethics. McCormick's analytic eye was keen, his dismantling of the illogical or specious argument unhesitating. He was always in touch with lively and contentious debates and with recent developments in church practice, medicine, and law. McCormick's choice of the *Directives* as a framework for the formulation of his bioethical proposal shows how seriously he and other Catholic moral theologians took theological and moral tradition, the importance and propriety of change, the essential nature of close and careful thinking in moving from theology to practice, and the indispensable role of practical experience and testing in regard to bioethical verdicts.

The CHA continues to have as a main function and concern the interpretation of the *Directives* for its members, and the negotiation of practical meaning and application in dubious, contentious, politically volatile, or novel cases. The social presence of theological bioethics through the CHA and Catholic health care institutions is discussed further in following chapters.

This chapter investigates some tools of moral analysis provided by Catholic tradition and used extensively and centrally for many years by McCormick and other Catholic moral theologians, as well as some Protestant theologians and many medical practitioners. These tools—double effect and the distinction between ordinary and extraordinary means of life support—were devised as responses to concrete moral dilemmas in medical care. In fact, they may best be understood, not as pure products of logic or theology, but as guiding ideas that rely on centuries of cumulative practical experience, considered in light of both a Christian worldview and the exigencies of social life. Double effect is a tool to guide decision makers through conflictual situations in which every alternative seems to have a cost, and no solution is problem-free. Ordinary and extraordinary means is a distinction meant to recognize the fragility of life, the importance of integrating decline and death with other human and social values, and the ultimate acceptability of death as the human end no one can avoid.

Ordinary and Extraordinary Means of Life Support

Gerald Kelly's 1958 commentary on the then-current *Directives* provides a succinct formulation of the difference between permissible and prohibited ways to bring about the death of a seriously ill patient. All "positive means to end life" are forbidden, for example, an overdose of drugs. Writing so shortly after the atrocities of Nazi medicine, Kelly would have had clearly in mind a social setting of euthanasia that was the direct termination of individuals who are judged useless to society. However, when considering whether indefinite prolongation of life is always necessary, he focuses on the good of the individual as a reason to cause death indirectly. To indirectly cause death is to withdraw or refuse technologies or other means that could possibly prolong life but do not offer a reasonable hope of benefit to the patient or involve excessive "expense, pain, or other hardship to oneself or others." Such optional means are called "extraordinary," a term that came to mean measures that could be used at the discretion of the patient.[9]

To determine the moral character of decisions to use or refuse means, the context must be examined. For one thing, a means that is virtually useless or very dangerous in one era of medical practice may improve in efficacy as time goes on. Similarly, what is not tolerable or effective for one patient may be reasonable and useful for another. Moreover, the patient considering the acceptance of death must sometimes take into account the "common good," for which he or she may still have a responsibility.[10] This would also seem to be true of decisions to use certain resources, at least in some circumstances. An essay on the ethics of allocation decisions begins with a "medical record note" from an acute care hospital:

> Long-stay patient died in intensive care unit with multiple systems failures. Patient utilized exorbitant resources—staff time and numerous tests, drugs, and interventions. (Staff believed early on that most of the patient's treatments were useless.)[11]

Was such care truly in the interests of the patient? Did it balance individual good with the common good?

In 1980, the Vatican restated Catholic tradition on these points, but in a tone of greater recognition of the fact that sometimes a mercy killing can be motivated by concern for a suffering patient. "By euthanasia is understood an action or an omission which of itself or by intention causes death, in order that all suffering may in this way be eliminated." The wrong is not found in the goal of ending suffering or in the fact that it is known that death will ensue. Rather, it derives from the fact that an action is done that directly results in death as its primary effect; the primary goal of the agent is to bring about death. "Euthanasia's terms of reference, therefore, are to be found in the intention of the will and in the methods used."[12] According to the *Directives*, "Euthanasia is an action or omission that of itself or by intention causes death in order to alleviate suffering. Catholic health care institutions may never condone or participate in euthanasia or assisted suicide in any way."[13] Official Catholic teaching, most Catholic theology, and actual practices in Catholic-sponsored health care remain resistant to widespread acceptance of euthanasia, preferring instead to set care of the dying within the reciprocal relations of the common good, including the spiritual and social support systems vital to a good death.[14]

Means to prolong life may be declined or removed if they are "disproportionate." In making a judgment, the agents involved must take into account not only the risk and benefits of the treatment but also its availability and cost, as well as the "physical and moral resources" of the sick person, his or her "reasonable wishes," and those of the family. "Excessive expense" is a consideration not only in relation to the finances of the patient but also in view of the resources of the community.[15] In 1995, the Committee on Doctrine of the National Conference of Catholic Bishops (U.S.) developed a revised *Ethical and Religious Directives for Catholic Health Care Services*.[16] Important changes in presentation include much greater attention to the social responsibilities of health care givers and to the gospel values motivating health care, and especially the mission of Catholic institutions to care for the poor. The prerogative of the patient to freely refuse burdensome, useless, or excessively costly treatment is reaffirmed.[17] Effective pain management is stressed as part of appropriate care.[18] However, the intention of causing death is rejected, even when measures are taken that ensure death will follow. The intention must always be focused on relief of suffering, with death as a foreseen but unintended secondary effect.[19]

In this context, the *Directives* address an ongoing controversy about when and why artificial nutrition and hydration must be provided to permanently comatose patients. Stating that the Vatican has taken no detailed position on the issue, the *Directives* assert that there should be a presumption in favor of providing such means to sustain life, "as long as this is of sufficient benefit to outweigh the burdens involved to the patient."[20] The document also identifies the issue of whether artificial feeding provides such a benefit to patients in what is termed "persistent vegetative state" (PVS) as "requiring further reflection."[21] The underlying debated question is whether indefinite existence in a state of PVS is a benefit or burden to a patient; must suffering be conscious suffering, or can persons suffer by being subjected to the indignity of being maintained technologically in a sort of living death?

In March 2004, John Paul II, at an international Vatican conference for physicians and ethicists, delivered an oral statement (an "allocution") that seemed to indicate that artificial nutrition and hydration for PVS patients are morally obligatory.[22] The main concern expressed by the pope is clearly that vulnerable individuals with greatly reduced function will be pushed aside by selfish family members or a utilitarian society and lose the respect that should be accorded every member of the human race. He mentions "psychological, social, and economic pressures" that can result in "discriminatory and eugenic" decisions and social policies.[23] Even those in PVS "retain their human dignity in all its fullness." "I feel the duty to reaffirm strongly that the intrinsic value and personal dignity of every human being do not change, no matter what the concrete circumstances of his or her life."[24] Every sick person still has "the right to basic health care."[25] In fact, societies must offer sufficient resources to support families in maintaining patients in a state of PVS and should establish "a network of awakening centers with specialized treatment and rehabilitation programs" for those who cannot be maintained at home.[26]

The pope wants to bring artificial nutrition and hydration under the aegis of basic health care, thus taking away any idea that there is no obligation to provide it to those who have indefinitely or permanently lost consciousness. Therefore he redefines tube feeding as an ordinary and natural means of providing food and water. He asserts, "the administration of water and food, even when provided by artificial means, always represents a *natural means* of preserving life, not a *medical act*." On this premise, he concludes that it "should be considered, in principle, ordinary and proportionate, and as such morally obligatory"—that is, "insofar as" it "consists in providing nourishment to the patient and alleviation of his suffering."[27] In other words, no matter what the quality of the patient's life, it is still worthwhile to provide artificial feeding from the point of view of the best interests of the patient, as long as it can supply an essential condition of biological life.

The statement provoked extensive press coverage and quick analysis by Catholic theologians. Some agreed. Richard Doerflinger, deputy director, secretariat for pro-life activities of the U.S. Conference of Catholic Bishops, applauds the speech for defining artificial nutrition and hydration as "normal" care, though he does not regard it as declaring an absolute obligation to provide such care in all cases.[28] Many demurred in stronger terms.[29] To these it seemed that the newer, apparently more restrictive teaching was not demanded by or even consistent with the principle that a means can be considered extraordinary or disproportionate if it does not offer a reasonable hope of benefit and threatened to upset the mission of Catholic health services to care humanely and holistically for all patients.

Though the pope's concern about diminishment of respect for those unable to assert their own right to medical resources is well warranted, it is paradoxical to assert that tube feeding is not "a medical act." To claim that artificial feeding is "natural" is to normalize technology and to medicalize and "technologize" the most basic human needs and the relations of interdependence through which they are met. Illness and decline should be placed in a larger picture of human relationships and in light of the horizon of personal, interpersonal, and transcendent meaning that includes individuals in their relations to God, their neighbors, and their communities.

As Thomas Shannon, James Walter, Kevin Wildes, and others have argued, no absolute distinction can be maintained between the quality of ongoing life as a whole and the burdensomeness of means used to preserve it. The goal of preserving biological life as such is not an adequate criterion.[30] Quality makes a difference, not in terms of social utility to others but in terms of the "worth" of continued existence to the individual living it. Biological existence has a purpose, and that purpose is to permit the person to seek spiritual and interpersonal goods, in solidarity with others with whom he or she shares community. These larger purposes were taken into account in traditional discernments of when a means of life support has become "extraordinary," but they seem to have fallen out of the evaluative matrix of those who insist on tube feeding at any length and at all costs.

In the words of Ron Hamel, director for ethics of CHA, and Michael Panicola, vice president of ethics of SSM Health Care in St. Louis, "in the majority of cases involving decisions to forgo nutrition and hydration or any other means of preserving life, the traditional teaching and a comprehensive palliative care strategy will be effective Christian witness to our basic understanding of life and death."[31] The overall condition of the patient, and not only the possibility of prolonging biological life, helps determine what is appropriate, humane, and morally praiseworthy care. The Christian horizon leads us to understand that removal of life-sustaining means can signify "acceptance of the human condition" in a spirit of care and solidarity, not "abandonment" of the patient.[32]

Further, it does not undermine human dignity to consider that individual lives, illnesses, and deaths have concrete implications for the common good, as part of dignity consists in humanity's social nature. Interdependence and participation in the common good are intrinsic components of dignity. On the one hand, it is certainly true that the worth of individuals should not be simply subordinated to an estimate of benefits or burdens for the community or society to which they belong.[33] On the other hand, however, to approach protection of vulnerable categories of persons simply by means of an inflexible approach to their individual rights is to bypass important questions about what participation in the common good really signifies and entails. This is particularly true when basic rights are articulated in terms of advanced technologies available only to the most prosperous categories of persons in the most prosperous societies of the world:

> It could be argued that consideration of distributive justice, responsible stewardship, and the common good would require dedicating our health-care resources first to rectifying some of the fundamental inequities in the current structure of access to health care in this country, before dedicating any resources to "awakening centers" that may or may not have any impact on outcomes.[34]

Specific allocations of health care resources need to be made in the context of variations in the resources available for medical care and, ultimately, in awareness of the need for redistributive justice in meeting basic needs of persons in less advantaged societies before providing relatively expensive or exotic life-prolonging technologies to those in more privileged circumstances, for whom benefit is at best questionable.

Recent discussions in the United States and interaction between Vatican spokespersons and U.S. bishops and theologians elucidate not only the practical nature of casuistry and its integral relation to structures of care, ecclesial relations, and social-political concerns but also the principle of subsidiarity. The major Vatican position paper on euthanasia and permitting to die remains the *Declaration on Euthanasia* of 1980.[35] The *Declaration* forbids direct killing, but does not exclude the possibility of seeing artificial nutrition and hydration as disproportionate in some cases.

> One cannot impose on anyone the obligation to have recourse to a technique which is already in use but which carries a risk or is burdensome. Such a refusal is not the equivalent of suicide; on the contrary, it should be considered as an acceptance of the human condition, or a wish to avoid the application of a medical procedure disproportionate to the results that can be expected, or a desire not to impose excessive expense on the family or the community.[36]

In the last two decades, various bishops' conferences and theologians have debated whether the removal of artificially provided nutrients is permitted under Catholic teaching, which would require viewing it as in some cases a disproportionate or extraordinary measure under the terms of the *Declaration on Euthanasia,* at least in some instances.[37] It is likely that the recent papal intervention (which in any case would be regarded as having a moderate level of authority and certainly not as "infallible") was prompted by concerns on the American scene that the Catholic pro-life mission was under threat from pluralism on this issue.

In any event, interpretation and application of the pope's allocution quickly devolved to the local level, with even a top official and spokesman for the pro-life office of the U.S. Catholic bishops (Doerflinger) maintaining that it still permits room for judgment, and the CHA referring members back to the 2001 *Directives* of the USCCB as the proximate arbiter. This guide asserts that "there should be a presumption in favor of" providing medically assisted nutrition and hydration, but the obligation holds only as long as the measure "is of significant benefit to outweigh the burdens involved to the patient." Whether tube feeding is a burden to a comatose patient is the debated issue, with some arguing that mere survival is an adequate benefit and that feeding must be considered nonburdensome if the patient cannot express resistance. Others argue that being maintained indefinitely in a comatose state is an offense against human dignity and that physical survival alone is not an adequate value in light of the psycho-spiritual nature of the person. The pluralism of interpretation remains, with actual practices determined at the local and institutional levels, as the USCCB did not move immediately to adopt a more restrictive stance in response to the pope, nor did the Vatican itself follow up with reinforcements. In fact, the Roman more than the Anglo-American legal mentality has typically been inclined to see norms and directives as prophetic ideals rather than as requirements to be enforced rigidly.

Double Effect

Behind all of these analyses of euthanasia, physician-assisted suicide, and provision or refusal of treatment lies the principle of double effect. The permissibility of refusing life supports when it is known that death will follow and the line drawn against direct killing both depend in part on this principle. Essentially the principle of double effect holds that acts with both good and bad effects may be justified under certain conditions, especially when the good outweighs the bad, and the bad is not directly intended or caused. An act that relieves suffering but also hastens the death of the patient may be justified if it is a last resort and is "indirect," for instance, the removal of a "useless" treatment rather than an overdose of drugs. In such a case, the primary aim and the direct focus of intention is relief of suffering, with death as a secondary and "indirectly intended" result. However, if the means omitted is "ordinary" (useful and not too expensive or burdensome), then the resulting death is regarded as directly intended, that is, illegitimate and immoral.

The roots of this principle go back to the middle ages, but for the operative modern formulation, Gerald Kelly is again instructive. Kelly lays out the four standard conditions of double effect in the following terms. "1) *The action, considered by itself and independently of its effect, must not be morally evil* ["intrinsically evil"]. . . . 2) *The evil effect must not be the means of producing the good effect*. . . . 3) *The evil effect is sincerely not intended but merely tolerated*. . . . 4) *There must be a proportionate reason for performing the action, in spite of its evil consequences*." Kelly then adds, "In some cases the difficulty of estimating the proportionate reason is so great that even the most eminent theologians may disagree in their solution" and further states that proportionality must be assessed in view of "the total picture." He allows that double effect is not only a "complicated principle," but is perhaps best understood as "a practical formula" that requires common sense and experience for its application.[38]

In the 1970s, this principle came under sustained attack by moral theologians who perceived that, despite Kelly's caveats, double effect had been applied to cases like a mathematical formula. It had been employed in an aura of certainty about results that is undermined when those results are more thoughtfully and critically considered in relation to circumstances. Moreover, the provisions of the principle, when subjected to sustained scrutiny in light of the ambiguity of real moral situations, seemed arbitrary and disjointed, even incoherent.

Criticism of double effect focuses on two major areas. First, does the category "intrinsic evil" make sense? How can a physical act, abstractly defined apart from circumstances, be known in advance to be morally evil? Does not morality almost by definition imply circumstances in which a conflict among goods is resolved by choosing one over another? In that case, moral evaluation would depend on knowing whether the right choice was made and the higher or more urgent good chosen. Second, is it so easy to distinguish and separate an outcome that is intended from one that is merely "foreseen" and "tolerated"? And even if there is a legitimate distinction to be made between direct and indirect intention, can this distinction bear such heavy and decisive moral weight in making a moral judgment in complicated circumstances?

Critics of double effect tend to place more importance on the total balance of good effects over harmful ones and to argue that a proper intention was implied by the very fact that the criterion of proportionality was satisfied in the outcome of the act. Acts cannot be judged "intrinsically evil" apart from an assessment of proportionality in concrete situations; and if an "evil" effect or aspect of an act or choice is counterbalanced by the overall good, then it is relatively unimportant whether the harm caused was prior to the good, subsequent to it, or even part of the means of accomplishing it.[39] In fact, the principle of double effect only makes sense as a practical generalization about relational factors that impinge in complex ways on any particular occasion of choice. As Richard McCormick rightly observes, morality may be "objective," but moral decision making can still be ambiguous. The discernment of a proportionate reason for ambivalent actions is inductive, the possibilities of conflict resolution multiple, and judgments often "rationally untidy."[40]

The area of making decisions in times of acute illness, approaching death, psychological and spiritual as well as physical suffering, possible scarcity of resources, and family stress is replete with quandaries that illustrate this point. Arguing from a personal experience, Margaret Farley makes the case that, although there is a "profound difference" between the "moral experience" of accepting death by removing barriers and the experience of actively, directly taking life, this difference is not enough to decide the issue of morality. First of all, "indirect" causation and intention are still causation and intention. The agent still provides an occasion of death and hastens death by a particular action. Moral responsibility for death cannot be avoided, even if the means is omission and the choice is evaluated to be morally good.[41] Going further, it is still a question whether "direct and active intervention with the intention to kill can ever be justified."[42]

> For example, for those who believe that God is their ultimate destiny—their beginning and their end, their holder in life and savior in death—is it not conceivable that profound "acceptance" of death, acknowledgment of an ending that is indeed God's will, can be expressed through action as well as through passion, through doing as well as being done unto?[43]

Those who die in the hope of "communion" with God will remember that "in communion action and passion, giving and receiving, embracing and letting go, become two sides of the same reality."[44]

Experience erodes the lines seemingly drawn by double effect. As a physician, Timothy Quill has felt morally compelled to support patients in their active choice of death, because the absence of other options has brought him to the point at which to do otherwise seems a failure of his duty to be "a midwife through the dying process."[45] One of his more excruciating accounts involves a man with a brain tumor who was beset not only by pain, but by agitation, sleeplessness, and hallucinations when he would feel fearful of and threatened by those around him. In his moments of clarity he pleaded for death, and on one occasion fled his house on the shores of Lake Ontario to try to drown himself in its icy waters. Eventually it became clear that taking him off one medication would allow death to occur within a couple of days—but, then again, what if this did not happen?[46] Moral theologian Margaret Farley poses essentially the same question when she asks, "If it is possible that an individual can be in such dire straits that her very integrity as a self is threatened (by intractable pain, ravaging the spirit as well as the body), is it not justifiable in such circumstances to end one's life, to surrender it while it is still whole?"[47]

One option in such cases, still short of the line of direct killing, is "terminal sedation." According to the principle of double effect (and Catholic medical ethics), it is permissible to give large amounts of barbiturates or other painkillers to the point of unconsciousness if necessary to relieve suffering and despite the probability that death will come more quickly.[48] Some opponents of euthanasia see terminal sedation as a preferable route, one that can manifest appropriate care and solidarity with the suffering person, yet avoid direct killing. Zbigniew Zylicz, the Dutch hospice director, argues that for the few patients who would otherwise die in "excruciating pain," terminal sedation is a good option. One cancer patient in his care was a former addict and thus did not respond to the usual opioids. Finally, "a dose of barbiturates was infused intravenously . . . he fell asleep and died two days later."[49]

Zylicz does not elaborate on the precise cause of death. Quill makes the point that most patients who are terminally sedated present the question of whether to continue to provide fluids and nutrition intravenously after they are unconscious and cannot eat. In such cases, should prolonging life be a goal? If not, then is death a goal? And does that violate double effect? Ordinarily, it is accepted by the health care team (and presumably the patient and family) that "terminal sedation" is a phase of dying that will not be unnecessarily prolonged. The patient is in the dying process, and death is the expected outcome. Yet Quill remarks that, in most cases, terminal sedation has the "disadvantage of requiring that the patient dehydrate to death over several days in an iatrogenic coma."[50] This situation could be justified under the rubric of "withdrawing extraordinary means." But is it correct and honest to say that the intentions of the participants are not oriented toward death as one goal among others (primarily relief of suffering)? "We must learn to ask hard questions about all potentially life-ending treatments and not assume that some categories are inherently safe and others are immoral by definition."[51]

The purposes behind acts like "providing terminal sedation" or withdrawing life support systems are not always clear and unidirectional. Rather, in light of modern psychology, one must admit that "human intention is multilayered, ambiguous, subjective, and often contradictory."[52] Indirect action to cause death is still responsible causation, and even with indirect killing, the attitude toward death may be ambivalent. Far from diminishing responsibility for our actions, this realization works to hold us accountable for foreseen consequences of actions and not only those we centrally desire to occur. Therefore proportionality—not intention—is central in evaluating the causation of bad effects. In Quill's view, the only proportionate reason for ending life, directly or indirectly, is to end patient suffering. "The specific method used is much less important than the process of caring, excellent palliative care, and joint decision making that precede it."[53]

Certainly the consensus of Christian tradition is that directly killing patients (or any weak or debilitated person) does not respect human dignity and the need for integrated spiritual, physical, and social support for those in difficulty. Instituting general practices of killing in such cases is a detriment to the common good, both because it endangers individuals in similar circumstances and because it undermines the social commitment and resources necessary to come up with more satisfying and less desperate responses to suffering.[54]

The motive of relief of suffering in decisions to end life might diminish in proportion to the motive to save costs. In Oregon palliative care is on the rise but medical practice in the Netherlands has been slow to utilize palliative care expertise. Indeed, physicians increasingly provide euthanasia for those unable to make autonomous decisions. "If this is true in a nation with universal health care coverage, how much greater the danger in a society in which [a large percentage] of the population is uninsured and concern for rising costs dominates the health care agenda."[55] There is a special danger to economically marginal populations, especially those without health care, and particularly to women. Women live longer than men, have been socialized to be less assertive and to have less sense of entitlement than men. Women often define their own interests as subordinate and feel they are responsible for the welfare of others. They are also less frequently regarded as full participants in decision making, by either families or clinicians.[56] Therefore, even in the event that women might "choose" to end their lives, their access to alternatives, and the pressures that shape their intentions and decisions, might not add up to autonomy or even prudence.

The best response to the movements for suicide and euthanasia of the ill and dying is to create a social ethos that accepts dependency and decline as part of the human condition and that employs the best medical knowledge to ameliorate physical and emotional suffering, while drawing on spiritual traditions and guidance to offer patients and caregivers hope in transcendent meaning beyond their present condition. Social justice as inclusive practices and theological bioethics as participatory transformation should work toward the creation of social practices and expectations that ensure that life-enhancing care is effectively provided to all in need.

Providing good care might eliminate most of the argument for direct killing, but not necessarily all. In a poignant personal statement, Frank Davidoff, MD, reflects on the problem of assisted suicide, and he distances himself from such a drastic alternative. Yet he, like Margaret Farley, still declines to state absolutely that care and love could never result in a justifiable and compassionate decision to cause death. His insights are compelling because they do not stem from professional expertise alone, but from the death of his twenty-six-year-old son from bowel cancer. Toward the end, says Davidoff, his son "was working so hard to deal with intractable symptoms—unrelenting intestinal obstruction, uncontrollable ascites, unrelenting hiccoughs, violent waves of nausea, weakness, wasting—that it would have been entirely understandable and, perhaps, acceptable to us if he had asked to be helped to die sooner than he did."[57] Davidoff believes, like Farley, that if the "medical imperative" for doctors is "always to relieve patients' suffering," then no one should "be shocked or surprised" when some doctors agree to assist the rare patient with ending "a life that has become, irreversibly and intractably, intolerable."[58]

Given the medical, psychological, and moral ambiguity surrounding the distinction between "allowing" death to occur and intentionally causing it, it may be difficult if not impossible to formulate a definitive argument that there is a clear, nontransgressable boundary between "direct" killing on one side of a moral divide and "indirect" killing on the other. The most significant arguments against euthanasia may derive from the prospect of its acceptance as a social practice, and the likely direction such an institution would take, given the trends present in every society for custodians of social resources to conceal exploitation under a rhetoric of the common welfare. Though naming euthanasia as a violation of God's will, a usurpation of divine dominion over human life, an abrogation of human rights or the sanctity of life, and so on may be successful as part of a social strategy to keep it out of bounds, coherent theoretical backing of an absolute norm against euthanasia is elusive.[59]

This does not mean, however, that theologians cannot or should not resist direct killing of the elderly or ill, especially when it is proposed as a legally protected social institution. Direct killing of any human being (even when "necessary" in conflicts of life with life) compromises respect for human life and erodes the solidarity to which we are called as Christians and as fellow human beings. Direct killing of patients not only undermines the traditional role of the medical care giver as healer but also uses medical measures and technologies to circumvent the difficult, profound problem of maintaining meaning and consolation in and for suffering life. From a Christian standpoint, this problem is better resolved through human relationships of love and compassion and through spiritual sustenance. I agree with Allen Verhey that the best and most effective counterargument to euthanasia is the availability of adequate care and support for patients and their families—medical, social, and pastoral. All the more vital, then, is the role of theological bioethics as participatory in underwriting health care practices that marginalize euthanasia by making other options more widespread, successful, and attractive.

Forced Choices, Adverse Virtue, and Social Justice

It is important to realize that most of the cases considered by Quill, Farley, Zylicz, and others who ask for a reconsideration of "exceptional" euthanasia, as well as those mandating artificial nutrition for PVS patients, and those resisting euthanasia in favor of "comfort care," involve patients with access to medical resources, therapies when possible, and palliative care when not. As we have seen, one of the most pressing ethical tasks of modern bioethics is to advocate for the implementation of palliative care and hospice programs. When very ill and dying persons with inadequate medical options, due to economic constraints, are brought into the picture, the state of the moral question changes.

The health care situation for disadvantaged populations is worsened by poverty and constraints on resources in the community as a whole; for individuals, it can also be exacerbated by communal expectation that the welfare of one should give way to the needs of the family. As we have seen, this can create a bias against the lives of the elderly or the debilitated as they lose function and the ability to contribute.

An example from the Philippines illustrates that even the most wrenching decisions about the fate of terminal patients in the United States take place within a much narrower array of negative constraints than in most of the cultures of the world. In the Philippines, a largely Catholic country, direct killing of terminally ill patients is not an acceptable option, especially in view of religious beliefs about the expiatory and redemptive value of suffering.[60] But decision making in the event of serious illness looks very different than in Western Europe and the United States. In one case, a seventeen-year-old boy, "Mr. C.," was paralyzed from the neck down in an automobile accident. His mother practically lived at the hospital ward in order to care for him, but hospital bills mounted to an intolerable level. He was the oldest of six children. His mother was a laundrywoman, his father a writer who made little income. The boy had supplemented the family resources by selling newspapers. The family was told that the boy would have to be maintained on a respirator for the rest of his life. At this news, "Mr. C. looks sad. After a few days, he requests that the respirator be removed."[61]

According to the analysis accompanying the case, the respirator can be considered extraordinary because it imposes an inordinate financial burden on the family. The mother is understandably torn between wanting "to give what is humanly possible" to her son, and the need to provide for the rest of her family. "She should be reassured . . . that although the withdrawal of treatment is a painful decision, it is the best for Mr. C. and the family."[62] The son may well have made the right decision in giving up his life for his family; it may be correct that the mother should be "reassured."

But is there or should there be a larger referent of the decision-making process? There are, no doubt, other people in the Philippines who could not have enjoyed even the level of care that this boy had. In the United States, however, there are few instances in which a respirator would not be provided for an individual, especially a minor, who both wanted to live and had family support. This case projects forward to the coming discussion of health care resource distribution worldwide.

In the present context, it helps raise the question of what counts as morally right and virtuous action in conflict situations. Quill, Farley, and Davidoff have presented the possibility that, even when moral intentions are there and all that is "humanly possible" to assist a patient in his or her suffering has been done, circumstances beyond human control can produce irresolvable conflicts. Doing "the right thing" might entangle agents in decisions, actions, and social practices in which neither moral approbation nor condemnation is clearly warranted. The case of Mr. C. poses the even more difficult possibility that agents must choose courses of action within adversity that is created and sustained by human actions, policies, and institutions, and not only by burdens of illness as such. The choices thus constitute a form of cooperation with the injustice that has perpetrated the adversity in the first place, as Mr. C.'s mother was no doubt desperately aware. Reassuring her on the basis of "double effect" seems not only futile but inhumane. What "choice" did she have? Using double effect to "resolve" the situation seems almost like a self-deceiving abdication of responsibility for the larger factors of unjust resource distribution that forced her choice.

Perhaps another rubric is needed to understand the moral character of forced choices. When choices represent human attempts to act with integrity in the midst of unavoidable conflict and adversity, they illustrate what might be called "adverse virtue." Such choices are not virtuous in the sense of finding just the right mean or balance between extreme alternatives, nor are they virtuous in the sense of being reasonable or of being fulfillments of all that human beings are meant to be. Yet neither are they necessarily best understood as forays into "sinning bravely"—into doing what one "knows" is wrong, but trusts will be forgiven. Nor are they "exceptions" to moral rules that can be clearly defined and justified in light of specific excusing circumstances, fitting neatly into a predictable worldview where their scope and repeatability can be controlled. To deem such choices essentially sinful is to undervalue the difficulty, worth, and courageousness of human attempts to discern the best way through impossible situations.

Yet to call such choices truly virtuous is to minimize the ambivalence that Quill has rightly surfaced in his discussion of direct and indirect intention. They may be better termed "exercises of adverse virtue."

Nevertheless, to regard acts of adverse virtue as "acceptable" social practices is to accept the causing circumstances, underwrite the practices that may have helped cause the adversity, and create social institutions and policies that facilitate their repetition in the future. To call life-saving measures "extraordinary" in the case of the poor but not the rich helps explain the virtue of the proximate decision makers, but it excuses the vices of those who benefit from the system.

Making a Difference

Has the Christian message or worldview made any difference in enhancing the opportunities to participate in one's communities throughout the process of living and dying, and in bringing solidarity with and care for all human persons in the process of decline and death? The evidence lies in participatory theology, Christian action, and the meshing of faith-inspired ventures with other invested groups and communities in the public sphere. Participatory theological bioethics constitutes a "counterargument in practice" to euthanasia and an "argument in practice" for the possibility of meeting illness, suffering, and death virtuously and humanely without it.

Modifying social practices toward wise and just solidarity with the dying demands the imaginative and practical introduction of a new horizon of meaning regarding these life experiences and events. Religious persons, churches, and theology can contribute by means of witness, advocacy, and action. In the week before his death from cancer in November 1996, Cardinal Joseph Bernardin wrote a letter to the Supreme Court urging it not to accept physician-assisted suicide. The last several months of Bernardin's life were a witness to Christian meaning making in the face of death, as he refused any treatments that would end his ministry to the Catholics of Chicago or his attempt to bring understanding and unity to an American church often polarized between tradition and change. His defining theological and episcopal contribution was the "consistent ethic of life," in which he broadened Catholic opposition to abortion and euthanasia to include positive "quality of life" ventures—including care of the dying, and access to health care for the uninsured—in support of society's marginalized.[63]

Christian practices of hospitality and care for the sick and dying, especially the poor, have always reached out into their social environment and made a difference. Specific liturgies for the sick and dying have always been a part of Christian sacramental traditions, breaking the isolation of illness and the grinding-down of suffering with communal presence and an opening to the experience of God.[64] New versions incorporate prayer for those making decisions about withdrawal of life supports.[65] A newer expression of participatory theological bioethics is the cooperation of Christian health care organizations, parishes, churches, and service agencies to develop programs that serve the aging and chronically ill, sometimes under the aegis of "parish nursing."[66] The institutionalization of parish (or congregational) ministries to the sick and dying respects human relationality, integrates decline and death with other aspects of communal life, and provides everyone who serves with preparation for their own dying process.[67]

Examples of participatory theological bioethics with even greater social presence and effect are the hospice movement, efforts of the CHA, and international networks of care for those dying of AIDS. The international hospice movement takes its name and origins from early Christian practice and in the twentieth century took on new life under religious leadership. The CHA brings together the multiple dimensions of the public presence of theological bioethics in regard to end-of-life care in the context of ongoing services. Although the AIDS crisis will also be treated more extensively in chapter 5 as a violation of just access to resources, here it will verify the global potential of participatory theological bioethics in relation to life-threatening illness.

Hospice is generally considered to be a program for those already in the dying process, whose care is shaped by medical needs and resources, even though neither cure nor prolongation of life is anticipated. However, today, hospice has expanded its mission to integrate care for the dying and the chronically ill with broader social goals and services. The CHA is more explicitly religious in identity and goals, and it too seeks a large perspective on decline and dying, whether due to illness or age, and on the social vulnerability that decline brings. Both the hospice movement and the CHA connect the quality of aging, decline, and dying with access to multiple relationships and resources, and both partner with other religious and nonreligious civic and governmental organizations in order to accomplish outcomes. Both—but especially the CHA—use the Internet to magnify and further their presence in civil society and to advocate for government policies that reflect their vision. More overtly than the hospice movement, the CHA provides a field for the transformative work of participatory theological bioethics. It adopts an "expansive" theological discourse that is tied to clear and specific social goals and policies. This discourse is being carried ever more firmly into the global arena through the agency of Christian nonprofit organizations and networks, such as those ministering to persons with AIDS.

Hospice and Palliative Care

The founder and mentor of the hospice movement, Cicely Saunders, recalls that hospice was religious in inspiration. In 1879, the Sisters of Charity opened the Hospice for the Dying in Dublin, taking the word *hospice* from early Christianity, as a word to describe a place where hospitality was offered to pilgrims and travelers, as well as the sick and destitute. In 1905, the Sisters opened St. Joseph's Hospice in a deprived area of London.[68] Saunders, a medical doctor, worked at this institution, which had made customary the then-unusual practice of giving patients oral doses of morphine in frequent enough intervals to keep pain at bay. When Saunders opened St. Christopher's Hospice in London in 1967, there was already an informal palliative care network through which pain researchers, social workers, psychologists, and sociologists cooperated to learn how to manage terminal pain, especially in cancer patients.[69] The first hospice program in the United States was started in Connecticut, in 1973, and was added as a benefit to the Medicare program in the 1980s.[70] In 2003, there were around 3,200 programs in the United States alone.[71]

In the United States, however, professionals' lack of expertise and interest in providing hospice or palliative care remains alarming. As of 1995, only 5 of 126 medical schools, and only 26 percent of residency programs, offered courses on care of the dying, and only 17 percent of training programs offered hospice rotation.[72] A four-year investigation of death in American hospitals, SUPPORT, whose results were published in 1995, found that physicians communicate poorly with patients, may overtreat with ineffective measures in lieu of communicating the real prognosis honestly with the patient, are ignorant about control of symptoms, and are unfamiliar with national guidelines for appropriate palliative care.[73] Despite a major four-year, two-phase educational and practical intervention program implemented by SUPPORT, involving nine thousand patients in five U.S. teaching hospitals, physician behavior was unimproved. While various explanations could be offered for this failure,[74] it is more than obvious that "much more effective patient-centered interventions" need to be established in hospitals, and that as things stand, it is much better for patients to die elsewhere. "We must put much more effort into hospice care and home care, both of which place the patient in the center of the enterprise."[75]

In 2003, a project sponsored by the Hastings Center and the National Hospice Work Group began its report with the statement "Too many Americans approach death without adequate medical, nursing, social, and spiritual support."[76] About 38 percent of those facing an anticipated death from cancer and other chronic diseases receive hospice care, though many of these receive it for such a brief time before death that they are unable to profit from all that hospice could offer. Patients in hospitals are usually surrounded by all the latest technological ways to detect and assault disease, but when they are declared terminal, they receive only the most rudimentary palliative care.[77] In fact, a review of the unavailability of adequate end-of-life care to most patients makes it clear why accusations that defenders of physician-assisted suicide like Quill, Compassion in Dying, and others are just abandoning patients or absolutizing autonomy are overwrought and facile. Patients seeking control over a final "way out" are understandably reacting to the possibility, even likelihood, that they will be subjected to technologies they do not want and pain and suffering they have no reasonable way to bear.

Beyond endorsing more flexible and cooperative forms of hospice services, the hospice care report makes the case that "social justice and equity, or fairness" demand that access to health care be improved across the socioeconomic spectrum.[78] Historically, hospice has served relatively few people of color, and people of color often mistrust the health care system. Good palliative care needs to be community-based and integrated in a continuum of care that meets community values and needs.[79] Equity in hospice care should be accomplished by making more people eligible for admission to hospice and for insurance or Medicare coverage, by referring people to hospice earlier, and by maintaining good stewardship of resources without sacrificing high quality of care.[80]

One commentator on the project, Daniel Sulmasy, is a physician and a theological bioethicist. He makes the case for health care justice by accentuating values of human dignity, compassion, and solidarity and invoking the common good. The components of human dignity and the claims dignity makes on others are notoriously hard to define. Sulmasy offers three elements that clearly reflect his theological commitments, but that are also philosophically attractive, particularly from a perspective that values autonomy, but places it within a communal context. First, human beings are "naturally social," yielding a "principle of social solidarity." Second, human beings are finite, which implies that the inevitability of death must be taken seriously. Third, "human beings have a radically equal intrinsic worth or dignity that commands the respect of others, independent of our preferences."[81]

Finitude results in the needs of human beings, and the fulfillment of those needs is essential to their flourishing. Social solidarity and equal respect create obligations to meet needs, although decisions about the use of scarce resources have to be made in the process. In order to do that justly, Sulmasy proposes six considerations: degree of individual need, prevalence (size of the group affected by the need), prospect of success, availability of alternatives, cost, and the common good. More than a way to summarize the first five criteria, the consideration of the common good refers to the quality of community itself. What is the quality of social relationships that will result from a certain practice regarding the fulfillment or denial of human needs?

> The opportunities for interpersonal reconciliation, caring, and solidarity that are afforded by hospice redound quite substantially to the common good. . . . Hospice can claim, in justice, significant medical resources vis-à-vis other medical interventions. Human flourishing is well served if people do not die miserable deaths, both for the individuals themselves and the community with which those individuals are in solidarity.[82]

The commitment to provide palliative care has emerged socially and culturally as a compelling alternative to euthanasia and physician-assisted suicide, and not just within the churches. Although there may be some cases of extreme mental or physical suffering that cannot be resolved by improving the social and relational circumstances of patients, there are many that can. It seems clear from the Dutch and Oregon experiences that many pleas for a quick death originate from despair, or even from physical symptoms that more expert or attentive care could well alleviate. It is the first and foremost job of caregivers and community to bring to the ill and dying the imaginative resources to envision their ongoing lives with realistic hope about the possibility of love and spiritual meaning, if not longevity. It is the job of medical professionals to make sure that the barriers of physical pain and struggle do not make it virtually impossible to know the joys of friendship and love. The health care professions can also enhance the settings in which care is received and integrated with personal relationships, whether at home or in a hospital, hospice, or long-term care institution.

Although the contemporary hospice movement began in the foundation of special homes to offer comfort and pain relief to terminal cancer patients, "hospice" services today can be provided in hospitals, in nursing homes, at home, or in hospice care facilities. Hospice no longer assumes that no further life-prolonging measures will be provided, nor even that the patient has reached the dying process. "Palliative care" is a comprehensive term that applies to all these settings and has as its goals "the alleviation of suffering, the optimization of quality of life until death ensues, and the provision of comfort in death."[83] Hospice has come to mean the coordination of services for patients and caregivers, including attention to social services as well as to more traditionally "medical" needs. Hospice care has been extended to dying newborns and their families and to dying prisoners and has tailored programs for faith-based Muslim, Jewish, and Christian populations. It also reaches out to the bereaved, including children and teenagers, parents who have lost children, those who have lost family members to suicide, and communities that have suffered catastrophic events.[84]

Hospice has grown into an international movement whose effect is reflected in the growing recognition that humane care of the seriously ill and dying must include effective palliative treatment.[85] Sociotechnical change is creating an unprecedented global context in which hospice operates. First, populations are destabilized, and hospice not only must operate amid frequent economic stresses but must respond to an ever greater array of subcultures in any one region. Second, the global economy opens the door both to entrepreneurship and to bureaucracy in the hospice movement. But, third, all parts of the globe are now linked by satellites, the Internet, faxes, transportation lines, and visual media that permit the spread of new ideas and a more rapid learning process.[86]

The hospice movement, with religious inspiration and often under religious auspices, has grown to a worldwide phenomenon and has an important role to play in linking the dying process with other social conditions that favor the ability to face decline in a humane way. Religious leadership can help make these connections. A figure like Mother Teresa and her Sisters of Charity, in establishing homes for those dying in abject destitution, have challenged cultural assumptions and so have become icons of the religious commitment to provide every individual with a sense of worth in solidarity with the poorest of the poor. Mother Teresa's vision was intentionally interreligious, as she pulled on resources and goodwill throughout each setting in which she undertook her work, often manipulating publicity and politics quite expertly to do so. Through her example, social structures have been challenged, even without explicit advocacy on her part for broad cultural change.[87] However, more systematic organization and partnership is needed on the part of religious institutions to carry the mission of hospice into the international arena and connect it more effectively with global policies on health care and on intergenerational responsibilities. Some movement in this direction can be seen in the work of Christian transnational organizations, which are discussed in a subsequent section.

Catholic Health Association

As we have seen, the CHA is not just a service and activist organization, it is dialectically attuned to Catholic teaching and contemporary theology and theological bioethics, both Catholic and Protestant. Theologians are invited to present at the annul CHA assembly, to participate in study and advisory groups on a variety of topics, and to contribute position papers to CHA educational and service publications. Theological and clinical bioethicist Ron Hamel is the CHA senior director for ethics. CHA president Michael Place is a Catholic moral theologian, a priest of the archdiocese of Chicago, and formerly a key advisor and assistant to Cardinal Bernardin.[88]

In 1994, the CHA published *Caring for Persons at the End of Life: A Facilitators Guide to Educational Modules for Healthcare Leaders.*[89] Several task forces contributed to the project, and many theologians served on these. The theological framework of the project relies on several basic religious insights. First, suffering is in itself an evil, but, with every other aspect of human life, it can be transformed in Christ. "The Risen One, surrounded by all the saints, goes with us, accompanies us into death, and invites us to participate in the resurrection."[90] Second, life is sacred and should be respected and supported, yet preserving life is not an absolute obligation.[91] Third, humans should exercise responsible stewardship over human life, not assuming absolute control and realizing that there are limits on life that humans must accept, in the hope of eternal life.[92] Fourth, direct killing is prohibited, especially the life of the innocent and vulnerable. Disproportionately burdensome treatments and futile treatments are not obligatory. This can include artificial nutrition and hydration.[93]

The project and its framing documents refer to cultural factors, such as the fact that most Americans die in institutions, the influence of individualism, "the technological imperative," and the fact that Catholic health care operates in a pluralistic setting. Political issues such as the movements for a right to die, advance directives, proxy decisions, and the legalization of physician-assisted suicide are treated. Sustained attention is given to pain, pain management, and hospice care. Finally, the implications for Catholic health care are voiced in terms of priorities to be set in creating an atmosphere in which Catholic teaching can be respected and patients and families well served in "a virtuous community of interdependence, care, and hospitality."[94] Collaboration with other communities that aim to serve the dying is affirmed, along with outreach to the patient's total network of support.

A decade later, in 2004, the CHA website had expanded with multiple theological and practical initiatives to advocate, stimulate, and coordinate care for the dying, in concert with advocacy for basic health care services, long-term care, support for the aging, and health care access reform. The issue of care for the dying has been increasingly integrated with related social, political, and theological-ethical concerns. Even more significantly, it has been placed to a much more significant degree within a program of broad social, political, and economic intervention that targets the needs of the vulnerable and underserved, especially the elderly.

The CHA's Continuing Care ministries include a theologically informed practical initiative, "Supportive Care for the Dying: A Coalition for Compassionate Care."[95] This coalition unites Catholic health care and service providers "dedicated to promoting cultural change" that makes "a better death" possible. It provides research, a "toolkit" to implement practices, membership benefits, videotapes, training opportunities, grant and award opportunities, information about how to form an interdisciplinary team and enroll patients, network with existing community supports, and use feedback from patients and families, including focus groups, to improve performance. It lists eleven member institutions in nine states.

Decline, Dying, and Global Solidarity

In July 2003, a colloquium for representatives of international Catholic bioethics institutes was held in Toronto to discuss care of the elderly and the dying. A consensus statement reflected Catholic teaching about end-of-life decisions, but took this tradition into the context of globalization and highlighted access and justice issues in a new way.[96] Signatories included forty-two persons, mostly Canadian, with representation from the United States and from Europe, some from developing countries in Latin America and Asia, and one from Africa. In regard to Catholic social teaching, the statement urges that "the alleviation of material, social, and spiritual poverty of the frail elderly is a fundamental obligation that Catholic health care and Catholic bioethics must address, according to the preferential option of the poor." "Globally, discussions about the care of the frail elderly and the dying must involve the participation of less affluent peoples and societies."[97] In the name of solidarity, subsidiarity, the common good, and the preferential option, the statement defines a responsibility of "the world community" to provide not only health care but basic goods such as water, police protection, and education. Specific practices regarding access must be defined locally, according to cultures and their specific needs.[98]

Christian NGOs aim to construct transnational infrastructures to collect and transfer resources from wealthy to poor constituencies and to influence cultural and political circumstances in the communities they serve. They integrate care for the dying and the aged with community services, seeking out social settings of general deprivation and violence. The AIDS crisis makes health care and related needs in these settings especially urgent. Although the loneliness and isolation of the elderly, along with reduced income, are the most visible social problems for European and North American populations, the aged and the chronically ill can face much more drastic exclusion and suffer lack of more basic needs on other continents, especially Africa. Because of the magnitude of the AIDS crisis, the fact that it strikes the poor most acutely, the fact that discrimination against persons with AIDS is prevalent, the fact that in most of the world access for all to life-saving drugs is absent, and the fact that those dying of the disease are thus often marginalized and without resources to meet death in a peaceful manner all make it evident why Christian care of the dying globally would focus especially on victims of this disease.

For example, Christian Aid, a British Protestant evangelical and service organization, has prepared an education program to be implemented in AIDS communities where victims are poor, often ostracized, and often orphans. The program features stories of individuals from South Africa, Congo, Uganda, Zambia, Jamaica, and Tanzania who, living with AIDS, have found community and church support and have access to resources to help with expenses, medical care, and education.[99]

Catholic Relief Services (CRS), a U.S.-based organization with programs in sixty countries, actively seeks to draw upon international resources to serve the aged and ill, especially AIDS victims, within their communities. One clinic in Ghana receives support from St. Sabina Parish in Chicago, Illinois, and Catholic Relief Services. This support allows the clinic to offer free medical care to the poor, including surgical operations, outpatient and inpatient treatment, and terminal care. The clinic also supplies free services such as medical care and hospice for HIV/AIDS patients, Meals on Wheels, support to abandoned elderly women, medical care and meals to prisoners, and interest-free loans to women for income-generating activities.[100]

In Guyana, CRS works closely with the Sisters of Mercy and St. Joseph Mercy Hospital, who are currently implementing a project to test for HIV/AIDS on at least 150 individuals free of charge, with a special focus on young women of childbearing age and women with infants. Those who are tested will be counseled, provided with needed drugs, and monitored through the hospital. The country suffers from the second highest incidence of HIV in the Western Hemisphere.[101] In Jamaica, CRS cooperates with the church's Good Shepherd Foundation in Montego Bay, which provides hospice care for HIV/AIDS patients. Government response to these social issues is limited due to lack of resources (Jamaica pays 65 cents of every dollar to service its foreign debt). The general decline in government social spending has forced civil society to lead the response on principal issues such as HIV/AIDS, social services provision, and education.

AIDS will be addressed more extensively in the following chapter. However, these few examples will suffice to show that when Christian participatory bioethics moves into the global arena, the subject of decline and dying has a much different aspect than in North America. In the ethics of death and dying globally, social justice and access issues come to the fore. Beyond the efforts of international relief agencies, however, political movements are emerging that advocate for a realignment of international as well as national structures through which the goods related to health are distributed. Religious vision, voice, and action are contributing to the momentum, paving the way for participatory theological bioethics. The role of theological bioethics in increasing access for those excluded from the goods of health care will be addressed in relation to health care access reform and to the uses of genetic knowledge and biotechnology.

For the present, it is evident that the modern Western approach to decline, terminal illness, and death has been assimilated to a medical model.

These human realities are ethically assessed in terms of individual-oriented values such as control, autonomy, dignity, and rights. While these are not necessarily bad in proper proportion, a balance of individual dignity and communal solidarity, in a context that is attentive to a rich array of human values, is what is often missing in the bioethics of decline and dying. In the African scenarios painted by CRS, moral and legal debates focused on physician-assisted suicide and tube feeding seem beside the point, if not ridiculous. Yet the intellectual tools used to advance those debates—extraordinary means and double effect—contain the seeds of a more social and contextual perspective. Sometimes decisions are complex mixes of good and evil; proper responses to mortality and suffering have to take into account concrete options and limits. A renewed insight for the twenty-first century is that human beings are responsible not only for their own choices but for the patterns of social relationship that constrain the choices of others. This is especially true when human beings lack the essentials of a good life and face death without any confidence that they have a share in the common good.

Participatory theological bioethics can mediate between a Christian worldview—emphasizing a transcendent horizon of meaning, solidarity, and special attention to the most vulnerable—and the social practices and institutions that determine the concrete experiences of decline and dying. Participatory theological bioethics keeps in view the larger picture of which these experiences are a part, such as the cultural significance of aging, networks of social services, and the practice of modern medicine. Participatory theological bioethics can and does give rise to practical initiatives to respect, serve, and empower the elderly, the ill, and the dying within communities of support and belonging, from neighborhood to city, region, nation, continent, and globe.

CHAPTER

5

NATIONAL AND INTERNATIONAL HEALTH ACCESS REFORM

A BASIC LEVEL OF HEALTH is key to a person's ability to function in his or her social and physical environment. The opportunity to enjoy good health is essential not only to individual well-being and fulfillment but also to one's participation in and contribution to the communities in which one lives. Thus health is a basic human and social good, necessary to the common good of local and global communities, a good that could even be considered a "right." Yet at least 45 million people in the United States lack health care insurance, resulting in many thousands of unnecessary deaths every year. Numbers continue to rise. Millions more lose health insurance for periods of time. Even so, public spending on health care for low-income people has slowed down in recent years.[1] Although the United States leads the world in spending on health care, it is the only wealthy, industrialized nation that does not ensure basic access for all citizens. The prestigious Institute of Medicine of the National Academies urged in 2004 that consistent, universal, equitable, and high-quality health coverage be achieved by 2010.[2]

Around the world, a large majority lack what most Americans would consider "adequate" access to the conditions of a healthy life. In many cases, this is because they are without even basic necessities such as food, clean water, and freedom from war and other types of violent social conflict. Global poverty kills more than 150,000 children every month from malaria alone. In 2000, the United Nations' Millennium Declaration[3] set as global goals the greater achievement of peace and security, the reduction by half of the more than one billion people living in extreme poverty by 2015, and the reduction by the same percentage of those who have no safe drinking water. It also aimed by 2015 to have reduced maternal mortality by three-fourths and infant mortality by two-thirds. It aimed to halt and start reversing the spread of HIV/AIDS, malaria, and other major diseases; to help children orphaned by AIDS; and to promote empowerment of women as an effective way to combat poverty, hunger, and disease, including AIDS. In January 2005, only five donor countries had made significant levels of progress toward promised amounts of aid, while the United States continued to give the smallest percentage of national income among the major donor countries.[4]

The problems of uninsured Americans can seem insignificant compared to those for whom pregnancy and birth are ordinarily life-threatening processes and whose families and communities are constantly ravaged by deadly disease. Nevertheless, U.S. citizens have an obligation to seek equity and universality in access to the goods necessary for health in their own national community, especially because people who use the latest innovations live in the same cities and towns as those with no ensured medical care at all. Some members of racial and ethnic minorities in America are little better off than the poor in other lands, at least as far as diseases such as AIDS and health care exclusion are concerned.

The problem of health care reform in the United States provides an opportunity to examine the ways in which technological development, market economics, and disparities of race and class affect health and health care. It will open a window through which to view how government and civil society, including religious groups and theologians, can cooperate to change unjust patterns of health, disease, and health-related benefits and goods. This chapter reviews some realities of health care access in this country, some basic proposals for reform, and the role of theological and religious voices and actors on the health care reform scene. Then the window will be thrown open to the global horizon. A target area for the consideration of global health inequities is the AIDS crisis. Religious organizations and theologians have been active at the global level, especially in response to the AIDS crisis. They have met with some significant successes, although it is undeniably true that global patterns of disease and death manifest the same dark fissures in solidarity that have always disrupted the relations of peoples and nations worldwide. There is important work for participatory theological bioethics to do.

Inequities in Access to U.S. Health Care

Whether one approaches the dilemma of health care justice from a communitarian, Kantian, Rawlsian, liberal, Catholic common good, biblical covenantal, discipleship-healing, or "liberationist" perspective, there is unanimity at the theoretical or philosophical level that conditions should change.[5] The question is not whether, but how, when, and to what degree. American voters, politicians, and policymakers, however, have been slow to come into line with the theoretical consensus about the universal access that justice requires.

Michael D. Reagan astutely diagnoses the origin of this recalcitrance in the contradiction in two assertions widely held by Americans:

- Everyone should have the best of whatever health care is needed, *but*
- government should keep out of it and market choices (mostly by employers) should determine the availability of coverage.[6]

Universal medical care will never be accomplished by the market alone. As the Institute of Medicine report asserts, there must be a federal role—in "leadership and dollars"—if reform is to occur.[7] As numerous critics have observed, markets are good at meeting demand efficiently, but not at equity, if equitable access to a resource is defined as access according to need. "Markets will distribute goods based on the distribution of purchasing power; they will not redistribute to or cross subsidize lower income people."[8]

The role of U.S. employers in selecting and conveying marketed health care is purely accidental. During World War II, the economy rose as a result of industrial production, but wage and price controls were put into effect to prevent inflation. Therefore, unions bargained with employers for fringe benefits, and health care coverage (through private plans invented during the Depression) was a beneficiary.[9] Other countries, such as Germany and Great Britain, responded to the modern development of more effective and therefore more expensive medicine by instituting forms of national insurance in the late nineteenth and early twentieth centuries.

Today, there are three basic models by which health services are provided internationally, at least in relatively wealthy western countries. One is the "private insurance model" (U.S.), in which individuals and/or employers buy health insurance coverage, and in which the production of health services and products is privately owned. Another is the "social insurance" model (Germany), in which universal health coverage is compulsory and is financed by employers and employees within a framework like Social Security, with production owned both privately and publicly. (Like the first model, this model has proved vulnerable to high unemployment and rising health care costs.) Some Western European countries (like the Netherlands) and Israel, on a variation of this model, guarantee coverage to all, but remove health insurance from the context of employment. Instead, individuals buy from competing health insurers who have an incentive to cut waste and maximize services. (Set coverage and competition help control costs, but a two-tier system could develop to accommodate the preferences of the wealthy with more money to spend.)

A third basic model is the "national health service" (Great Britain, Canada), with tax-based universal coverage and national ownership and/or control of services.[10] (Here costs can be kept down through federal administration, but popular dissatisfaction and complaints can lead to either a rise in national health expenditures or a two-tier system, where the wealthy buy services on the private market, either in or outside of the country.) A comparison of these systems forces the conclusion that some governmental role is necessary to redistribute the resources to buy health care from the more to the less well-off members of society. No society guarantees health care access to everyone unless all contribute according to ability to pay and abide by the principle of "the cross-subsidization of the sick by the healthy and the lower income by the higher income earners."[11]

The United States today has a mixture of private and public programs and plans that provide insurance to some segments of the population, but not to all. Employers are still the main source of coverage, though small businesses and employers of part-time workers are not legally obligated to provide this benefit. Since World War II, health care and health insurance have increasingly come to be organized around a system known as "managed care." Managed care has largely supplanted the traditional fee-for-service, physician-patient relationship.

> The term "managed care" refers to a variety of continually adapting and developing arrangements that involve four groups. These groups, which have been labeled by the world of business, not health, are the "consumer" (once patient), the "provider" (the physician and other health care professionals), the "insurer" (the reimburser for any care), and the "purchaser of care" or the primary buyer of health services (the large employer organization).[12]

Between 1988 and 2000, the membership in managed care plans rose from 27 percent to 92 percent of those who were insured through their employers.[13]

Some managed care plans pool talent, knowledge, and resources to provide high-quality care economically, with cost containment being a benefit rather than a major goal. Others, however, try to make a profit by cutting costs and risks, recruiting only healthy patients, and making expensive or intensive care difficult to obtain. Managed care as a system is not in itself ethically objectionable, but rather the fact that some plans are run by for-profit corporations that compensate executives handsomely while they frustrate providers with paperwork, bribe them with financial incentives to cut costs, and endanger the health of members.[14]

However unsatisfactory the health insurance opportunities for most Americans, there are millions of others with no opportunity at all. Some are unemployed. Yet eight out of ten uninsured persons belong to working families. Their employers either do not offer insurance, or the employees decide that they cannot afford the premiums that they would have to pay. In fact, in 2004, despite a growing economy, health care costs for employers averaged $3,000 per employee and were rising at more than three times the rate of inflation.[15] Therefore, in order to avoid paying exorbitant sums for this benefit, more employers were choosing not to add full-time positions. Others increased employee premiums or deductibles, dropped care for dependents, dropped the health plan altogether, or tried surreptitiously to hire only younger workers. The cost of products like cars also rose as employers tried to recoup health care expenses, driving such goods even further out of reach for workers who had to cut back on other purchases in order to cover their health care premiums and uncovered expenses.[16] Family members can also lose coverage through divorce, retirement, the death of the policyholder, or in the case of dependent children, when they reach the age of nineteen and are no longer full-time students.[17] A large number of the uninsured are adults without children, especially young adults.

The uninsured typically resort to charity care in hospital emergency rooms, where only about 35 percent of care billed to them is actually paid. Much of the rest is absorbed by taxpayers, in the form of subsidies to hospitals and clinics.[18] This does not mean that the care received in this manner is adequate. The uninsured usually delay visits, make fewer visits, arrive in more acute stages of illness, and cannot afford follow-up care and medications. They incur more long-term effects of illness, a lower quality of life, and ultimately the need to utilize more costly health resources than would have been necessary to fund preventive measures or early interventions.

If those not insured through employment cannot afford to buy insurance privately, they may qualify for one of the strictly limited federal programs available to the poor, to the elderly or disabled, or to children. In 1965, Medicaid and Medicare were introduced to cover lower income persons and persons over sixty-five, respectively. The poor and retirees are among the most likely to be unable to afford private coverage. These programs are paid for jointly by federal and state funds, but states have wide discretion in establishing eligibility rules. Most states set their income eligibility levels for Medicaid very low, often excluding those who work full-time at a minimum wage job and whose income falls well below the poverty level. It is easier for parents of children to get coverage through Medicaid than childless adults. In the great majority of states, adults without children are ineligible for Medicaid, unless they are elderly or disabled.[19] According to a 2005 report of the National Governors Association, even with these limits, Medicare places unsustainable burdens on state budgets and needs to be trimmed further.[20] Many of those whose employers drop health insurance because it is too expensive apply for Medicare, so that states are forced to assume a larger share of the burden. Meanwhile, adjustments in Medicare coverage to add a prescription drug benefit resulted in decisions by some businesses to eliminate this feature from their own pension plans for retirees.[21]

In 1997, the State Children's Health Insurance Program (SCHIP) was enacted, bringing good-quality, basic health insurance to millions of children. It is widely regarded as a policy success. SCHIP offers federal matching funds to states that offer coverage to children in low-income families. Although enrollment increased during the recession that began in 2001, millions more eligible children remained uninsured, because states erected barriers to enrollment in the form of onerous appointments and documentation, or even froze enrollment in SCHIP.[22] Nevertheless, these programs provide a needed safety net for many low-income children, persons with disabilities, and seniors.

It is evident that the U.S. system already includes some role for government in insuring the least well-off. But incremental coverage for disadvantaged populations has still not closed the health care gap. In fact, Medicare and Medicaid are seeing cutbacks and constraints. The number of uninsured is far too great, and health care costs continue to escalate, endangering those ensured by both private and public plans. Causes include the development of expensive new drugs, advertised directly to consumers; new diagnostic tests that require costly equipment; a reaction against managed care plans that have in the past attempted to limit costs by refusing tests and treatments advised by doctors; and the graying of the "baby boom" generation that is consuming ever more medical resources and depending more on Medicare. Despite its apparent zeal for medical technology, the health care establishment has been slow to invest in communications technology that could enhance both efficiency and consistency of patient care and follow-up.[23] When better communication and more efficient systems do permit doctors to improve care while reducing time and waste, for example, by computerizing records and communicating with patients by e-mail, the savings often go to insurance companies rather than back into enhanced services.[24] Insurance companies and companies that manufacture the new technologies constitute powerful lobbies against reform.[25] In the words of Steven Schroeder, former president and CEO of the Robert Wood Johnson Foundation, "Health care is 14% of the GDP. It's a $1.4 trillion dollar industry [as of 2004]."[26] The prospect of big profits provides incentives to maintain and increase hi-tech tests and treatments and militates against preventive care, which is ordinarily low-tech and relatively low cost, yet has more beneficial results for the long-term health of recipients.

Racial and ethnic bias in health care adds a dimension that is often neglected in discussions of health care deprivation and reform. Disparities in health and health care among racial and ethnic groups, disparities that particularly affect African Americans, have long been acknowledged. However, most of the time these have been attributed to unemployment and lack of medical insurance and the need to rely on Medicaid or emergency care or to do without. Certainly these factors do account for poor health outcomes among many minorities. In addition, distrust of a system that is unfamiliar with and unsympathetic to cultural differences, and that is at least perceived to be part of the systemic exclusion of blacks and other minorities from participation in the "common good" of a white-supremacist society, is another reason for underutilization of medical services and medical advice.

Yet a study by the Institute of Medicine revealed that racial and ethnic minorities tend to receive lower-quality medical care than whites, even when they come from comparable income and insurance levels. Racial differentials in treating heart disease, cancer, diabetes, and HIV infection especially contribute to higher mortality and morbidity rates for minorities.[27] For example, they are less likely to receive bypass surgery, transplants, kidney dialysis, or medications for pain and are more likely to have a leg or foot amputated as a result of diabetes. They are less likely to receive sophisticated treatments for HIV, which could delay or prevent the onset of AIDS. Although health care providers may not be overtly biased, they apparently fall back on unconscious stereotypes and on expectations about a patient's condition based on race, ethnicity, or economic condition, especially when under time pressure or when symptoms are not clear-cut.

Moreover, even though racial bias is evidenced when minorities are not poor, minorities are still more likely than whites to be economically disadvantaged and thus more likely to be enrolled in lower-cost health plans that place stricter limits on coverage and require higher copayments.[28] Beyond the specific issue of access to medical services, poverty in itself is a cause of ill health, disability, and premature death. The poor face chronic deprivation of food, housing, and education; exposure to environmental toxins, for example, in substandard housing; physical threats to health and safety, for example, from crime; unsafe jobs at low wages; and chronic psychological stress. These effects are magnified in regions where there is a great deal of income inequality—where the poor are not "average," but clearly disadvantaged in relation to community standards.[29] In fact, one's prospects of life and health or sickness and death are patterned according to social class, even when there is universal health insurance, and particularly when there are vast social disparities in the amount of wealth enjoyed.[30]

Reform Prospects

Fundamental reform in the national health care system has been on the political table since at least the early 1990s, when President Bill Clinton established a task force to propose changes that could help curtail costs while bringing all Americans under the health care umbrella. Proposed in 1993, the Clinton Health Security Plan was legislatively dead by 1994. Although considered "radical" at the time, the Clinton plan was far from a government takeover of health administration and financing. Large employers, as well as "health alliances" made up of consumers and small businesses, would have been the purchasing agencies for a standard benefits package as defined by the government. The alliances would have been government sponsored and would have functioned rather like the benefits office of a business or a university, offering a few plans from which members could select. Employers would have been required to insure employees and would have paid 80 percent, compared to workers' 20 percent. People would have been able to sign on through employers, or individually if not employed, with subsidies enabling even people with the lowest incomes and small businesses to participate. The system would still have been mostly employment based, with competition among health plans to get businesses and alliances to sign up, based on quality of service in relation to cost. The government would have set a ceiling on insurance premium rises, however.[31] The need to compete within specified cost parameters would presumably have enhanced efficiency and reduced waste and unnecessary technologies, while bolstering quality. Although the prospect of change was popular at the time, the Clinton plan failed, for several possible reasons.

Among the most important are that the plan was presented in terms that were too complex for most of the public to grasp easily, and that the involvement of government, particularly the capping of costs to buyers, was rejected by the health industry as inimical to its interests. As Michael Reagan acerbically notes, "One might suppose people would see that as a good thing, but a ceiling on payments for some people is a ceiling on incomes for others—and those whose incomes are at stake are politically better organized."[32]

Perhaps equally important was the fact that, in 1994, the need for massive reform was not sufficiently evident to most middle-class voters. The American public apparently bought into the myth that the uninsured will be able to get the care they need free, tended to assume that the poor were poor by desert, did not regard the health care of the average family as seriously at risk, and was manipulated by the public opinion campaign of the antireform lobby. More than a decade later, some incremental increases have been made in federal programs such as Medicare, though these could turn out to be more expensive than voters bargained for and lead to a health care reform backlash. According to a study sponsored by the Robert Wood Johnson Foundation, the best-case scenario by 2010 is a reduction in the number of uninsured to 30 million, and the worst-case alternative, an increase to 65 million.[33]

Reformers debate the extent to which change should rely more on market competition and incentives—the path of least resistance—or on government intervention, even a single-payer health system. Both history and the Clinton failure have shown that, whatever its merits from a justice perspective, anything even approximating the central administration of health care by the federal government is a nonstarter for U.S. citizens. Some critics believe that reform should be promoted by increasing competition among providers. Consumers (individuals and employers) are already becoming better informed through the Internet and are increasingly assisted by "report cards" on physician groups, health care plans, and hospital systems issued by advocacy organizations, insurance companies, and analysts hired by employers.[34] Better informed choices among consumers may improve efficiency in supplying what they want at a cost those with money or insurance are willing to pay. However, it can never fully resolve the problems created by inequities in the economic resources with which people try to address their health care needs in the first place.

From the family's point of view, the greatest disadvantage of the employer-based system is that it ties insurance to one particular job.[35] As insurance costs rise, full-time jobs are harder to get and keep. Moreover, workers may be paying a higher percentage of their premiums than they think, in the form of lower take-home pay.[36] At the same time, health benefits for workers are subsidized by tax exclusions (wages that go toward health premiums are not taxed), which is even more unfair to the unemployed and to low-end workers who do not qualify for benefits.[37] Worst of all, in a context of globalization, financial pressure on corporations may drive some of them to take jobs to environments in which health care is not mandated.[38]

In *Insuring America's Health*, the Institute of Medicine argues that everyone living in the United States should have health insurance, that all members of society should contribute financially (through taxes, premiums, and cost sharing), and that basic health care for all should include preventive services, prescription drugs, specialty mental health care, and outpatient and hospital services.[39] Although a major expansion of public programs and a new tax credit for those buying insurance would be least drastic and would encourage some reforms, it would be unlikely to result in full coverage. A single-payer model would be most likely to eliminate gaps in coverage, but would also require the most radical change, and is thus least likely to be acceptable to the American public and even less so to American business.

Two middle options would be for the government either to mandate individual coverage and give tax credits (or refunds to the unemployed) to cover a substantial amount of the cost, making care virtually free for the poor, or to mandate individual coverage and also employer coverage, again with subsidies to some employers and individuals and with public programs for the unemployed. These middle options would ensure more affordable care and a reliable source of funding (the federal government, especially if subsidies or credits were funded by taxes) and would allow government leverage in defining a basic benefits package.[40] Such benefits would have to be supported by taxpayers, and there would be limits on expensive beneficial care. Though this strategy would put in place a transparent system of tax and transfer, it might also result in a two-tier system in which "adequate" insurance for the currently uninsured does not add up to the same benefits enjoyed by those who are employed and who are able to select on the market among newly competitive plans seeking their health care dollars.

Mark Pauly, an economist, poses a difficult and vexing ethical question, one that is sure not to go away any time soon. "What is to prevent the bad outcome in which citizens are unwilling to give philanthropic donations and are unwilling to support higher taxes that are needed to make greater public transfers?"[41] This, he acknowledges, would represent a political and moral failure. It is a failure that can be avoided only by political action, organization, and advocacy, because ultimately the government will be able to elect and sustain policies only if these are persuasive to voters. "Some wrenching social decisions—how much quality is enough, how much do we care about our fellow citizens, how much residual uninsurance are we willing to tolerate?—need to be posed and addressed."[42]

Organization and advocacy imply the vital role of civil society in shaping health care ethics and policy. Bioethics institutes such as the Hastings Center, private foundations such as the Robert Wood Johnson Foundation and Kaiser Family Foundation, and nonprofit advocacy groups such as Families USA have all taken active roles in forming public opinion and seeking institutional change toward greater equity in health care. The perceived openness to change that made Clinton feel he had a mandate to reform the system, the national debate that his administration inspired, and the continuing and increased restiveness of the American public around health care issues a decade or more later are evidence that these efforts have had some effect. In 2004, a survey conducted by National Public Radio, the Kaiser Family Foundation, and Harvard's Kennedy School of Government found that most Americans consider coverage for the uninsured to be an even more pressing public priority than helping the elderly buy prescription drugs.[43]

The next task is to consider what role religious organizations and theologians have had and could have to give momentum to change in the health care scenario in America. What models do they provide or suggest for the engagement of participatory theological bioethics in bringing about health care reform and equity?

Religious and Theological Engagement

Like philosophers, virtually all theologians and churches believe that the current maldistribution of health care in the United States offends against morality and justice. Various denominations have taken public stances on the matter, of which the efforts of the U.S. Catholic bishops have been perhaps the most visible (with the exception of the 2004 national elections, when they kept a low profile on this issue). Their "Resolution on Health Care Reform" was published at the time the Clinton proposals were being crafted and unqualifiedly endorsed the idea of access for all.[44] The Presbyterian Church in the USA published a similar resolution in 2002 that detailed its past statements and also outlined views and activities of other churches and representatives, including the Union of American Hebrew Congregations, the CHA, the United Methodist Church, and the Evangelical Lutheran Church.[45] But just as for philosophers, the question that must be addressed by the churches and by theological bioethics is not merely what is right or wrong ideally or in the abstract, but what difference the chorus of voices on behalf of health care justice has made or can make in the future.

The terms and content of ethical claims on behalf of universal coverage are not irrelevant to the chances of making a difference, of course. Depending on the size of the denomination and the prominence of its representatives, the analysis they offer becomes a part of the cultural debate and has potential to influence the way others envision the issues. Religious speakers typically refer to symbols and narratives from religious traditions and authoritative writings, in order both to form their own communities and to exert a prophetic influence in the culture at large. They also refer to economic and social data that help form the basis on which religious beliefs are applied to the current situation. In addition, they express their commitments in terms that are likely to have wider currency in their local, state, and national communities.

Yet equally important is whether a religious tradition or theological-ethical claim can give its worldview and its moral commitments social "traction" by enacting them within the social infrastructure where religious persons and groups join other expressions of civil society and become involved in shared institutions, public discourse and action, and political activity. Roman Catholicism may have a certain advantage in this regard, in that its health care ministry has had a significant institutional presence in America since at least the nineteenth century.[46] Another advantage is that the national bishops' conference, and other fairly comprehensive and wide-reaching expressions of Catholic identity, such as the CHA and the Catholic university network, provide vehicles for the interaction of health care practice and theology as well as a public voice for Catholic advocacy of health care reform.

This potential was tragically underutilized in the 2004 U.S. presidential election season. "Progressive" Catholic theologians and bioethicists tended to focus on scholarly debates and elite policy discourse. In this, they were like the theological bioethicists in other "mainstream" denominations. Nonetheless, theological discourse in conjunction with episcopal teaching, health care institutions, institutions of higher education, Catholic voluntary organizations, and a national and international network of parishes and dioceses constitutes a very fertile field on which the seeds of future health care reform could be sown and cultivated. Both more cautious or conservative and more progressive or radical theologians can turn up on national advisory bodies, and both have educational institutions and other scholarly fora in which to refine and voice their views. However, at least in the recent past, the more socially conservative theological bioethicists have been better tied into or backed by local activism and coalition building that prioritized issues such as abortion and stem cell research, rather than widening access to health care. Very unfortunately in my judgment, this has also been true of the Roman Catholic Church.

The circumstances could and should be different, given previous teaching. In their resolution of 1993, which remains a landmark, the bishops assert as a basic principle that "Every person has a right to health care. This right flows from the sanctity of human life and the dignity that belongs to all human persons, who are made in the image of God." Moreover, they invoke "the biblical call to heal the sick and to serve 'the least of these,' the priorities of social justice and the common good," the "virtue of solidarity," and "the option for the poor and vulnerable." The "value of stewardship" demands better use of resources and the cutting of excessive costs that drive necessary funds away from other social goods such as housing and education.[47] This is theological bioethics operating in the narrative and prophetic modes.

Turning to ethics and policy, the bishops call on the government to assume a role in ensuring that all are guaranteed universal access to quality care and comprehensive benefits (no two-tiered system), that the poor receive priority attention, and that the values of religious providers and health care facilities be respected in a pluralistic society.[48] Three aspects of their stance are notable. First, the religious values cited are, for the most part, used to back views and potential policy options that are not exclusive to Catholicism, but have been advanced by many other analysts, including those cited earlier. However, the religious language and indirect references to biblical narratives, such as the Creation story in Genesis 1 and the parable of judgment in Matthew 25, are effective ways to invoke a larger horizon of meaning and value and to challenge others to consider what are the highest values at stake and the most honorable actions before the American public.

Second, the bishops issued a "prophetic" call without really delving into the hard questions of specific policy. Their emphasis on equality and inclusion, their insistence that health care is not a "commodity," and their appeal for government intervention lean in the direction of a single-payer system supported by taxes. Yet they do not assert this directly. Nor do they address whether good "stewardship" of resources will be enough to cut costs and provide universal high-quality care, without making hard choices about types of care provided or the priority of health care compared to other social goods. In this regard, the bishops could be accused of naiveté, and even a certain degree of moralistic thinking.

However, and third, the most important dimension of this statement is undoubtedly its repeated insistence that health care policies be evaluated in light of the plight of the most vulnerable members of society. Here their prophetic role is carried into ethical analysis and policy. Their call goes far beyond enlightened self-interest, and even beyond simple equality or equal respect. It takes to heart the Christian message about a moral society and projects it outward as a challenge to all who are invested in the common good of America. In other words, religiously based social teaching is, in this case, reaching for broader relevance and persuasive power and trying to meet the challenge that is obvious to philosophers and even to economists: "What is to prevent the bad outcome in which citizens are unwilling to give philanthropic donations and are unwilling to support higher taxes that are needed to make greater public transfers?" The answer given by the bishops is that they and other moral leaders should insistently and repeatedly hold up before the American public the ideal of solidarity in the common good. Disappointingly, the Catholic bishops have not unambiguously advocated for this ideal in U.S. legislative and electoral politics, preferring to sacrifice the cause of health care justice to the cause of prohibiting abortion and embryo research.

In the real world of participatory bioethics and politics, progress cannot always be made by insisting that ideals be perfectly matched by policy. The practical expression of religiously transmitted and theologically defended values such as the value of unborn life and the value of health as a basic good will have to be negotiated at the ground level, as well as in midlevel policies and general principles. Insofar as some of the outcomes represent compromises that are the best that Christians or other religious believers can achieve in particular circumstances, they yield "middle axioms." An example would be advocacy for a reform of the insurance system in which some employment-based measures were combined with government funds and subsidies and in which the market controlled some portion of costs and availability. The framework of solidarity and the preferential option for the poor might theoretically be best represented by a single-payer system, in which poor and wealthy have the same treatment in all cases. But given the historical and political realities, this best option might not be a realistic option for America. The same holds true for the negotiation of policies on stem cells, for example, that must be accountable to diverse values, such as the good of scientific research, the value of the embryo, and the value of maximizing the benefits of health expenditures for the least well-off. (Stem cell research will be considered more extensively in the next chapter.)

Insofar as it assumes that the formulation and application of policies at the local level must be sensitive to particular circumstances, theological bioethics respects the principle of "subsidiarity." What it means to achieve "equal access" or make an "option for the poor" in a particular state, city, or health facility must be honed in the more particular setting in which care is received. Theological bioethics respects subsidiarity in that its detailed requirements cannot be settled a priori, abstractly, or comprehensively. Conversely, concrete applications will refine and often challenge the initial bioethical analysis. And insofar as decision makers as individuals, families, or care teams must determine what is the best course of action for a given patient in view of the resources available, local policies in place, and the needs of the patient and his or her family, the process of decision making is a form of "casuistry." "Virtue" is the integral disposition of an individual, group, or even an institution to seek the welfare of all according to practical demands and in light of the common good. And to the extent that conflict, chance, or injustice excludes good options, agents are constrained to practice adverse virtue.

Leadership in Practice

The power of persuasion must rest on more than a clarion call. It requires a track record, an example, and some evidence that the would-be persuader has the experience and integrity to affirm convincingly that the course of action urged is possible and will bear fruit. The theological and ethical analysis must be participatory. The audience of the appeal must see the speaker not only as someone who voices a vision of the future. The most persuasive moral call comes from someone who in the listener's own experience has demonstrated the truth of his or her words by actions and with whom the listener has even shared some steps along the way. Participatory theological bioethics engages, persuades, and changes patterns of social behavior by involvement with others in practices that represent values and commitments coherent with a religious worldview, but that also gain influence and respect in the "real world" of health care and biomedicine.

From the early 1980s until his death of cancer in 1996, Cardinal Joseph Bernardin of Chicago strove to form Catholics and Catholic health care in the practice of what he called "a consistent ethic of life."

> Those who defend the right to life of the weakest among us must be equally visible in support of the quality of life of the powerless among us: the old and the young, the hungry and the homeless. The undocumented immigrant and the unemployed worker. Such a quality of life posture translates into specific political and economic positions on tax policy, employment generation, welfare policy, nutrition and feeding programs, and health care.[49]

In a lecture commemorating Bernardin, Michael Place, as president of the CHA, observed that the consistent ethic of life

> calls us to be a stronger witness of Gospel values to the wider public. It calls us to a deeper concern for all people, particularly the weak and vulnerable, whose dignity is threatened and whose potential is squelched by unjust situations, conditions, and laws that exist today.[50]

This expression of the basic principle of Catholic health care ethics is meant first of all to call Catholics to a more clear recognition of their social responsibilities. But it is also a way of introducing Catholic values into the political context and urging that a more compassionate approach to health care prevail generally. Bernardin did not specify exactly what "consistency" would look like in detail, leaving room for casuistry, subsidiarity, and middle axioms. Place, who stands professionally at the center of many quite fractious debates about the relative priority of the items on Bernardin's list within Catholic health care, and about how Catholic facilities are to relate to the general legal, political, and moral environment in aiming to put their principles into practice, necessarily has experience with such tensions. Just as in the culture at large, the practical application of even agreed-upon general values can be tendentious within Catholic ethics and within Catholic health care systems and dioceses, for example, on specific reproductive services.

Bernardin served more as a source of moral and spiritual leadership in health care ethics than as a policymaker. In the last few months before his death, Bernardin became a public spokesperson for the possibility of a hopeful approach to death and trust in a loving God. Bernardin demonstrated another way to meet terminal illness, an alternative to the panoply of modern medical armaments. His choice also comports well with the need to balance health care resources within a comprehensive social and spiritual perspective.

In Catholic theological bioethics today, the practical sociopolitical counterpart to the bishops' ethical analysis and Bernardin's personal example is the institutionalization of health care under Catholic auspices in the United States. Taken together, Catholic healthcare facilities are the biggest private, nonprofit provider of care in the United States and regard so-called charity care as an essential part of their mission.[51] The distinctive religious ethos of the United States encouraged voluntary hospitals, sponsored by medical colleges and religious denominations, to flourish alongside state and city institutions.[52] Congregations of religious women furthered this mission throughout the United States; especially important religious orders in the establishment of Catholic health care were the Ursulines, the Sisters of Charity, and the Sisters of Mercy.[53]

Today two thousand Catholic health care sponsors, systems, facilities, and related organizations serve across the continuum of care; one in six Americans is cared for in a Catholic acute care facility; and the Catholic health ministry is the largest not-for-profit provider of health care services in the nation.[54] In a summary of the Catholic health care mission, Michael Place has asserted that, in the absence of a firm national commitment to guarantee health care access for everyone, Catholic providers

> will not allow access to our health care system to depend on one's individual circumstances, such as the good fortune of working for an employer who provides adequate insurance, or the happenstance of qualifying for Medicaid or Medicare. No. *Universal access to health care will be a central tenet of*

> *our health care system.* That system will guarantee an adequate level of care to all.[55]

Many analysts depict public hospitals, especially public teaching hospitals in large cities, as the primary providers of "safety-net" care in the United States.[56] The Institute of Medicine has defined core safety-net providers as those that "by legal mandate or explicitly adopted mission . . . maintain an 'open door,' offering access to services to patients regardless of their ability to pay," and for which "a substantial share of the patient mix" is "uninsured, Medicaid, or other vulnerable populations."[57] Catholic facilities fit this description, but are often neglected in national data about safety-net providers. The volume of care provided by Catholic hospitals should not be measured only by comparing individual facilities to individual urban hospitals. Catholic health care should be viewed overall as an inclusive network. Until the 1970s, Catholic hospitals were operated as independent entities, even though several might be staffed by one religious order. In the 1970s, most religious communities joined their facilities into unified health care systems, either a national system for orders with fewer hospitals, or, for those with a larger number, a regional system.[58] Taken together, the role of Catholic facilities is significant. A special feature pertaining to charity care is that health systems sponsored by religious orders are often able to spread losses over several facilities. More importantly, the systems to which the safety-net providers belong allow them to access capital at significantly reduced interest rates, based on the credit reliability of the whole. In addition, some of the larger systems provide internal charitable donations, often used as seed money for targeted programs.[59]

The CHA commissioned a study by the Georgetown University Institute for Health Care Research and Policy to better define the role of Catholic health care in maintaining the U.S. safety net. This study, *A Commitment to Caring,* found that Catholic hospitals serve diverse communities in diverse ways, sometimes being the main safety-net provider, and sometimes sharing that responsibility with public hospitals or other not-for-profits. The combined percentage of publicly insured and uninsured patients in the hospitals studied ranged from 64 percent to 86 percent.[60] Catholic hospitals provide free in-patient care and also contribute to primary care services through clinics and medical outreach services. "Their safety net mission is very much a part of their history, heritage, identity, and organizational culture."[61]

Catholic hospitals are more likely than other types to offer a variety of services, including trauma care, neonatal intensive care, and HIV/AIDS care, that are most likely to be used by the poor. They also provide social services and community services funded directly out of their operating budgets. Examples include community-based programs for elders, gang rehabilitation and leadership programs, teenage pregnancy prevention programs, and other educational programs. They may also provide transportation, clothing, and housing support.[62] This, of course, does not mean that Catholic nonprofits can or do provide limitless care to the poor. Sometimes their mission commitment creates a precarious financial situation that ultimately leads to the closing of a hospital, and hence a reduction of services to the community.[63] The report commissioned by the CHA echoes the Institute of Medicine report in calling for a federal initiative to support core safety-net providers.[64]

The extensive need for and presence of Catholic charity providers, along with other key providers in the safety net, attests, however, that much more drastic reform is needed than to bolster their capacity. In fact, enhancing and further institutionalizing charity care as an access route to health services reinforces the dependency of those otherwise excluded. It enables other members of society to assume that the poor do not need guaranteed equitable access, because they will somehow be able to get essential access when they need it. This is both untrue and a form of injustice. Providing charity care is an expression of adverse virtue, in that it discerns as the best practical option a strategy that enables society to escape responsibility and keeps the poor in a dependent, demeaning, and health-reducing situation. The provision of charity care is a moral obligation for religiously based health care services in view of the common good; yet it is also a form of cooperation in and even perpetuation of conditions detrimental to the common good.

African American theologian Emilie Townes, a Protestant, utters a cry of lament for the suffering of her people and for all those deprived of human compassion and basic needs. But she urges Christians not to concede too readily "that true justice and equality will never be a part of the fabric of living in our lifetimes."[65] She urges her readers to have hope, fractured as it may be from the impact of discouraging experience, and to take the risks to which hope will lead. "When we truly believe in this hope, it will order and shape our lives in ways that are not always predictable, not always safe, rarely conventional. This hope will lead us to protest with fury the sins of an inequitable health care system."[66] Michael Place echoes her vision when he affirms "that life is full of possibilities, and that together we must establish the conditions that allow all to share in life's possibilities" in a health care system that, without denying death and limits, upholds the flourishing of every person and the health of the whole society.[67]

These two advocates are hardly alone in the new priority they give to social justice as a component of bioethics. Documents of the Catholic bishops on health care consistently sound this theme. Andrew Lustig does not overstate the case when he generalizes that, in post–Vatican II Catholic social teaching, "access to health care is seen as a positive right, i.e., a justified entitlement claimable by individuals against society."[68] Part one of the 2001 edition of the *Ethical and Religious Directives* is devoted to "The Social Responsibility of Catholic Health Care Services," an emphasis that was unheard of in 1949.[69] Catholic ethicist Philip Keane, in a major study of justice and Catholic health care, grounds the concern with distributive justice in Catholic social teaching and asserts that "if health care is a common good issue, health care can never be understood as a mere commodity . . . without consideration of the deeper good of both individuals and society."[70] Whether or to what extent it is appropriate to view health care as a commodity is a debated issue,[71] but it is far less debatable that persons have rights to essential goods that extend beyond their ability to pay the market price and that the common good requires mechanisms beyond the market to allocate such goods.

As Allen Verhey puts it, "When the contemporary Good Samaritan invokes the standard of justice embedded in the larger story of Scripture, she encourages people to test policy recommendations not just against a standard of impartial rationality but against the plumb line of 'good news for the poor,' including especially the sick poor."[72] The common good tradition matches these prophetic biblical ideals with an ethical vocabulary that calls all members of society to be responsible for their neighbors, especially the most disadvantaged, and to reform social institutions that militate against fair access. The compassion of the privileged is indeed good news for the poor, but not as good as structural justice.

From Vision to Advocacy to Implementation

The normative vision of a just and inclusive health care system ultimately returns theological bioethics to the means and ways of reform. On the one hand, philosophers, theologians, and important national bodies such as the Institute of Medicine all call for universal coverage. On the other, the Clinton overhaul was roundly rejected by the public and legislators. Though

SCHIP has made a big difference to children, subsequent incremental reform of Medicare has been piecemeal and unstable and has arguably served pharmaceutical companies more than the poor. The spokespersons of neither major political party are making daring proposals for resource reallocation. Will the religious prophets always be voices crying in the wilderness?

Not necessarily. Religious denominations and organizations have mobilized advocacy for policy changes; perhaps more significantly, they have mobilized already to enact different real patterns of access to care. This is true of both Catholic and Protestant denominations and agencies, but it is especially true of Catholic health care, with its pervasive presence in civil society and its partnering with other organizations and with government. Though Christian advocacy and action have not achieved wholesale "conversion" of the national moral will or the national health care system, they are a significant leavening agent. They have done more to convert practices "on the ground" than would be evident by inspecting legislation and the health care "reform" platforms of national political candidates. The purpose of surfacing specific examples is to motivate theological bioethics in general to turn its attention more firmly to social ethics and to practical grassroots, midlevel, and nongovernmental expressions of its values and capacities for change.

Examples are numerous in Christian (especially Catholic) health care, which does far more than provide a safety net within the present deficient biomedical establishment. Religious groups are strong and loud advocates of changes both in policies and in practices. They have developed means to organize their own members, other groups, and individual citizens around their policy reform agendas. Going beyond public advocacy for different, more equitable health care policy and practice, religious groups take representative, cutting-edge action in their own institutions and in their communities to begin to implement the vision they hold out as a societal ideal.

Once more, the CHA has perhaps the most extensive advocacy presence, going far beyond lobbying by its Washington office. It aims to catalyze a political movement to change practices at the grassroots level and to demand policy change by government. Its website links to position papers, policy status reports, and advocacy opportunities too numerous to mention. In 2000, the CHA board of trustees approved *Continuing the Commitment: A Pathway to Health Care Reform* to establish a vision for a Catholic reform initiative.[73] Acknowledging the failure of the health care debates of the early nineties, the board and president of CHA called for renewed resolve by "the Catholic community, Catholic health care facilities and other system stakeholders, government and elected officials, and, ultimately, the general public."[74] Citing its history of crafting documents and proposals and engaging in grassroots advocacy, the CHA planned to wage a national communications and education campaign to put sequential extensions of coverage and eventually global policy changes on the agendas of physicians and caregivers, legislators, faith communities, and the general public.

The position of CHA is that all persons living in this country should be entitled to medically essential services, as well as those necessary to meet special needs, and that a supplemental package should be available for purchase. In 2000, it recommended that employer coverage be encouraged by federal subsidies, that the insurance program for federal workers be expanded to cover the unemployed, that Medicaid and SCHIP be expanded, and that Medicare be reformed. CHA recognizes that sequential reforms will have greater political viability than wholesale reconfiguration of the health care system. The steps it recommends are examples of middle axioms that represent the best practical opportunities for Christian values of inclusion, service, and empowerment of the poor to begin to permeate U.S. health care policy. Using the strategies of participatory democracy and deliberative democracy, CHA joined forces with other groups in civil society, such as the Health Insurance Association of America and Families USA, which are often on opposing sides of reform issues, but in this case came together in recognizing the need to broaden insurance coverage.[75]

By 2004, some expansion of federal programs had been achieved, but without funding adequate to guarantee their viability for the future. The unemployed remained without coverage, and employers were cutting down on rather than expanding health benefits. CHA, together with the American Hospital Association, developed a new legislative proposal to provide universal coverage for children, premium support through tax credits, a tax credit for insurance purchase by small employers with a low-wage workforce, and tax credits for low-income persons to purchase insurance individually or through the workplace.[76]

CHA is renewing efforts to create public awareness and support for change, in partnership with organizations like the Robert Wood Johnson Foundation, sponsor of a national coalition to cover the uninsured.[77] Through a "Cover the Uninsured Week," CHA publicized and participated in interfaith events; educational forums and press conferences; educational sessions at medical, nursing, and public health schools; seminars for small businesses to obtain insurance coverage; "health and enrollment fairs" at malls, churches, and hospitals; a major targeted effort to enroll more children in SCHIP; and counseling for the uninsured. The major aim of this campaign was to build the public awareness and support without which policymakers will not seriously consider innovative or broad-reaching solutions.

The CHA website[78] provides links to dozens of related items, including proposed federal changes to Medicare, a CHA commendation for the Department of Health and Human Services' Rescue and Restore campaign, and a CHA "advocacy alert." The latter encourages ministry to submit comments on the implementation of new regulations regarding Medicare prescription drug benefits; comments on proposed federal funding of emergency health services to undocumented aliens; comments on the impact of pending legislation on rural hospitals; and comments on federal budget proposals, as well as in support of expanding Medicaid; and a letter urging Congress to carefully balance budget enforcement legislation with our societal responsibility to support the most vulnerable. The website also provides links to CHA Internet services and networks, including "Washington Update," "Advocacy," "eAdvocacy," and CHA print publications and "Toolkits." Ensuring health care access for all remains a key advocacy priority of CHA; it calls for "a social movement that is driven by a fundamental conviction to improve the access to quality health care for all." The CHA is aware that "real, sustainable health reform will require an extraordinary demonstration of public and legislative will to succeed," and it is highly invested in producing that will.[79]

At the end of 2004, CHA and the Catholic health ministry launched a campaign "focused on fomenting a national movement—a demand for social reform—that will transform health care delivery and ensure that every person in the United States can obtain necessary health care services."[80] CHA and the American Hospital Association collaborated on a proposal to cover 27 million of the uninsured, partly by mandating coverage to all children under the age of nineteen. The CHA board committed its organization and members "to begin by working with others, building effective coalitions, conducting public dialogues both to raise awareness of the issues and to find strength through collaboration."[81]

Possible signs of hope are that surveys attest a growing concern in the United States about the health care crisis; dissatisfaction with the system and its services; anxiety about losing coverage; more attention to health care by national organizations, policymakers, and campaigning politicians; and increasingly visible collective efforts of thousands of organizations and individuals.[82] Some of these are the members and governing bodies of other religious denominations, especially the Protestant churches.[83]

Meanwhile, Christian health care leaders are not waiting for official initiatives from the federal or state level. They seek and try innovative approaches to care on the basis of subsidiarity. Care for the uninsured is provided not only in religiously based hospitals but increasingly in community settings, where preventative, long-term, and cooperative health support can be better maximized. Faith leaders and organizations are discovering that collaboration is essential to improving care for the uninsured and underinsured. In its report on "Catholic Ministries as Catalysts for Healthier Communities," CHA offers standards, software, workbooks, think tanks, a member consortium, a strategy action group, and a publication on forming partnerships with other religious, nonprofit, governmental, and health care institutions in pursuit of its approach to collaborative activities toward community health improvement. It also offers seven case studies of facilities and systems that are examples of "best practices."[84]

The 2003 CHA Assembly featured three speakers from different local communities that presented the results of collaborative efforts to expand care. One described a medical center in Michigan that sponsors six clinics serving the elderly, AIDS patients, and ethnic communities. It makes a concerted effort to involve the surrounding community and neighborhood groups. A second speaker introduced a health care network in Texas that serves the uninsured in three counties of the fastest growing area in the state. It is a collaborative effort between many public and private providers. A third, from Colorado, spoke of the integration of mental health services into health care provided by clinics. Enabling factors are the sponsorship of a Catholic hospital, volunteer efforts of medical and dental students, and agreements with pharmaceutical companies to secure resources. All these facilities assist the underserved and reduce the need for acute care and longer hospital stays.[85] Catholic health facilities often combine forces with Catholic Charities to provide a variety of services that are important to health, such as housing, long-term and nursing care, and social services.[86]

There are plenty of non-Catholic parallels to the activities of the CHA and other Catholic networks such as Catholic Health Initiatives. The Carter Center is an Atlanta-based institution founded by former president Jimmy Carter. The Carter Center's and Emory University's joint Interfaith

Health Program challenges all faith traditions to make health care more equitable, in collaboration with each other and with public structures that share their goals. According to Carter, "The most exciting opportunities are not found in high-tech cures, but in new ways of preventing disease and promoting wholeness. These opportunities demand the full energies of religious organizations of all faiths."[87]

The Interfaith Health Program's *Strong Partners* advances this vision with theological and practical commentaries and with case studies of several foundations that realigned health resources from hospitals to community-based interventions and services. In recent decades, a number of religious hospital sponsors have opted to sell their facilities, rather than compete with for-profits in an environment where acute care facilities may not provide the optimum community health benefits. Many have devoted the proceeds to collaborative, community-oriented care. This is true of both Catholic and Protestant sponsors.

According to William Foege, a preventive approach requires the partnership of three types of entities: community organizations, religious congregations, and government.[88] The social roles of private, public, profit, and nonprofit structures are being renegotiated at local, state, regional, and national levels, which presents a window of opportunity for innovation. In one case, Wesley Medical Center, a prospering Methodist-owned hospital in Wichita, Kansas, was sold in order to convert assets and talent into community care. Proceeds from the sale of the hospital were invested in the Kansas Health Foundation, with ties to the Methodist Church. In the decade following the sale, the foundation has "supported community health assessments, parenting education, childhood development, research, nutrition education and substance abuse prevention programs, as well as served as an advocate for public health in many other areas." It has also supported health care education.[89]

Gary Gunderson points out that approximately 75 million people attend worship services more than once a month. Health organizations list a high number of their employees as active in religious traditions. This confluence of faith and practical expertise in health care offers a largely untapped resource to develop "more neighborhood-level health promoters, more parish nurses, more health committees, more professionals working part time and as volunteers, pushing the knowledge and services down into the health frontier: local communities." Obviously, this would also require a realignment of payment systems, fund-raising systems, training systems, health and religious systems, and career-track systems.[90] Perhaps new problems can bring "new connectional forms," facilitated by new communications technologies, especially the electronic exchange of documents and consultation by email.[91]

Advancing the concept of "boundary leaders," Gunderson calls on religious groups to take advantage of the spaces between organizations, structures, and groups, interstices where conditions are in flux, and power and relationships are being negotiated.[92] It is at the boundaries that "webs of transformation" have the chance to emerge. Webs of transformation form "at the confluence of opportunity and concern," after practical demands become so overwhelming that action and solutions simply cannot be avoided.[93] According to Gunderson, boundary leadership in creating transformative webs "is a claim against the obvious momentum of 'the powers.'"[94]

This discussion of religious and theological creation of transformative webs in health care practices is essentially a way of displaying how theological bioethics can connect normative analysis with social justice in a society that is pluralistic, not uniformly committed to equity, and certainly lacking in national political leadership to enact legislative change, and even leadership in national ethical advisory bodies to tackle the access issue. The message is not just that religious people and churches should "get involved" to help their neighbors and build up the common good. It is also that theological bioethicists should think and theorize differently about what scholarship in their field is and does. One task of theological bioethics is to connect faith traditions with applied ethics theoretically. Theological bioethics must make the case that certain values constitute the moral heart of a tradition; it must also connect these values to decisions and practices in as clear and critical an analysis as possible. But theological ethics is not only a matter of scholarship and argument. Theories of theological bioethics must envision it as *participatory* discourse, in which the narratives, theological explanations, and ethical theories of religious traditions are always interactive with their context. Theological bioethics is not merely the *product* of contextual shaping; it *interacts* critically with its contexts, and it must face the responsibility to *intervene* in those contexts through "transformative webs" of discourse and practice.

AIDS, Bioethics, and Religion

When the emerging AIDS crisis first rose to public consciousness in the 1980s, U.S. bioethicists, like the public at large, perceived it as a problem affecting gay males and intravenous drug users. The ethical issues emphasized were homosexuality, sexual promiscuity, the use of condoms to prevent transmission, and whether clean needles should be provided free to people engaging in an illegal activity. Another issue was the confidentiality of medical information, as infected people could transmit HIV, the virus that causes AIDS, to sexual partners who might be unaware of their exposure. Mandatory testing was also posed as a public health issue, for example, testing of newborns whose mothers have HIV. As research on treatments progressed, the ethics of enrollment in drug trials became part of the ethical picture. In some cases that picture was expanded to other cultures, where drug trials (e.g., on the prevention of mother to child transmission) were conducted with fewer legal restraints than in the United States. With improvements in treatment of HIV/AIDS, the disease has been redefined for many in "first world" countries to a chronic, manageable illness, rather than a death sentence. Unfortunately, disproportionate rates of infection and relatively poor access to treatments still plague black Americans. Among gay men, the risk may be returning due to the misimpression that AIDS is no longer a worrisome danger.

With very few exceptions, however, "mainstream" bioethics in the United States has approached and still approaches AIDS as a sexual issue, and as an issue raising ethical concerns mainly around sexual autonomy versus risk to others, and around the individual's right to informed consent to participation in research. And those issues no longer have a high profile in the main bioethics journals. The frameworks of distributive justice, the common good, and justice in health care access globally are rarely brought to bear on a disease that remains a horrendous plague on other continents. In fact, those continents are rarely part of the moral analysis of mainstream bioethics at all.

The approach is different in theological bioethics, however. Theologians have by and large caught onto the fact that AIDS is about poverty and sexism, and poverty and sexism are ethical issues. They have a place in bioethics, and when the question of AIDS arises, they have a central place. In a recent essay creating an overview of Catholic responses to AIDS, a Catholic moral theologian and a Catholic physician—both priests—note this paradigm shift. They conclude that "human rights" is an appropriate conceptual framework for AIDS, that socioeconomic conditions contributing to AIDS must be studied, and that it is essential "to galvanize the political will to respond effectively to these conditions."[95] Methodist theologian Donald Messer concludes a study of AIDS by saying that "Christian hope demands our political involvement in matters of social justice and to envision a world without HIV/AIDS."[96] Catholic theologian Maria Cimperman urges that the ministry of Jesus, the cross, and the common good all demand engagement in a process of transformation of the levels of poverty and oppression that create the devastation of AIDS.[97] Edwin Vasquez uses the case of Brazil to connect Catholic social teaching to local action to make antiretroviral therapy available to all, despite inaccessible pricing set by the major drug companies.[98]

As expressed in a report for the South African Catholic bishops on care for children affected by AIDS, "When you sit at the bottom of the pile and seek to attend to the needs of the millions of children, women and men who, through life's circumstances, find themselves in a wretched place, you can't help but ask yourself what it is that can, must and should be done to make a difference?"[99] Unfortunately, there are all too many people and societies who find it easy not to ask that question, especially among those who are not themselves sitting "at the bottom of the pile." Theological bioethics can analyze the reasons why Christian and human values should lead to action against AIDS, but unless it finds ways to engage social practices so that motivations and actions change, the analysis will be ineffectual, as well as unaccountable to those who are truly "in a wretched place." The report itself outlines many community-based programs and interventions under the sponsorship of or in partnership with the bishops' conference that "show just how important grass roots initiatives are to the lives of people marginalized by poverty and disease."[100]

In addition to the social conditions that facilitate the spread of AIDS, religious thinkers, especially church representatives, give a good deal of attention also to the use of condoms to prevent HIV transmission.[101] However, theologians are increasingly aware that poverty and sexism play major roles in condom availability and use and that addressing the social conditions of the spread of the disease is more important than addressing this one means of prevention in and of itself. When marginal populations, including women, are educated and economically viable, they will make their own decisions about sex, abstinence, and condoms. In fact, theological debates about condoms are as much politically as ethically motivated.

The condom issue has been most inflammatory in the Catholic Church, following on Catholicism's absolute teaching against the use of artificial birth control (*Humanae vitae,* 1968). However, as many theologians have argued, condoms used to prevent HIV transmission could easily be justified by the principle of double effect. Contraception may be viewed by some as a bad effect, but it is not the object directly intended and is a side effect rather than the direct effect of using condoms to avoid AIDS. Moreover, there is certainly a proportionate good at stake: human life. Whether condoms would encourage promiscuity is a valid question, but the risk of an eventual social danger does not outweigh immediate risk to life. In any event, a "slippery slope" argument is contingent and not absolute. However, authority and loyalty in the Catholic Church have been defined in relation to the birth control question since the 1960s. "Hardliners" therefore refuse to yield on this issue, even though lives hang in the balance.[102] The contribution of theological bioethics is essential to render AIDS a social ethics concern; the contribution of participatory theological bioethics is essential to close the gap between analysis and change.

In July 2004, the Fifteenth International AIDS Conference met in Bangkok. At that point, 40 million people were infected with HIV worldwide, thirty million of whom lived in the developing world. However, just 400,000 of those with HIV in poorer countries were receiving anti-AIDS drugs.[103] By mid-2005, 12 million children in Africa had been orphaned by AIDS, along with 3 million on other continents. Orphan girls are often pressured into sex to support themselves and siblings, thus risking HIV infection themselves. AIDS as a justice issue concerns the social relationships that help spread HIV and fail to alleviate AIDS, relationships of power and vulnerability that are in violation of equity, the common good, and the preferential option for the poor. HIV infection is spread through individual behaviors, especially multiple sexual contacts and drug abuse; these are morally objectionable and deserve to be addressed. However, these behaviors are strongly influenced by social, cultural, and economic conditions. Similarly, the ability to choose different behavior patterns—such as sexual fidelity in marriage to an uninfected spouse and a healthy lifestyle—depends on being in social circumstances that make such choices real possibilities.

Most of the people in the world infected by HIV live in developing countries, where the great majority lack not only consistent access to basic health care but also education, nutrition, and sanitation. The fact that poverty and poor health are linked needs no argument. When people are deprived of access to the basic means of subsistence, their physical and social well-being declines. Poverty denies people social access to the means of deterring specific health threats. This includes their ability to avoid contracting or spreading HIV/AIDS.

People living in poverty not only suffer a general loss of well-being but are forced to adopt "survival strategies" that expose them to health risks.

This is especially true of women, who may already be disadvantaged by patriarchal customs mandating very early marriage of girls to older men, inability of girls and women to make their own decisions about marriage or sexual activity in general, and little ability to influence a spouse's sexual practices, including whether he is monogamous or wears a condom. Married couples may be split apart when men leave traditional agricultural work to seek waged employment in urban areas or with international corporations.[104] They may meet women who, even more desperate economically, have either turned to prostitution or are willing to enter a more long-term arrangement in which they trade regular sexual access and emotional support to a man in exchange for financial support for themselves and possibly their children.[105]

A report from Lesotho, a tiny country with the world's fourth-highest infection rate, describes young women garment workers who resort to "transactional sex" because they cannot support themselves on 70 cents an hour. Their sexual partners pay rent, offer transportation to work, provide food, or help with bills. The women's employers sometimes extort sex. In Lesotho HIV infects one in four men between the ages of fifteen and twenty-four, but one in two women.[106] UN officials say that young African women are three times as likely as young men to become infected with HIV. Worldwide, 48 percent of those with HIV are women, an increase of nearly a third in twenty years.[107] In Africa, women have been reported to account for 67 percent of those infected.[108]

AIDS is proliferated in different ways in different cultures. Gender discrimination is undoubtedly a key factor in the transmission of AIDS. In many cultures, not only in Africa, women have less power in sexual relationships than men and fewer opportunities to make a living wage. In the United States, overt homosexual activity has played a large role, combined with the fact that men who have AIDS not infrequently have sex with women who are unaware of their partners' HIV status. In some social sectors, drug use has exacerbated this problem. In Thailand, 50 percent of new infections are due to intravenous drug use, and rates are higher in Eastern Europe.[109] In Africa and Latin America, homosexuality is taboo, making it secretive but not nonexistent, just a greater threat to heterosexual women as well as to gay or bisexual men. Attitudes permitting men freedom to have more multiple sexual partners than women also increase women's vulnerability. In India as in the United States, at least in urban areas, sexual variety is more openly pursued and exhibited, and homosexuality and transsexualism are more tolerated. In other countries, such as Russia and the United States, the prison system is a major vector of HIV/AIDS.

In all these cases, men who contract HIV/AIDS pass it on to women at disproportionate rates. In virtually every culture where AIDS takes hold, it is acknowledged by most observers that women are generally at a disadvantage in setting the terms of sex or abstention from sex. Faithful, respectful marriage may be the normative setting for sex—but it is a setting more idealized than realized for many women. For example, a Catholic religious sisters' group (Sisters for Justice of Johannesburg) criticized a South African bishops' pastoral letter on AIDS (Message of Hope[110]) because it counseled chastity and fidelity as a solution to the AIDS crisis. "Phrases such as 'the beautiful act of love' and 'equal and loving partners' seem to us to direct the Message of Hope to people who are in fairly healthy and stable marriage relationships, but not to people, usually women, in abusive, oppressive or desperate relationships or circumstances and who are very much at risk of being infected by the HIV."[111] A "pastoral response" by theologians and AIDS activists gathered at a conference on the campus of St. Augustine College in South Africa (2003) sought to overcome the preoccupation with condoms and change the perception that the Catholic Church was a liability rather than an asset in the fight against AIDS.[112] Instead they recommended embodying "responsibility" through a number of practical and institutional forms, such as inculturated ministry to indigenous tribes, public education, better formation regarding the crisis in seminary and religious education, outreach to women and girls, and dispelling cultural myths and taboos regarding the origin and transmission of AIDS.

An African author enumerates cultural practices such as prostitution, genital cutting, polygamy, and lack of education for women, along with the encouragement of a nonassertive, submissive role for women, as contributing to the spread of AIDS—and these are practices not limited to Africa.[113] AIDS in some cultures still carries such a stigma that the victims are blamed for their own illness and ostracized. Women are rejected by the husbands who infected them. They are thrown out of their marital homes, and are sometimes no longer accepted even by their natal families, who fear the disgrace of AIDS will destroy their honor and reputation. Gillian Patterson, an advisor to Christian Aid, calls for interfaith cooperation in fighting AIDS, and particularly in seeking "the economic, social, educational and legal empowerment of women and girls" as well as women's access to safe and reliable means of protection under their own control.[114]

Beyond injustice to women, the social results of rising rates of women's infection with AIDS are dire. As local cultures and resources disintegrate under the impact of AIDS, there are fewer and fewer women to perform their age-old role of surviving in adversity and providing for community needs. Farming, which is the backbone of the social structure in traditional societies, and in which women play a key role in Africa, is on the point of collapse on that continent. Health care systems that were never robust are forcing more triage and more desperation as doctors and communities alike are forced to redefine what medical professionalism means and what moral commitments demand, and "adverse virtue" gives way to resignation.[115] Traditional healing arts, especially as cultivated by women, are unable to cope with the magnitude of AIDS. And there are few remaining caregivers for the millions of AIDS orphans, many of whom are already surviving on their own or in child-headed households.[116] The social contexts and consequences of AIDS worldwide burst the individual-oriented paradigm of western bioethics and show that the decisions of elite governing bodies are only a small part of the solution, proving the need for a multidimensional ethical analysis and social-political campaign.

In 2001, a UN special session issued a "Declaration of Commitment on HIV/AIDS."[117] It defined AIDS as a human rights and security issue, called on international cooperation and resources to address it, and named the empowerment of women, care of AIDS orphans, the monitoring of drug prices, and AIDS education among its priorities. The WHO began an initiative to provide AIDS retroviral drugs to 3 million people by 2005 (the "3 × 5 initiative"). In 2001, the Global Fund to Fight AIDS, Tuberculosis, and Malaria was established under the auspices of the WHO.[118] Headquartered in Geneva, the Global Fund is a multilateral, public-private entity and solicits and redistributes international donations to local programs, rather than devising and implementing programs under its own authority. By announcing the Fund, UN Secretary General Kofi Annan hoped to attract $10 billion a year in donations, an amount of which the annual contributions of about $1 billion annually have fallen far short. In 2004, about $5 billion was invested annually worldwide in the fight against AIDS, but $12 billion was the estimated need for 2005, with $20 billion called for by 2007.[119]

Although in the first three years of the Global Fund the United States was its largest contributor, the totals donated still fell short both of the need and of what the United States had originally promised ($15 billion over five years). Although Congress nearly tripled the president's 2005 budget request for global AIDS, the amount allotted to the Global Fund, $2.5 billion, suffered in comparison to more than $100 billion spent on military operations in Iraq.[120] Moreover, in his 2003 State of the Union address, Bush promised $15 billion to the global campaign against AIDS, but then refused to give most of this to the Global Fund. He established instead a separate fund under U.S. authority that would negotiate bilateral agreements with countries willing to comply with Bush administration policies such as the preferences for abstinence education over condoms and for expensive and profitable brand-name drugs. As of 2004, the U.S. fund was serving 15 countries, the Global Fund 130. At the 2004 International AIDS Conference, U.S. representatives were the targets of extensive criticism.

Nevertheless, Peter Piot, the executive director of UNAIDS, introduced a moment of optimism in Bangkok when he announced in his concluding speech that for the first time he felt that there was "a real chance to get ahead of the epidemic."[121] Five years earlier, the global AIDS crisis was hardly on the political or bioethical map in regions with enough resources to address it, with no semblance of an organized global response visible on the horizon. Worldwide consciousness and efforts were catalyzed in large part by a debate over the availability of costly AIDS drugs to the world's poor, set off by the decision of the South African government to openly buck the patent system set up by the rules of the World Trade Organization. After the mobilization of AIDS activists, religious leaders, NGOs, advocacy groups, UN officials, competitive generics companies, and diverse media voices, trade agreements were relaxed, beginning at the 2001 meeting of the World Trade Organization in Doha, Qatar, and continuing in negotiation to August 2003. Countries experiencing an AIDS health emergency are now more easily permitted the manufacturing and importation of much cheaper antiretroviral drugs, in forms simpler to administer and monitor, and so begin to bring meaningful treatment to those dying for lack of access to advanced care.[122] The problem is far from resolved, however. Some countries fear reprisals in the form of trade barriers if they use generics, others are unable to afford even lowered prices, and still others could not effectively deliver drugs to the neediest even if they were available.

Yet AIDS is on the international moral agenda to a degree that could barely have been anticipated less than a decade ago. The development of the question of AIDS and the practical resources being marshaled to meet it manifest the crucial role of many networks and agencies in both government and civil society in changing the status quo. "Webs of transformation" constituted by entities as diverse as citizen groups, nonprofits, corporations, foundations, governmental agencies, and religious traditions, whether local, national, regional, or transnational, are needed to accomplish social change.

Participatory Theological Bioethics and AIDS

Participatory theological bioethics addresses AIDS at the point at which theories of Christian discipleship, the "preferential option for the poor," justice, and the common good come together with practical realities that challenge the theories, induce the theories to be responsive to practices, and offer the chance for visions and theories to make a difference in the way the real world is imagined and engaged. This nexus of ideas, concerns, and actions is also a place in which different, even seemingly opposed, worldviews and theories find common ground in addressing mutual problems. This is true of faith traditions working together on AIDS and of strands within traditions that are in some ways at odds with one another.

For example, while the highest-level teaching of the Roman Catholic Church has been adamantly opposed to condoms, it has been outspoken and clear about the evil of stigmatizing persons with AIDS, about the mandate to minister to AIDS patients, and about the injustice of withholding essential medical care from those too poor to pay the going rates in "first world" nations. A Methodist theologian gives the Catholic Church credit because it "probably offers more hospices, hospitals, orphanages, and parish programs providing care for people with AIDS and their families than any other religious organization." Indeed, "the Vatican speaks out for increased international spending on AIDS care and treatment. Pope John Paul II has attacked the international pharmaceutical companies for excessive and sometimes even exorbitant costs of AIDS drugs."[123] In a statement calling for international solidarity, long before most other leaders were invested in the crisis, the pope insisted that

> AIDS threatens not just some nations or societies but the whole of humanity. It knows no frontiers of geography, race, age or social condition. The threat is so great, indifference on the part of public authorities, condemnatory or discriminatory practices toward those affected by the virus or self-interested rivalries in the search for a medical answer, should be considered forms of collaboration in this terrible evil which has come upon humanity.[124]

In a statement to the United Nations in 2001, a Vatican representative upheld sexual control and morality, but continued,

> An important factor contributing to the rapid spread of AIDS is the situation of extreme poverty experienced by a great part of humanity. Certainly a decisive factor in combating the disease is the promotion of international social justice. . . . The Pope reminds us that the Church has consistently taught that there is a "social mortgage" on all private property, and that this concept must also be applied to "intellectual property" [patents]. The law of profit alone cannot be applied to essential elements in the fight against hunger, disease and poverty.[125]

Among the specifics identified in this statement are care for AIDS orphans (mentioned twice); education about sexuality and AIDS; increased treatment centers, along with "a maximum reduction in the price of antiretroviral medication"; the prevention of mother-to-child transmission; assistance, without neocolonialism, from the industrialized countries; the equality of men and women; and the end of sexual exploitation, including sex tourism, through which the wealthy prey on the vulnerable. In 2003, John Paul II reiterated that "humanity cannot close its eyes in the face of so appalling a tragedy!"[126]

The Vatican program of action on behalf of social justice in regard to AIDS is exemplified in a concrete way by the work of Jesuit priest Angelo D'Agostino, a psychiatrist with more than two and a half decades' experience in Africa. The dynamic created by D'Agostino, the Vatican, pharmaceutical suppliers, World Trade Organization rules, secular and religious news outlets that have captured his story, and the Christian bioethicist who appropriates it theologically amounts to an exercise in participatory theological bioethics. D'Agostino heads an orphanage and clinic for children with AIDS (called Nyumbani—"home" in Swahili) in Nairobi, Kenya.[127] D'Agostino's physical and spiritual care of these children is of course an expression of Christian discipleship and a "preferential option for the poor." He has been honored nationally and internationally for his work on behalf of exploited children. Beyond this vocation, however, D'Agostino is a tireless advocate for AIDS victims and, in light of Catholic norms of social justice, for a transformation of patterns of global power and economics that lead to the suffering of his young charges and of their families. Not mincing words, he indicts "the genocidal action of the drug cartels who refuse to make the drugs affordable to Africa even after they reported a $517 billion profit in 2002."[128]

D'Agostino is one link in the network of theology, ethics, politics, and action that has begun to transform access to AIDS drugs. Testing international law, he announced in 2001 that Nyumbani would order AIDS medications from an Indian generics manufacturer, Cipla, which was among the first to support South Africa in its World Trade Organization challenge. This permitted Nyumbani to treat an additional twenty children every month, but brought the organization into direct conflict with the Kenyan government and international drug companies. Shortly after this decision, and in response to similar acts of resistance on the part of other care providers and activists, drug companies such as GlaxoSmithKline announced sharp cuts in prices to nonprofit organizations and eventually in prices to poor countries in general.[129]

At a 2004 news conference marking the pope's Lenten message on behalf of the hardships of children, the Vatican called on the world's Catholics to help fund the campaign against AIDS and announced the issuing of a Vatican postage stamp, the proceeds from which were designated for Nyumbani. At the conference, D'Agostino defined drug prices as an injustice manifesting the lack of conscience of major pharmaceutical companies and was supported by other Vatican spokespersons who likewise called for further reductions in price.[130] The story was picked up by *America,* the Jesuit magazine, and from there made its way into theological reflection on bioethics and the common good.[131]

Numerous Christian organizations and networks, Catholic and Protestant, as well as interfaith organizations, are active in the struggle to change the global conditions of AIDS. These include Catholic Relief Services, Caritas International, the Jesuit Refugee Service, the Jesuit African AIDS Network, Christian Aid, and the Global AIDS Interfaith Alliance.[132] The Community of Sant'Egidio's effort in Mozambique provides retroviral therapy, assistance to pregnant women with AIDS and their newborns, a support network for AIDS patients, with funding from diverse public and private, Christian and nonreligious sources, including the donated time of Sant'Egidio member physicians. In communities affected by AIDS, Sant' Egidio projects go beyond treating victims; they educate and inspire them to become local leaders in education, health improvement, mobilization of women, and community support.[133]

Embodying the importance of subsidiarity in defining needs and seeking solutions to health crises,[134] local, national, and regional church bodies are also organizing politically against AIDS. Locally, they provide funding, treatment, and spiritual and social support to those afflicted. The African Catholic bishops are not only funding retroviral treatment in church-sponsored centers, but, reflecting a theological bioethics challenged by "participatory" engagement, some individual bishops and bishops' conferences have taken the initiative to advise married couples to follow their consciences in deciding about condom use.[135] Of course, this does not necessarily resolve background social issues, such as poverty and gender inequality, that contribute to the spread of AIDS and make it difficult to use condoms even if "approved." Essentially, the more permissive casuistry on condoms does not remove the necessity for many to exercise adverse virtue, whether that means to use condoms to reduce the effect of an already unjust disease burden or to live with the risk of disease when one cannot obtain a condom, persuade one's partner to use a condom, or refuse sex.

The Church of South India, the Salvation Army in India, the National Council of Churches of India, the Anglican churches of Africa, the Inter-Religious Council of Uganda, and the Methodist Church of Southern Africa sponsor parallel Protestant initiatives.[136] More flexible Christian approaches to condom use and needle exchange also move theological bioethics toward "middle axioms," in the sense of endorsement of AIDS-fighting public measures such as AIDS education, promoting condom use, or needle exchange programs.

A "local to global to local" religious movement to empower women against AIDS has taken shape under the leadership of Sisters of Mercy Margaret Farley and Eileen Hogan. Farley, a feminist theologian and bioethicist and Yale faculty member, sought funding from USAID to begin the Yale Divinity School (YDS) Women's Initiative, which became a springboard for cooperation with African women theologians. Out of this was born the All Africa Conference: Sister-to-Sister, which seeks funding and support from international congregations of religious women and other donors to partner with African Roman Catholic sisters. The object of three conferences to be held in Africa is to enable African women to come together to share wisdom and devise strategies suitable for their own communities.

Farley's commitment to AIDS was prompted by an invitation to speak at a White House summit on AIDS, as well as by a nephew's death of the disease. Her experiences widened her religious imagination and theological concepts. She in turn has relied on faith traditions and theology to warrant and advance a "web of transformation" in response to AIDS. Members of the YDS Women's Initiative have communicated with theological peers in the American Academy of Religion and the Society of Biblical Literature, as well as with feminist and womanist scholars in institutions of higher learning across the United States. They hope to inspire similar projects in other universities and in relation to Asian, Latin American, and North American communities.[137] *This* is participatory theological bioethics.

Theorizing action and holding up the transformative interstices of action, belief, and theology are essential tasks of theological scholarship in bioethics. It is an antidote to the stifling rhetoric of a "neutral" and "secular" public sphere in which theology is silenced. Although it is difficult to hope for significant change in the face of intransigent inequalities worldwide, judgment upon injustice and work to increase compassion, hope, and solidarity are integral to the mission of theological bioethicists. Forming moral understanding by ethical and policy analysis, forming the will to act by narrative and prophecy, and forming structures of change by participatory political engagement, theological bioethics is a transformer of culture and not just its adversary.

CHAPTER

6

REPRODUCTION AND EARLY LIFE

ABORTION LAW in the United States has been permissive since the 1973 Supreme Court decision in *Roe v. Wade.* Although the decision established landmark protections for "a woman's right to choose," the resulting rates of elective abortion have been high. Religious and theological responses to abortion are notoriously mixed and divisive, as absolutists on both ends of the spectrum refuse to compromise their defense of either women's rights or the rights of the unborn. Meanwhile, social programs that could offer meaningful alternatives to women who would prefer to birth and raise their children have been cut back in the name of "welfare reform."

Reproductive technologies are also used liberally in this country. They picked up speed in 1978 when the birth of Louise Brown marked the first successful in vitro fertilization. Such technologies have moved from a way to help infertile couples bear children from their own eggs and sperm to spawn a sizeable and virtually unregulated trade in eggs, embryos, wombs, and highly sophisticated clinical expertise. While many religious voices and activists continue to uphold the norm of procreation only by partners to a heterosexual marriage, and while religious objections to the sale of parts of the human reproductive process are loud and clear, technologies to assist reproduction enjoy wide cultural acceptance. Like abortion, they are promoted (and paid for) under the moral shelter of beneficence and free choice.

This chapter considers the appeal of these practices from the standpoint of the values they represent, especially the equality of women and the self-determination of women in issues related to parenthood. These values, as well as the value of early life, are affirmed by theological bioethics. Yet it is necessary to ask whether liberalism, science, and the market have channeled interventions into human reproduction in a way that is inconsistent with the genuine well-being of human persons, and with the common good, as including basic health access for all. Once again, the discussion will direct the focus away from federal legislation and judicial decisions in examining the role of religious and theological influence in shaping and changing practices. Instead, projects, processes, and coalitions in civil society provide spaces in which polarized cultural debates about abortion, and the lack of any real debate about reproductive technologies, can be alleviated.

On the issue of abortion, the challenge to theological bioethics is to affirm and advance gender equality in practice as well as in theory, while providing positive alternatives to women and couples for whom pregnancy is a threat to well-being. On reproductive technologies, theological bioethics can and should join the multiple other voices calling for regulation, while placing the value of having children in a larger worldview that includes the just use of medical resources and the value of care for already existing disadvantaged children.

Abortion

In 1973, the U.S. Supreme Court ruled that states may not prevent women from having abortions during the first six months of pregnancy. Six months coincides roughly with the time of "viability," the ability to survive outside the womb. States are permitted to prohibit abortion during the last ten weeks of pregnancy, but not when abortion is necessary "to preserve the life or health of the mother." This stipulation in effect creates a permissive abortion policy, "abortion on demand," as threats to psychological health can be construed very broadly. In 1992, the Supreme Court, in *Planned Parenthood v. Casey,* granted to the states some right to regulate abortions, even if not to forbid them. States may require physicians and abortion clinics to provide women seeking abortions information about the procedure, as well as about fetal development. They may impose a twenty-four-hour waiting period for an abortion; they may require girls under eighteen to obtain the consent of one parent or a judge in order to have an abortion.[1]

In 2003, Congress passed a bill against a procedure called "partial-birth abortion," a means of intervening in the birth process by destroying the head of a fully formed fetus. The law is being challenged, because some maintain that the procedure is in rare instances necessary to save the mother's life. However, the debate about the procedure and the general disapprobation it incurs even from many who otherwise support abortion rights has underlined the fact that many Americans do not believe the right to abortion should be totally unrestricted.[2] In fact, polls over the last twenty years have shown that while most Americans, both Protestant and Catholic, support women's legal right to choose abortion, they do not believe that all abortion decisions are morally the same. In fact, many believe even the legal right should be restricted to the "hard cases." In 2004, a Zogby poll showed that 56 percent would accept significant restrictions on abortion rights and that numbers favoring restriction were strong in the eighteen to twenty-five years age group—60.5 percent.[3]

In practice, abortions number more than a million annually in the United States, having leveled off after a surge to 1.5 million in the years following *Roe*. This accounts for about half of all unintended pregnancies, and about a fourth of all pregnancies. Recent data indicates that around 80 percent of abortions are to unmarried women or girls, half of whom are under twenty-four.[4] Each year, approximately 19 percent of young black women, 13 percent of Hispanic, and 8 percent of white, aged fifteen to nineteen, become pregnant. The rate is highest for young women who have sexual partners six or more years older than they. Among teenage pregnancies in 1994, 55 percent resulted in birth, 31 percent in abortion, and 14 percent in miscarriage.[5] Ninety percent of abortions take place in the first trimester, and only 7 percent involve rape, incest, severe fetal defects, or a serious risk to the health of the mother.[6] Many abortions are performed for reasons related to the social circumstances and relationships of the pregnant woman or girl, such as education, employment, financial resources, degree of support from husband or partner, maturity, and ability to care for a child.

Mainline religious denominations, academic theologians, and theological bioethicists reflect trends in the general population toward acceptance of abortion as in some cases justifiable. Yet theologians tend to portray justification in terms of fairly severe burdens of childbirth and motherhood, or in terms of significant and irremediable medical problems for the newborn—even though these factors do not characterize most abortions. For example, Allen Verhey, a biblical theologian, concludes that in some tragic situations, goods conflict and evil cannot be avoided, leading to the sanctioning of abortion. Abortion is acceptable, in his view, in cases of sexual violence, serious threat to the life or health of the mother, congenital abnormalities that would be fatal or amount to "torture," and social or economic conditions that entail "very great hardships."[7] Some evangelical Christians and the leadership and official theology of the Roman Catholic Church take a stronger stand against abortion.[8] Feminist theologians, including Catholics, tend to view abortion as a tragic necessity in some cases. Catholic feminists, however, are less likely to focus their feminist self-understanding on abortion as a "right" or as an item of first importance in seeking the equality of women.[9]

A major encyclical of John Paul II, *Evangelium vitae* (*Gospel of Life*),[10] discusses at some length the evil of abortion, taking as its point of departure the Second Vatican Council's listing of abortion among a series of "infamies" that injure human life and can do so increasingly with the help of modern technology.[11] "Today there exists a great multitude of weak and defenceless human beings, unborn children in particular, whose fundamental right to life is being trampled upon."[12] John Paul II views abortion as an instance of the domination of the weak by the strong. This is true in a double sense. Adults attack vulnerable life in the womb; women seeking abortions are often unable to access the resources to continue a pregnancy and raise a child.

John Paul II adds a couple of new notes, in comparison to traditional theological condemnations of abortion. First, he names solidarity as a virtue necessary to address the problem of abortion,[13] attributing violence to life, including children's lives, to unjust distribution of the world's resources.[14] Second, he does not condemn women who have abortions as sinners, nor does he even single out women as the agents of abortion.[15] Instead, he views women who have abortions as acting under duress and as lacking other options. He portrays women who continue hardship pregnancies as rising to a level of exceptional moral virtue.

> There are situations of acute poverty, anxiety or frustration in which the struggle to make ends meet, the presence of unbearable pain, or instances of violence, especially against women, make the choice to defend and promote life so demanding as sometimes to reach the point of heroism. All this explains, at least in part, how the value of life can today undergo a kind of "eclipse."[16]

John Paul II grants that uncertainty can mitigate the moral responsibility of individuals involved in abortion and goes on to identify the denial of solidarity and structures of social sin, in which power is abused, as creating a climate in which abortion is approved and sought as a last resort by women.[17] Sustaining the lives of the unborn may be a special duty of parents, but they require social supports in order to do that: "the task of accepting and serving life involves everyone."[18]

Feminist theologians who advocate for abortion rights would not see eye to eye with John Paul II on the characterization of abortion. In their view, abortion is not best seen as a victimization of women by society, but as liberation of women from patriarchal control and oppression, particularly from control over sex and reproduction. Abortion may not be a good in itself, but it is a necessary step and option in reclaiming women's bodies and spirits from gender-unequal social institutions that are often violent toward women. Although feminist theological supporters of abortion might agree with John Paul II's analysis of structural sin, they would see abortion as a means of securing women's welfare in a time in which that sin has not yet been overcome, solidarity with women is rarely practiced, and social and financial resources to contend with problem pregnancies are all too inadequate. In the words of Beverly Harrison, "Even to imagine a society that would function to prevent a trade-off between fetal life and women's well-being is difficult. . . . We do not live in a society that cares very much either for the well-being of women or for most of the children women actually bear, much less one that values fetal life."[19]

It has been more than two decades since Harrison wrote those words, and young women in North America have made great strides toward social equality. The rightful equality of women is, in fact, reflected in the way abortion and other matters of sex, parenthood, marriage, and family are today presented in papal teaching and magisterial assessments of these issues. In his "Letter to Women," preceding the 1995 UN Conference on women in Beijing, John Paul II praises "the great process of women's liberation."[20] However, women still have not attained full equality with men in society or the family, and patterns of sexual behavior often reflect this fact. Moreover, the discrepancy between men's and women's roles in organized religion, particularly in the Roman Catholic Church, is striking. Therefore, it will be important to test the value of John Paul II's words against current social practices, and especially against the practices associated with types of theological bioethics that offer critiques of abortion. Do those voicing such critiques enact gender equality at the practical and social levels? How far do they attempt to put into practice meaningful alternatives to abortion?

In 1982, Harrison hoped that

> if together we recognize and embrace a broader positive social agenda for enhancing procreative choice, we may begin to find lines of strategy that will simultaneously bring about both less reliance on abortion and less resort to coercion of women and enforced childbearing."[21]

Since that time, the numbers of abortions and social approbation of abortion have apparently declined. But what alternatives are in place for women? Has theological bioethics participated constructively in remedying the situations that lead to abortion? While Harrison's liberal emphasis on "choice" is not the most adequate framework for analyzing gender or reproductive issues from a common good perspective, her fundamental observation of the need for a "broader social agenda" is well taken. Harrison is well aware that choice is meaningless unless resources are adequate to offer a range of positive choices, choices that serve the well-being of the decision makers and respect their relationships and responsibilities as well as their freedoms.[22] Theological bioethics must place reproductive matters in the context of social practices, institutions, and policies and address the roles that religion and theology may have in making these more equitable and just.

Three fundamental issues in the abortion debate are the value of the fetus, the equality of women, and the proper role of law and policy. Whereas the pro-life movement prioritizes the unborn's right to life, the pro-choice movement prioritizes women's right to self-determination. Both seek to have their privileged value enshrined in laws that prohibit interference and punish infringement. Both the pro-life and the pro-choice movements advance their positions by what could be viewed as prophetic and narrative discourse, appealing to the imagination and solidifying group identity by the use of slogans and symbols such as "sanctity of life," "murder of the unborn," "our bodies, ourselves," and "reproductive choice." Visual images are important to both, whether of unborn babies or of women who have died from illegal abortions, whether of abortion clinic picketers or demonstrators in favor of abortion rights. These types of discourse function primarily as rallying calls for those who share the worldviews of advocates. Rather than building bridges to those of different convictions, narrative and prophetic discourse around abortion widen divisions, while reinforcing group bonds and goals.

The most vocal and visible activists in both constituencies move rather directly from narrative and prophetic modes of speech to policy advocacy, and not surprisingly, approaches to policy are combative rather than cooperative. Ethical discourse on this subject is often deeply rooted in practice.

Advocates are personally or politically committed to and active on behalf of specific social policies or laws that either adamantly protect or seek to overturn abortion policy since *Roe v. Wade.* They are engaged in and committed to gender and family patterns they perceive to be threatened by the "opposite" stance on the legality of abortion. Abortion has immense symbolic value both for supporters of the "traditional" heterosexual, nuclear, procreative family and for supporters of women's equality with men in the family and marriage and of women's right to seek public and professional roles outside motherhood and domesticity.

As Margaret Farley observed in the immediate aftermath of *Roe,* partisans on the extremes of the debate frequently disparage the values of importance to the other, while willfully ignoring the inconsistencies or gaps in their own positions. Pro-abortion advocates refuse to confront the significance of the fact that abortion destroys what is undeniably a developing human life. Anti-abortion advocates refuse to recognize that pregnancy can sometimes create or exacerbate devastating circumstances for women, circumstances that are not easily resolved by heroism or emergency aid. Partisans on both sides respond to different experiences of moral obligation to protect the unborn or to empower women. But if the resulting impasse "remains unresolved for long, . . . it can only contribute to a deepening moral anguish or a growing moral apathy, and to an overall societal fragmentation or self-deception."[23]

Farley's hypothesis turned out to be a prediction: women who have abortions may experience anguish, but the majority of the public today exhibits alarming apathy about the number of abortions performed a year, as well as about the conditions that lead women to resort to what is, after all, an undeniably violent measure. Meanwhile, pro-lifers deceive themselves that if abortion were outlawed, the conditions of women's and children's well-being would necessarily be improved; and pro-choicers deceive themselves that a right to abortion gives women access to true reproductive choice. The Catholic Church, a leading opponent of "abortion rights" and supposedly a defender of the social rights of women, has not put out nearly the amount of energy and effort to underwrite gender equality as a key plank in its social justice platform as it does to ensure that legal abortion is defeated in legislation and at the polls.

Much needed, in my view, is an ethical discourse that examines in a more thoughtful and consensus-building way the status of the fetus, the practical demands of enacting real equality for women, and the function of law and social policy in enabling creative solutions to unplanned pregnancy or to pregnancies in which the child to be born is threatened with serious illness. Most important, participatory theological bioethics must meet the challenge of encouraging or instituting practices that can provide the material base for rapprochement between the two warring outlooks. Theology and religion can and should endeavor to bring together women's well-being and the value of developing life in supportive practices that go much further than "pregnancy help."

In the words of a loyal critic of the Roman Catholic Church, Harry J. Byrne (former chancellor of the archdiocese of New York), a new kind of abortion politics and strategy is needed if religious leadership is to be effective, one that goes beyond "authoritative statements from on high" to grassroots discourse.[24] Such discourse should aim not only to convey the pro-life message (as Byrne suggests) but to convey and enable equality for women in matters related to sex, marriage, and family. Recent polls may be correct about an emerging consensus regarding the need to reduce the numbers of abortions, but continuing willingness to keep abortion safe and still available signals respect for the commitment to women's rights that often motivates pro-choice advocates. The American public needs and may be ready for innovative and consensus-building policies that respect the complex realities behind simplistic abortion politics.

Any adequate solution to the problem of abortion must recognize the importance of sexual responsibility and equality for women and men; the responsibility of both parents for children, born or unborn; and the responsibility of every community to ensure that no one chooses abortion because she lacks health care, housing, food, or necessary child care, or because bearing a child would sound the death knell of educational and employment goals and hopes. No position on abortion will have persuasive power or wide credibility unless it is verified in practices that respect and choose life equally for women and for children, born or unborn. Better policies would enhance the options of pregnant women rather than handing them abortion rights in the absence of more long-term, socially integral, and probably expensive measures.

The Status of the Fetus

The flagship claim of the pro-life movement is that the embryo and fetus not only are human from the time of conception but have the full moral value of a person. The ground of this claim is the genetic uniqueness and completeness of every newly created life and its intrinsic ability to develop into a baby if left undisturbed in its natural environment, the uterus of its genetic mother. Millions of pages of debate have been spent on the validity of this claim, and these will not all be rehearsed here. Three prevalent criticisms of the idea that the fetus is a "person" from "the moment of conception" have focused on the facts that an embryo can split into more than one individual until about two weeks after fertilization, that embryos and fetuses that do not survive until birth are not treated religiously or culturally as if they were babies, and that a potential state is not the same as an actual one.[25]

Although abortion has been condemned as a sin (against the goods of marriage and procreation) since New Testament times, the status of the fetus has been open to discussion, even within Catholicism, up until the nineteenth century. In the late nineteenth century, the Vatican condemned the equivalent of partial-birth abortion (craniotomy) and stated unequivocally that all direct abortion is wrong, even if both mother and child will otherwise die.[26] Although the prohibition of abortion to save a woman's life has never been formally retracted, official Catholic teaching today rarely if ever reiterates this point. In a 1987 *Instruction* on infertility therapies, the Vatican reinforced its protective view toward life in the womb (or the petri dish), but aimed its critique more against widespread social practices than against crisis medical decisions involving individual women. The *Instruction* also grants a degree of doubt about the "personhood" of the embryo or fetus.

> Certainly no experimental datum can be in itself sufficient to bring us to the recognition of a spiritual soul; nevertheless, the conclusions of science regarding the human embryo provide a valuable indication for discerning by the use of reason a personal presence at the moment of the first appearance of a human life: how could a human individual not be a human person? The magisterium has not expressly committed itself to an affirmation of a philosophical nature, but it constantly reaffirms the moral condemnation of any kind of procured abortion.[27]

The intransigency of the abortion debate is due partly to the fact that, although determining with precision and clarity exactly what status and value the fetus has as a member of the human species is key to a cogent moral analysis of abortion, this determination has never been made in a conclusive and persuasive philosophical argument. And it probably cannot be. The link between various facts of fetal development and moral status is highly dependent on the worldview and value system of the interpreter (as the Catholic magisterium acknowledges) and is, moreover, just as highly implicated in the moral practices in which interpreters already participate. As far as the status of the fetus is concerned, ethical discourse about abortion must proceed in the presence of uncertainty.

As Kevin FitzGerald has noted in relation to debates about embryo research, "too often the opposing positions in the . . . debate are presented in terms of the obviousness of the assertions they make." Yet "the reality that informs these assertions is much less clear and certain than the debaters themselves often recognize."[28] Abortion debate appears irrational and hostile precisely because opposing parties refuse to confront and accept this fact. Instead they resort to the tactic of falling back on narrative and prophetic modes of discourse that are concordant with their own worldviews and social agendas. Not infrequently, they co-opt the "feminist" or "pro-life" language of the opposition, reinventing its meaning within their own symbol system.[29] They fail to engage their interlocutors in empathetic dialogue toward mutually acceptable solutions. Instead, they proceed as if their own narratives—symbolically enshrining the sanctity of unborn life on the one side, and women's right to control their own bodies on the other—were a clear and adequate basis on which to enact policies that affect both fetuses and women.

In an analysis of abortion that unfortunately still holds true, Karen Lebacqz asserts that "the way in which this issue is commonly debated today is a dead-end street that obscures rather than clarifies moral questions."[30] She continues,

> There are insurmountable difficulties in choosing a time at which the fetus is "human" or a "person" with rights. Not only do reasonable people disagree about what this time would be, but the disagreement is built into the nature of the question precisely because it is a moral issue. In my opinion, the most reasonable time for the acquisition of human rights or protectable "humanhood" is sometime after the time of twinning but long before the development of lung maturation or current standards of "viability." Thus I would argue that most abortions done today are on fetuses that have acquired some minimum of rights.[31]

It is not in doubt that human embryos and fetuses are human and are alive, thus constituting "human life." The issue is what moral status they have in the early stages of development, a status to which reference is often made by means of the category "person." Though what constitutes personhood is exactly the matter of debate, the ethical valence of the term is to convey that those individuals who come under it should be accorded full rights, respect, participation, and protection within the human community of subjects.[32]

It may well be the case that there is no one "dividing line" at which a developing human life acquires a unique new status that was completely absent before that time. Even setting the line very early, such as two weeks (the time of final "individuation" and the end of the possibility of twinning), seems to imply that before that time the embryo has negligible value and immediately after it, a value equal to that of its mother.[33] Both seem implausible. The integral relation and interdependence of human embodiment and human identity recommend the conclusion that the moral status of developing life also develops. If the fetus has an incremental value that develops during pregnancy, this makes ethical analysis of situations in which the needs of mother and fetus conflict, or in which a good can be achieved only at the price of destroying an embryo, quite uncertain. Uncertainty is heightened by the fact that there is disagreement over and no clear criterion for deciding whether that developing value begins as fairly heavy and warranting restriction of interference from the outset or as fairly insignificant and warranting only attitudes of "respect" in the process of destroying it.

Christian tradition overall has seen life from conception as worthy of serious if not absolute protection. This hermeneutic has weight today as a "hermeneutic of suspicion" against the discourses of science and the market that aim to make embryos available for profitable technologies and against the discourse of political and economic liberalism that adopts the rhetoric of "choice" in order to promote abortion rights in lieu of social welfare rights. It is essential to seek solutions to crisis pregnancy that empower and support women and avoid the need for abortion. The precise status of the embryo or fetus remains uncertain. Problematic, puzzling, and uncomfortable as this uncertainty may be, ethical analysis of abortion (and of destruction of embryos in general) may have to coexist with it.

Creating Solidarity

How then to proceed? Conclusive ethical determination of the spectrum of justifications for abortion is unavailable, but the value of developing life and the value and equality of women should guide social policy regarding pregnancy, parenthood, and, when and if necessary, abortion. Key to moving abortion ethics, politics, and policy to a new and more productive level is the cultivation of an ethos of solidarity that can create and sustain practices that reduce conflicts of value and needs and mediate solutions when conflicts arise.

An ethos of solidarity is a contrast to the ethos of liberal individualism that currently pervades both the pro-choice and pro-life movements. The public advocacy of both focuses on individual rights that clash irremediably with the rights or needs of others. The feminist philosopher Sandra Harding characterizes modern western liberalism as a systematic worldview organizing the state, science, and the economy. In the liberal outlook or ethos, "human beings are essentially rational individuals possessing timeless and universal natural rights, and . . . when such rights conflict, they should be adjudicated through the free market of social contracts."[34] Debates over the personhood of the fetus are essentially about whether or to what degree fetuses can be considered "rational individuals." Such debates serve merely as a distraction from the fact that "liberal" society is in reality ordered so as to exclude from social viability many of those to whom full "personhood" is granted in the abstract. Harding believes that both pro-life and pro-choice feminists have a stake in refuting liberal assumptions, for both agree that women's full humanity is denied in the actual sexist, racist, and classist social order in which liberal values are implemented. Neither women nor fetuses are given equal recognition, nor do women have equal access to "contractual" solutions to their problems.

In a provocative study of American law, Mary Ann Glendon substantiates her claim that "we" in the United States

> lead the developed world in our extreme liberty of abortion, while we lag behind the countries to which we most often compare ourselves in the benefits and services we provide to mothers and to poor families, and in the imposition and collection of child support obligations."[35]

Most European countries ensure paid parental leaves, publicly supported child care for preschool children, and cash grants to families with children. "A Martian trying to infer our culture's attitude toward children from our abortion and social welfare laws might think we had deliberately decided to solve the problem of children in poverty by choosing to abort them rather than to support them with tax dollars."[36] The clash between the "rights of the unborn" and the "rights of women" comes across as a zero-sum game, skewed by the tacit belief of many that women in poverty, especially if they are members of racial and ethnic minorities, do not deserve assistance. African American theologian Traci West detects in the policing of black women's sexuality, through the stigmatization of "illegitimacy," a racist social program that excludes women and children from social welfare[37] (and makes abortion seem a more attractive or at least more accessible option). Clearly, abortion cannot be addressed apart from larger issues of social justice, issues that cannot be surfaced, much less resolved, on a liberal model of social relationships.

Although it may remain useful to employ the "rights" language that ordinarily structures the abortion debate, rights must be conceived within the contexts of sociality and community and adjudicated in a spirit of solidarity. Of particular relevance to the abortion dilemma is the fact that duties or obligations can bind humans to their counterparts in ways to which they have not explicitly consented. Such obligations find little room in the liberal outlook. In the liberal ethos that originated with the seventeenth-century social contract theorists, and that has shaped the American constitutional tradition, persons are seen as free and autonomous agents for whom society exists to protect mutual agreements based on self-interest.

But there are some moral bonds that can arise among human beings and within and among societies simply as a result of reciprocal relatedness, and not because of free consent. The mother-fetus relation is characterized by obligations of this sort, as are all parent-child relations. Beyond the specific focus of childbearing, members of communities have obligations to sustain one another, especially in times of urgent need or crisis, whether or not such obligations were intentionally undertaken or even foreseen. A theory of the common good begins with the premise that persons are by definition interrelated in a social whole whose fabric of reciprocal rights and duties constitutes the very condition of their individual and communal agency and well-being. The community is prior to the individual, and each individual is entitled to participate in the community and share in its benefits as well as obligated to contribute to the good of the whole and of fellow members.

The present cultural dominance of the idea that every woman has a right to decide for herself, and on the basis of her own religious and moral convictions, whether or not to have an abortion does have positive aspects, especially as correcting conventions of sex and reproduction that are biased against women. The pro-choice position represents positive recognition of the full humanity, dignity, and equality of women and the need to take women seriously as moral agents. On the twenty-fifth anniversary of *Roe v. Wade,* Frances Kissling, president of Catholics for a Free Choice, made an impassioned plea for resistance to "conservative" forces opposing abortion.

> Most of us worked for abortion rights because we had a deep and uncompromising commitment to the social recognition of women's moral capacity to make the most controversial and complex life decisions we could imagine. We believed that women had the right to decide when, whether, and how to bring new life into the world.[38]

Societal and legal protection of the freedom to control childbearing, through abortion if necessary, represents a challenge to those dimensions of marriage, family, and employment that continue to oppress and subordinate women. To leave abortion decisions to the discretion of the agent most directly and intimately involved is to acknowledge the individuality that attends every moral decision, especially decisions that are complex, filled with conflict, and even tragic. It also respects and restores women's agency in the sphere of reproduction.

However, and more negatively, an individualistic view of a woman as a self-determining moral agent can cut her off from the social conditions necessary to support meaningful choice among viable options. It also omits attention to the moral bonds that may arise between a woman and the dependent life she carries, bonds that are not only obvious but anguishing to many women seeking abortions. These bonds are represented by the pro-life position. The liberal ethos also downplays the bonds between such women, other members of the community, and the community as a whole and its institutions, bonds that demand responsive initiatives of support. By overemphasizing rationality and freedom, and by absolutizing "civil liberties," the liberal ethos neglects and even denigrates human embodiment, the relationships deriving from physical proximity and material interdependence, the material conditions necessary to well-being, and material welfare obligations.

Yet, from the pro-life side, insistence that Catholic politicians adhere to the anti-abortion stance of their denominational leadership is rarely matched by adherence to the Vatican's calls for socioeconomic solidarity with the poor. Where are the demands that Catholics defend and vote for domestic programs that would match the rhetoric of recent social encyclicals? Observing that "a human embryo can never turn out to be a cat or dog," Kenneth Woodward chides Mario Cuomo, Catholic and former governor of New York, for not taking a strong public stand against the legal right to abortion.[39] Woodward insists on the link between private conviction and public action, and he mentions that work, education, and lack of financial support are among the reasons for abortion. Yet he never addresses the need (and the "Catholic" obligation) to alleviate these causes or acknowledges that the programs favored by Cuomo and other Democrats may have done more to reduce the actual number of abortions than thirty years of mostly fruitless hammering against *Roe v. Wade* by social conservatives. Similarly, Germain Grisez asserts that Catholic politicians who support abortion funding "intend to promote the killing of the innocent." Leaving aside the question whether such politicians rather could be intending to deter illegal abortions or to reach legislative compromises in which other pro-life goals might be served, it should be noted that Grisez does mention supports for pregnant women, but thinks in terms of "diapers, cribs, and so forth."[40]

Cuomo's rejoinder, which consists, in part, of reflection on the role of law, voices the surmise that few Americans view all abortion as "murder" and includes reference to measures other than legal restriction that Cuomo instituted as governor. These programs aimed "to reduce abortions by reducing the number of unintended pregnancies" and to assure "a poor woman who did find herself unintentionally pregnant all the resources she needed to bring the fetus to term and then have the child adopted by a suitable parent or parents."[41] In a 1984 Notre Dame address on abortion, Cuomo explicitly tied such measures to episcopal teaching and called for pro-life and pro-choice cooperation on making them more available. His vision ranged widely, from prenatal care to education and job training.[42]

Abortion and Gender: The Credibility Gap

Unfortunately, in much of the Catholic self-presentation, anti-abortion polemics run far ahead of pro-woman advocacy, and the treatment of abortion as a moral dilemma is out of alignment with treatment of other types of just and unjust killing. An intricate casuistry, using the principle of double effect, is used to excuse the agent from sin if the abortion can be categorized as "indirect," but not if it involves the direct killing of the fetus, ostensibly even if the death of the woman will result. For example, the *Ethical and Religious Directives for Catholic Health Care Services* states categorically, "Abortion (that is, the directly intended termination of pregnancy before viability or the directly intended destruction of a viable fetus) is never permitted."[43] In this analysis, a pharmacological or surgical measure to remedy a serious threat to a pregnant woman's health is approved, even if it causes a miscarriage, and even if it is the uterus or fallopian tube that must be removed, for example, in the case of cancer. However, directly removing the fetus in order to decrease strain on the woman's cardiac function would not be allowed. Clear lines are thus drawn between moral culpability when direct killing is involved and lack of culpability when an action "indirectly" results in the death of the fetus.

As became evident in the discussion of euthanasia in chapter 4, the distinction between indirect and direct action and intention may well be unable to bear all the weight that traditional moral theology has placed on it. In existential experiences of highly conflictual or tragic decision making, it may even break down. In any event, it is facile to assume that double effect can neatly separate agents from the responsibility they bear for "indirectly" caused harms, and just as neatly determine moral blame even in the most difficult cases of situational pressures and dearth of acceptable alternatives. Although the category of "adverse virtue" might justly and prudently be employed in assessing borderline actions that result in human deaths, theological tradition and current official teaching do not acknowledge this fact consistently.

Christine Gudorf contrasts the approach to abortion as a morally simple problem with an approach to the taking of innocent life in war that leaves a wide margin for the determination of when such killing is really "direct" and that attempts to persuade rather than coerce military leadership and individual combatants. Though she (generously) does not attribute this discrepancy to sexism on the part of official church teachers, she does maintain that "the continuation of methodological inconsistency which discriminates against women as moral persons is possible only in a climate of misogyny," a social climate in which women are raped, beaten, objectified in medical care, and denied control over the reproductive capacities of their own bodies.[44]

An issue clearly related to abortion is sexual morality, and sexuality cannot be addressed apart from gender roles and relationships. In addition to the value of unborn human life, the "Catholic message" on abortion includes a theology of sex that asserts an intrinsic relation between sexuality and parenthood that affirms the shared responsibility of women and men in the family and the social participation for both women and men as a requirement of social justice.[45] Unfortunately, the power of this message on abortion, sexual responsibility, and justice for women is undermined by the Catholic Church's record on women's roles and by a continued teaching on sex that ties its purposes too closely to the procreative structure of isolated sex acts. Catholicism's ambivalence about both sex and women cripples its call to Americans to come together in support of the unborn. The moral courage to work out more demanding but less violent solutions than abortion is undercut in the absence of full political commitment to the reform of discriminatory social institutions and by the attitude that women do not really have a right to control their fertility or to seek roles beyond motherhood as equally important to their identities.

Ambivalence about sex, gender, and women's agency in resolving problem pregnancies is persistent. It is an obstruction to feminist theologians and theological bioethicists who want to avoid or discourage abortion while still fully supporting women. One Catholic woman who gave up her first child for adoption but opted to abort a second pregnancy recounts how as a student at a Catholic college she found it impossible to reconcile bearing a child out of wedlock with being a "good Catholic girl." Yet when she gave up her baby for adoption, she was emotionally devastated by the lack of preparation and ongoing support. Eventually, she also realized that she was not confronting her own sexual behavior, the emotional needs behind it, or its repeated consequences. Her Catholic education and "support system" had not furnished her with any personal or moral compass to guide imperfect behavior that did not conform to acceptable norms, to think through the prospect of motherhood and adoption maturely, or to imagine and construct a life with her child in a community of support.[46]

In 2004, Angela Senander followed up a recent statement by the Jesuit provincials of the United States in favor of support for the unborn by checking the websites of the twenty-eight Jesuit colleges and universities for support services for pregnant students.[47] She found that only seven schools offered pregnancy tests, four schools offered counseling, two offered campus ministry resources, one identified a women's center as a resource, and only three offered the possibility of deferring student loans. Notable exceptions are Georgetown University and Marquette University, both of which offer a comprehensive response through a single website.

Senander has also conducted an extensive analysis of activities of the National Conference of Catholic Bishops on behalf of pro-life causes.[48] Senander's own position is that liberation theology's "option for the poor" should be applied to girls and women in crisis pregnancies, giving rise to social action that can liberate from the need to choose abortion because there are no other alternatives. Senander also sees this objective as a way to unite pro-life and pro-choice feminists around common goals. She discerns interest in the pro-choice movement as well in moving past a single-issue focus on abortion and toward a more integral approach to abortion that would link it with health care access, education, employment, child care, and housing.[49] Catholic feminist Mary Segers, a political scientist, represents a correlative modification of the pro-choice position when she grants that the morality of abortion is at times questionable and that "education, health care and other non-coercive measures" should be used to reduce it.

> Catholic moral teaching has much to offer a secular society which can be casual and calculating in decisions about human dignity and life. In particular, Catholic teaching on social justice supports social solidarity and advocates the kinds of broad initiatives which would enable involuntarily pregnant women to genuinely choose to bring new life into the world.[50]

The ecclesial and theological leadership in the U.S. Catholic Church has not been very successful in advancing such objectives, however. In recent years, the NCCB (now USCCB) has moved past recitation of the Second Vatican Council's condemnation of abortion as an "abominable crime"[51] and toward recognition that women have abortions due to entangled circumstances for which responsibility is shared. For example, in the 1995 pastoral letter *Faithful for Life,* the bishops name and applaud the social and emergency services provided by Catholic Charities, by more than three thousand emergency pregnancy centers nationwide, by hospitals and medical centers, by adoption agencies, and by programs of emotional and spiritual healing in the aftermath of abortion. They also recognize that pregnant women and mothers need long-term support, such as housing, and pledge solidarity with women in seeking to augment such benefits.[52]

However, as Senander points out, the bishops have neither made these broad changes as visible a part of their pro-life platform as resistance to legal abortion nor been as vocal in seeking justice for women generally in society. Nor do they advocate equality for women in the church at a level that matches their recognition of women who are already serving in social leadership positions as government officials, judges, doctors, business executives, college presidents, and faculty in higher education.[53] Therefore, their practices and those of the Catholic institutions they lead do not match their theological rhetoric. The participatory side of the USCCB's theological bioethics is out of line with its ethical and policy analysis. The narratives of Catholic identity that the episcopacy has promoted around abortion, and the "prophetic" actions many bishops have taken, do not add up to practical solidarity with women in crisis pregnancies.

During election years, bishops are much more visible in support of candidates who favor retraction of the legal right to abortion as well as restrictive welfare laws than in support of candidates who accept the legality of abortion but want to expand health care and other social services. The fact of being pro-choice was enough to make some U.S. bishops state that they would deny communion to 2004 Democratic presidential candidate John Kerry, despite the fact that he sought to enact much more extensive national health care reforms than his Republican opponent, George W. Bush. Confirming the analysis of Christine Gudorf, none proposed to deny communion to Catholic officials prosecuting the Bush administration's war in and occupation of Iraq, despite the fact that by the time of the 2004 elections, it had cost thousands of civilian lives and had been condemned by Pope John Paul II.

The bishops, Catholic health facilities, and the CHA are also adamant in their opposition to any legal requirement that services under Catholic auspices provide access to family planning measures that violate Catholic teaching, including contraception, sterilization, and abortion.[54] In turn, pro-choice advocates attack Catholic health providers who avoid these services, even though those same providers may be aggressively seeking ways to provide health care and other services to underserved populations and to change state and federal policy to support women, children, and families in a variety of ways.[55] Moreover, while Catholic providers may not have formal policies endorsing steps such as emergency contraception or sterilization, practices may be more complex and flexible at the "ground level." Again, different sides of the abortion debate should come together more productively to seek means of avoiding unwanted pregnancy, support pregnant women, help families to cope with a hostile public welfare environment, and militate for more inclusive family-friendly policies.

A critical review of the effects of U.S. welfare reforms (The Personal Responsibility and Work Opportunity Act of 1996) shows that effects on poor single-parent families have been dire. This law "changed the nature of welfare, transforming it from an entitlement for low-income single-parent families funded by a federal matching grant to states into a block grant system that allowed states to impose an array of sanctions and even mandated time limits and a set of work requirements for fixed percentages of state caseloads."[56] The law also included reductions in other benefits, including food stamps, child nutrition programs, and grants for social services and support for disabled children.

An especially problematic aspect of the new policy is the so-called family cap, which is a policy of denying to families already on welfare an increase following the birth of another child. The 1996 law allowed states to implement a family cap, and twenty-three did so. New Jersey, through a federal waiver, had experimented with the family cap since 1992. Using data from 1992 to 1996, a Rutgers University study found that many women cited the cap as a reason not have additional children, and 14,000 fewer births did occur than would ordinarily have been expected in the target group. However, the number of abortions was 14,000 higher than expected in this same population. Moreover, 25,000 children had been denied benefits under the law.[57]

These findings galvanized opposition to the family cap. However, assaults on the resources available to single mothers and the poor continue. In September 2004, the Bush administration proposed cuts in the value of the subsidized housing vouchers to be provided to poor families in several urban areas, including Boston, New York, Detroit, Atlanta, Philadelphia, and Chicago.[58] Although Catholic organizations such as the CHA and Catholic Charities are tireless advocates for housing and other benefits, such advocacy needs to become a visible and integral part not only of the Catholic theological bioethics of abortion but also of all feminist ethics and bioethics that recognizes access to basic social goods as the precondition of meaningful decision making in relation to motherhood and family.

Sociologist James R. Kelly, who records the vagaries and nuances of U.S. Catholic abortion politics, detects at least a few issues on which activists from disparate points on the political spectrum have been able to form coalitions to work toward better policies and practical solutions. Granting that, in a reductionist political climate that worsens around election times, "a constructive contemporary politics of abortion is not likely," he still believes that "women and men of good will keep trying."[59]

For example, an abortion "common ground" effort was begun in St. Louis in 1990 by a pro-life lawyer, a past president of Missouri Citizens for Life, and the director and a staff member from St. Louis Reproductive Health Services.[60] The point of the project was not ideological conversion, or even conversation, but joint action to decrease the demand for abortions. Members banded together around better perinatal care, treatments for substance abuse, welfare reforms, day care, affordable housing, adoption, recruitment of foster parents, and job and educational opportunities and testified on measures before the state legislature. Yet the phrase "common ground" has rarely been adopted by national leadership on either side of the question and instead is criticized as too compromising. An exception was a national coalition of religious, civil rights, and women's rights organizations that issued a press release in 1995 rejecting the family cap. They included the American Civil Liberties Union, the National Organization for Women, Catholic Charities USA, and Feminists for Life.[61] As

Kelly concludes, "Diminishing state support for poor women, rationalized by a moralistic language of self-reliance, constitutes the most severe kind of challenge for the integrity of both movements." Right-to-life advocates must question their political alliance with fiscal conservatives; right-to-choice advocates must reexamine their focus on liberty apart from substantive understandings of the common good.[62]

The main priority in supporting a candidate or a policy is the effect on the total social context within which "reproductive rights" and the "right to life," inclusively considered, are advanced or demeaned. James Kelly illustrates the adoption by theological bioethics of a "middle axioms" approach to policy, in light of the overarching common good. He surmises that "the Supreme Court is most unlikely to recriminalize all abortions" and draws the conclusion that federal legislation will be most successful in enhancing the conditions of life "not when it directly attacks Roe, but when it emphasizes real choices and alternatives to abortion." In his view, only marginal groups support either any abortion or no abortion, and there is an emerging consensus in favor of lowered support for abortion as the fetus increasingly resembles a baby at birth. He hopes to draw agreement from counterparts on the pro-choice side of the equation about the connections among the different types of violence represented by war, poverty, and abortion. Together, they may move toward consensus policies that support women and families without abolishing the legal right to abortion.[63]

In the model of "deliberative democracy" discussed in chapter 3, policy agreement is enabled by discourse that includes substantive and not only procedural values. Such discourse envisions traditions and worldviews that can introduce comprehensive moral frameworks and conceptions of ultimacy while remaining respectful of differing standpoints. Social change toward consensus and toward better policies will occur through interventionist practices that are supportive and inclusive rather than competitive and adversarial. Although abortion is generally regarded as one of the most divisive and insoluble cultural issues in America, religious traditions and participatory theology can contribute to the creation of local networks of transformation through dialogue and experimentation with better alternatives.

Abortion and the Roles of Law

Extremists and national leadership on both sides of this vexing debate are captive to a dichotomous mentality focused on federal legalization or abolition of a "right to abortion." Some feminist thinkers and theologians, as well as grassroots and local activists for women's and families' welfare, are seeking more creative ways to deal with the problem and exert pressure toward incremental changes in social policy that reduce abortions without penalizing women and children.[64] It is not sufficient for the law to enforce "a negative moral obligation prohibiting the killing of the innocent" in the absence of equally strong and even more vital "positive obligations to assist the weak and the vulnerable."[65]

First of all, even the enactment of negative prohibitions requires a consensus adequate to a law's enforceability. Furthermore, not every aspect of the common good or morality can be prescribed or forbidden by civil law, but only those requirements that are necessary for public order. In the tradition of John Courtney Murray, the scope of law is limited, and prudent laws must be able to be enforced or they will earn disrespect and threaten to bring contempt for the whole system of law of which they are a part.[66] In the words of a Catholic politician who was threatened with excommunication by his local bishop, "Society has unfortunately demonstrated for centuries that abortions will be performed regardless of the law. That raises the question of whether it is truly moral to discourage respect for all law by passing laws that are unenforceable."[67] Good laws sometimes have to combine, if not wholly reconcile, the moral convictions and goals of differing parties, whose mutual coexistence and cooperation are necessary for the common good. Members of religious traditions and theologians should be able to support such laws, even if they do not conform in every respect to their platform of moral values.[68]

Cathleen Kaveny points out that there are special problems involved in overturning a law that has become an assumed part of jurisprudence, of cultural attitudes toward women's rights, and of the medical system. Even just changes in law can be socially destabilizing if they are too sudden or extreme.[69] Therefore more moderate adjustments such as a requirement of parental involvement in the abortion decisions of minors or a waiting period might induce serious reflection about abortion and the exploration of other options, without taking away the basic legal right to choose abortion in the end. I would add that, as in the case of euthanasia, the social institutionalization and legal facilitation of the occasionally necessary exercise of adverse virtue can normalize the conditions requiring it. What should be a rare and regrettable response can easily become the standard anticipated solution. It is clear that in the United States, permissive abortion policy has discouraged rather than required serious moral probing of abortion choices and serious social attention to the conditions under which abortion has become a widespread practice. It has also deterred a sustained commitment to other remedies, especially those that cost more money.

Although the law does have a legitimate restraining function of preventing harms, it also has a pedagogical function of inducing virtue in those who respect, and understand the reasons behind, just and effective law.[70] Good law awakens people to their moral and social responsibilities; sometimes law is bad law precisely because it enables such responsibilities to be ignored or circumvented. The Civil Rights Act, the Family and Medical Leave Act, and the Americans with Disabilities Act all gesture "toward a vision of how the citizens of the United States should live their lives in common." Citizens should move beyond mere compliance to share in "the broader vision of community" that the law seeks to encourage.[71]

In addition to Kaveny's functions of "law as police officer" and "law as moral teacher," a third role might be envisioned: law as social enabler. Law not only restrains public vice and teaches social virtues, it also enables transformative collaborative action by creating expectations and institutions in which these virtues are put into practice. Good laws and policies do not merely teach citizens at the level of beliefs or individual moral character what a just society would look like but also engage people and groups in ways of life that make it more possible to coexist justly and in solidarity. While some such practices may be instigated by federal legislation or Supreme Court rulings, others are the result of laws and policies at the local, state, even international level. Many of these policies will be enabling and supportive rather than restrictive. When hammered out collaboratively through compromise, they will also educate for and enable virtues of social life that make it possible for "culture wars" to be transcended in the name of the common good. They can be an exercise in participatory and deliberative democracy, to which theology contributes by analysis, by prophetic critique of the status quo, and by forwarding realistic practical alternatives.

Even briefly, recognition should be given to abortion policy as an international issue on which religious groups and theologians have played a role. As on other matters of health care access, there is no overall legislative or policy-setting body to supervise and enforce practices in this difficult area. Cultural practices are notoriously variable, and just as notoriously, equal respect for women in matters of sexuality and family is low in many cultures that have permissive or coercive abortion policies, as well as in cultures that take strongly punitive stands toward women having abortions.[72]

Over and above national laws and practices, the safety and availability of abortion, as well as its attractiveness in relation to other options, is determined by family planning and women's health care subsidies provided through the United Nations or NGOs. The same tensions and inconsistencies beset religious involvement at this level as at the level of policy internal to the United States. At the 1994 UN Conference on Population and Development in Cairo, and the 1995 UN Fourth World Conference on Women in Beijing, Vatican representatives attempted both to advocate for women's social and domestic equality and to exclude approval of and funding for family planning services that included contraception, sterilization, and above all, abortion. Although the western media frequently seemed to highlight and exaggerate the anti-woman bias of Catholic representatives and to stress the adversarial nature of the relation between women's rights advocates and Vatican delegates, it is undoubtedly true that the latter made common cause with some of the nations with the most restrictive views of women's place in order to combat abortion.[73]

Although the Vatican resisted "liberal" rights activists at Beijing as inadequately respectful of community and solidarity, in the analysis of Bridget Burke Ravizza, it did not base its own positions and recommendations on consultation with women.[74] This was especially essential, not only in view of the exclusion of women from the formulation of the teachings backing the Beijing stands, but also because women in different cultural settings have needs, outlooks, and social constraints or opportunities that European and North American spokespersons may not fully appreciate. In this sense, the activist groups were seen as much more empowering of "grassroots" women and more sensitive to their needs.

In the global realities of women's lives, it is important to be mindful that many women around the world do not in fact seek freedom from reproduction and domesticity, but have different, perhaps more urgent, goals: freedom from sexual and domestic violence and the ability to bear and raise children safely and with hope for their own and their children's future. To these women, papal words about the dignity of motherhood and obligations to the poor may represent a significant advance over the status quo. Unfortunately, restricting abortion access will do little to help women without access to health care or family planning information, with little control over marriage and sex and with severely inadequate resources to feed and clothe their families. Abortion, legal or illegal, may continue to draw some of these women unless education and access to income or comparable social goods can be improved. Religious leadership against abortion will only have oppressive consequences to such women, unless it comes in the form of strong, consistent advocacy for women's overall well-being, formulated in dialogue with women themselves.

The moral and social problems of abortion are clearly not such as can be resolved by elites at the level of comprehensive legislation, whether generated by the U.S. Supreme Court, or even in a more global and "participatory" way by UN conferences, where policies are debated by high-level representatives in varying degrees of contact with a grassroots base. In the United States, abortion continues to be a politically and ecclesially intractable issue, at least at the ideological level. At the practical level, some pro-family activists, advocates for social benefits, women's groups of different sorts, analysts with religious and denominational ties, and theologians are crossing the divide. Models of the law as teacher and enabler take the focus off its restrictive function. They evoke the participatory mode of theological bioethical discourse to arrive at middle axioms on abortion policy that bring together ideals and the ability to compromise, while working with others toward common goals.

In deliberative democracy, expansive discourse has an important place. Theologians rightly place abortion against a horizon that includes the value of all life, God's care and providence, and judgment on human sinfulness. In a common good perspective, such symbols and narratives will function prophetically to awaken a critical approach to cultural norms and social structures that undermine women's agency in sexual relations, perpetuate socioeconomic divisions, and preclude collaborative social agency in response to family needs. A focus on the procedure of abortion disenables the participatory process that could lead, locally and globally, to more fundamental and necessary changes. These are, above all, education and economic opportunities for women, the essential preconditions of equality in decisions about sex and parenthood.

Assisted Reproductive Technology (ART)

"Modern medicine" has developed many new techniques to enhance the freedom and choice of women and couples in the "first world" who want to become parents. From a global perspective, these techniques are sold and used in a rarified atmosphere of medical sophistication, consumer power, free-form family building, and for-profit health care. They are also parasitic on continuing gender norms in which parenthood is seen as indispensable to social adulthood, especially for women, and in which women's fulfillment and flourishing are closely tied to maternity. Although motherhood is a "profoundly meaningful" experience, and a desirable one for many, it should not be portrayed as an ideal that completely fulfills or exhausts the meaning of life.[75] At the same time, women's increasing access to public and professional roles has meant delay of marriage and maternity, as well as an increased frequency of sexual activity before marriage. These trends contribute to infertility.[76] While ostensibly holding up the goal of motherhood for women, modern U.S. culture has failed by and large to reorganize professional roles in a way that accommodates domestic and family responsibilities for both women and men. In many respects, assisted reproductive technologies are a medical solution to a complex set of social challenges.

The U.S. Centers for Disease Control (CDC) defines ART as any "fertility treatments in which the egg and sperm are handled in the laboratory" and offers detailed assessments of their varieties, frequency, and success on its website.[77] Although sperm donation has been widely in use for decades, the birth of Louise Brown in Britain in 1978 signaled a new era of medical intervention into the reproductive process, one in which both male and female infertility could be combated by techniques that unite sperm and eggs outside the human body. The viability of women's ova decreases with age, especially after thirty-five. While only about 10 percent of women under thirty suffer miscarriages, the rate triples for women in their early forties. Even in younger women, fibroid tumors in the uterus can interfere with pregnancy; endometriosis or pelvic inflammatory disease can cause blockage of the fallopian tubes. Pelvic inflammatory disease is caused by bacteria, is sexually transmitted, can be avoided by the use of condoms, and results in infertility for about 100,000 women per year.[78] Men over forty are more likely to produce damaged sperm that can cause birth defects. There is a slight decline in sperm quality and motility after men turn forty-five, but these ordinarily remain within normal limits until age seventy.[79] Assisted reproductive technologies, especially in vitro fertilization, are rapidly developing and popular ways to resolve infertility.[80]

In vitro fertilization (IVF) can compensate for dysfunction in a woman's reproductive system and allow for the donation of both male and female gametes. Either sperm donation or in vitro fertilization can enable "surrogate motherhood," in which a woman is the genetic mother of and carries the child of a man whose wife is unable to become pregnant, or carries the embryo created from the gametes of a couple in which the woman has eggs but is unable to carry a pregnancy. Sometimes unfertilized eggs and sperm or zygotes are transferred into the fallopian tubes within a day or two of retrieval. These are known as gamete and zygote intrafallopian transfer (GIFT and ZIFT). Another adaptation is intracytoplasmic sperm injection (ICSI) in which fertilization is in vitro but is accomplished by injecting a single sperm directly into the egg, a technique developed for couples with male factor infertility. ICSI may increase the incidence of birth defects by forcing fertilization with defective sperm.[81]

In 1989, preimplantation genetic diagnosis (PIGD) of embryos conceived in vitro was used for the first time to identify embryos that carry the risk of inherited anomalies and to select healthy ones to attempt a pregnancy. Diseases that can be detected include cystic fibrosis, fragile X syndrome, Duchenne's muscular dystrophy, Tay-Sachs disease, hemophilia, Marfan syndrome, and sickle-cell anemia.[82] This same technique can also be used to select for genetically based preferred characteristics (such as sex), and not only to eliminate disease. In some cases, preimplantation diagnosis has been used to create a sibling donor for a child affected by a genetic disease.

The number of infants conceived through ART almost doubled between 1996 and 2001. As of 2001, there were 421 ART clinics in the United States. In 2001, 29,344 women gave birth to a living baby as a result of ART, which accounts for approximately 1 percent of total U.S. births. However, the number of ART cycles required to produce this result was 107,587, meaning that ART has a success rate of about 33 percent, varying with the clinics in which it is performed. Since 1992, clinics are legally mandated to provide data on their individual success rates to the CDC, which makes reports on individual clinics available on its website.[83]

Pregnancies associated with ART and drugs that induce ovulation are more likely to result in multiple births. This involves pregnancy complications and increased risk for mothers. Moreover, multiple births of three or more children carry greater risks of prematurity and low birth weight, which result not only in the death of many newborns but in serious long-term physical and mental disabilities. The resulting social and economic burdens for families and for society are substantial. To maximize birth-rates, physicians who perform IVF often transfer multiple embryos, which increases the risk. IVF success can be improved with donor eggs from younger women. For slightly more than 89 percent of the ART cycles in 2001, fresh or frozen nondonor eggs or embryos were used.[84] Due to social trends toward delayed marriage and childbearing, the use of donor eggs has become common, even allowing women in their fifties and sixties to become birth mothers. The number of births to women aged 45–54 rose to 45,666 in 2000.[85] Thus far, the oldest woman to give birth was sixty-three.[86] In 11 percent of ART cycles, eggs or embryos were donated by another woman. The risk for a multiple-birth delivery was highest for women who underwent ART transfer procedures using freshly fertilized embryos from either donor eggs (42 percent) or from their own eggs (36 percent).[87] In many cases, physicians use the technique of "fetal reduction" to abort some fetuses and increase the chance of a healthy birth for the remaining one or two. Yet some studies have also shown that, despite improvement of techniques to produce good outcomes of ART, there is greater risk to all children born of IVF than to those conceived naturally.[88]

Meanwhile, "spare" or "leftover" embryos that are created but not used by a couple for IVF or PIGD are frozen for possible later use. The American Society for Reproductive Medicine has published guidelines stipulating that no more than two to five embryos should be implanted in a woman at one time, the precise number depending on her chances of achieving pregnancy.[89] However, in the vicinity of fifteen might be fertilized at once. Remaining embryos are cryopreserved and can be kept indefinitely, though some clinics have a policy of disposing of them after a determinate number of years. These embryos may also be donated to research or to other couples. Either destruction of spare embryos or their instrumental use raises ethical issues that are partly contingent on the status accorded the embryo, the meaning of respect for it, the costs and burdens that would be involved in continuing to preserve it or implanting it in someone's womb, and the comparative worth of benefits to be derived for others from its use or disposal.

Since 1997, it has become possible to create an embryo by cloning, that is, by inserting the nucleus of a cell from one person into the enucleated egg of another, creating an embryo and potentially a child who has only one genetic parent, of whom he or she is the genetic "twin." As of 2005, there were no verified births resulting from reproductive cloning. The great majority of ethical commentators and policy advisory bodies have taken a negative stance on this variation of ART. Many voice objections based on the problematic nature of the individuality of the resulting child (even though he or she could not literally be the "copy" of the parent) and on the high level of control this would permit parents over the genetic identity of their children. At a minimum, concerns about safety, such as birth defects and unforeseeable long-term health outcomes, as well as about the need to reduce these by "practicing" on children, have led virtually all to exclude such a means of reproduction.[90] The use of cloned embryos to create stem cells for research and therapy has been much more widely accepted. The ethics of stem cell research involves uncertainty about the status of the embryo, the likelihood and significance of potential benefits, and the issue of who will have access to those benefits (to be addressed in the next chapter).

This wide array of reproductive options is not available without a high cost, despite the 66 percent failure rate. Fertility pills and artificial insemination can run from $1,000 to $2,000, with treatments involving injected drugs costing up to $5,000. In vitro fertilization with a woman's own eggs runs from $12,500 to $25,000, while donor eggs can take the expenses up to $35,000.[91] In fact, couples advertise in campus newspapers for young women donors of specified physical appearance, IQ, and artistic or athletic abilities. Entrepreneurs recruit attractive young donors and advertise their "services" (including "donation" of their eggs) to desperate consumers in the market for infertility help. One web advertiser features photographs of fetching young women (some inappropriately and suggestively posed), along with the credo: "Beauty is its own reward. This is the first society to truly comprehend how important beautiful genes are to our evolution." A page offering sperm for sale "auctions" a male model, posed in briefs, muscles gleaming.[92]

Infertility therapy is expensive and not generally covered by medical insurance; thus it is not surprising that most couples who seek it are primarily white, well-educated professionals. This is not the population that is most burdened by infertility, however. The profile of the typical woman is someone who is black and has less than a high school education. Socioeconomic status is a defining condition of access to reproductive technologies, and the "medical marketplace" responds to the needs or wants of those with purchasing power.[93]

It is not uncommon for couples to spend in the hundreds of thousands of dollars in their quest to bear a child who is biologically related to at least one of them or to fulfill the woman's drive to experience pregnancy and childbirth. And the emotional and physical tolls are high; infertility therapies require an intrusive and rigorous regimen of drugs, medical procedures, and scheduled sex that can throw lives into chaos and put relationships under stress. Many who have experienced the process have written about the all-consuming nature of what becomes a single-minded focus on bearing a child and the seemingly irreversible momentum toward ever more extreme, exotic, low-success, or high-risk technologies.[94] The

United States, and some European countries such as Belgium, where the infertility industry is virtually uncontrolled by law, attract foreigners who are unable to access desired services in their own countries. Reproductive "tourism" circulates clients in search of egg donors, donors for women past menopause, insemination with a brother's sperm, insemination with the sperm of a deceased husband, preimplantation diagnosis for sex selection, surrogate mothers, and so on.[95]

The more responsible and socially conscious infertility experts worry about exploitation of the infertile couple. Partly due to the rise in obstetrical malpractice suits, physicians are branching out into subspecialties without adequate training. The new technology is developing "in an ethical and regulatory vacuum." And for-profit entities are advancing into the infertility arena.[96] Patient expectations become inflated when specific clinics advertise success rates that far exceed those substantiated in the literature; some clinics exclude patients who are unlikely to conceive in order to protect their rates.[97] One group of specialists in reproductive endocrinology and infertility observes, "Unfortunately, in a consumer-driven medical care system, the [ethical] physician is often in a precarious position of having to offer premature or indiscriminate therapy to those who demand it, or risk losing the patient to a more accommodating competitor."[98] "Desperate" patient demand is something that not all physicians resist, and some may even solicit and exploit it. To the contrary, and perhaps in a minority, these professionals assert, "our integrity as a specialty demands that we resist misdirected pressure applied by our patients and adhere to the most appropriate course of treatment."[99] What constitutes an *ethically* appropriate course of treatment for infertility remains, however, under debate.

Theological and Ethical Analysis

Early religious commentators tended to be cautious, if not alarmed, with a few exceptions.[100] However, they were much more ready to accept technologies used by married couples than donor methods (including sperm donation). Concerns about whether even ART in marriage reinforces patriarchal views of women's need for motherhood or male control over women's bodies, and about social injustice in access to these methods or in recruitment of donors, did not surface in the debates of the 1970s and even 1980s to the extent that they did later. Rather, the key concern was whether there is a created and thus "natural" unity of marital love and procreation that the introduction of a donor violates. From a biblical standpoint, and in a "classic" though typically convoluted statement, Paul Ramsey asserts that

> we procreate new beings like ourselves in the midst of our love for one another, and in this there is a trace of the original mystery by which God created the world because of His love. God created nothing apart from His love; and without the divine love was not anything made that was made. Neither should there be among men and women (whose man-womanhood—and not their minds or wills only—is in the image of God) any love set out of the context of responsibility for procreation, any begetting apart from the sphere of love.[101]

In other words, just as God creates out of love, so must human beings; it is the human body and not only our free intentions that image God. Human bodily procreation must remain within the sphere of love represented by marriage. It is not enough to simply decide or choose that a couple's parental love will take shape around an act of conception constituted by the physical (genetic) union of one spouse with a third party, via the meeting of their gametes. Ramsey is also concerned about the depersonalization of children and the possibility that the whole process of procreation will be invaded by technology and commercialization.

Richard McCormick concurs in this analysis:

> We are face to face once again with an all too familiar and destructive dualism, where persons love and care in many ways, but not in their sexual intercourse or procreation. Ultimately such an attitude is rooted in a principle that depreciates the body and disallows its participation in the specifically human."[102]

McCormick does not object to measures undertaken within marriage in order to support the fertility (and love) of the couple.[103] But, like Ramsey, he is worried about the "technologization" of marriage, the wasting of extra embryos, and possible risk to the children born of such a procedure.

Among feminist theologians, Catholics seem to have been more prolific in addressing the new reproductive technologies, probably because they belong to a church with an unusually vocal and dogmatic teaching authority, one that has frequently been associated with positions on gender and reproduction that assign women to domestic and maternal roles, even while narrowly limiting legitimate means to achieve pregnancy. Protestant and Jewish women had no such authoritative body against which to react and tended cautiously to follow the cultural trend to view such technologies as medical measures in the battle against infertility.[104] Writings by Catholic women around the time ART became common took aim first of all at the idea that "artificial" conception was immoral even for a married couple using their own gametes.[105] Margaret Farley granted provisional acceptance to technologies such as artificial fertilization as aiding "just and responsible procreation," if it is safe, conducive to the development of the child, and meets criteria of distributive justice.[106]

The stricter position adopted by the Vatican in 1987 continues to guide policy in Catholic health facilities. The *Instruction on Respect for Human Life* (*Donum vitae*) declared that all types of reproductive assistance that in any way destroy embryos, violate the procreative unity of the marriage bond, or separate sex from the process of conception violate the norms of natural law and should be prohibited by the civil authorities. This rules out even techniques such as IVF or artificial insemination using a wife's and husband's eggs and sperm. Interestingly, though, the Vatican acknowledges that homologous (husband-wife) insemination "is not marked by all that ethical negativity found in extraconjugal procreation; the family and marriage continue to constitute the setting for the birth and upbringing of the children."[107] Nevertheless, even in marriage, such technologies interrupt the union of sex, love, and procreation and deprive human generation of its proper meaning and function.[108] They also violate the dignity of the child and the relation of parents and child by establishing "the domination of technology over the origin and destiny of the human person."[109] The *Instruction* does allow space for therapies that do not circumvent fertilization by sexual intercourse.[110] Some justify procedures such as the supplementation of natural intercourse with insemination by the husband's sperm, or GIFT, in which the gametes are collected and placed in the fallopian tube, where fertilization occurs.[111]

In the past three decades, theological and ethical literature on these matters has been extensive.[112] Of note is the emergence of a more positive analysis, under the aegis of the idea that responsible human freedom includes the invention of ways to relieve human suffering by using technologies to personal and social advantage, even if they interrupt bodily processes and kinship relations that used to be regarded as "natural." Many contemporary readers will discern instead that neither the claims of Ramsey nor the claims of the Vatican are "clinched" by the arguments they offer. Both raise legitimate concerns, as does McCormick, about the ideal nature of parenthood in marriage, but they have not demonstrated conclusively that only one answer to the problems raised by birth technologies is persuasive and acceptable. McCormick may be right that more goes into the creation of moral convictions than "rational" arguments and that arguments that may appear rational often owe a large debt to premises that can be questioned.

As if to underline this point, subsequent authors, including theologians, have questioned whether the bond between the "spheres" of love and biological cooperation for procreation was as tight as these early analyses made it seem. Jean Porter does not regard it as "either possible or desirable to identify clear-cut, absolute prohibitions in the areas of sexual and reproductive morality, given the central importance of the affective and relational for this dimension of human life."[113] Paul Lauritzen defends donor insemination (and by extension other donor methods) on the basis that the love of a couple for a child is paramount, even if there is an asymmetry in their biological relation to it.[114] In the view of Ted Peters, "the explosion of progress in reproductive technologies is creating choice in a dimension of life we previously consigned to destiny, namely procreating children."[115] Developing what he calls a "proleptic ethics," Peters defines human dignity in terms of an eschatological future oriented by Jesus Christ. In this future, it is not biological kinship or genetics that defines human relationships, but spiritual unity. In the image of God, we are "created co-creators" who look optimistically toward the future and guide our actions by love, not biology.[116]

While Peters rightly incorporates the priority of inclusive love in his ethic of family and parenthood, a question not yet fully resolved is the role of kinship and biology in defining family relationships in the here and now, and in light of long-standing cultural and religious assumptions about family bonds as somehow related to sexually consummated, permanent male-female relationships and the offspring that result from them. Philosopher Thomas Murray maintains that

> control and choice—the values at the heart of procreative liberty—are not entirely out of place in the relationship between parents and children. But they are hardly the entire story, or even the most important themes, and excesses of control and choice can distort and destroy what is most precious in families.[117]

Few theologians today would absolutize biology or refuse to recognize families built in nontraditional ways, for example, through adoption. But insofar as humans are embodied and families are understood in some ways to reflect and respect sexual and reproductive embodiment, the challenge of explaining the importance of embodied relationship to the general definition of parenthood remains.

Many feminists have been concerned with the impact on women of the new forms of assisted reproduction and of new types of prenatal and preimplantation genetic testing. For theologians and others, women's self-determination is a major principle in the ethics of reproduction. In general, feminist theologians view reproductive technologies as enabling women's choices about pregnancy and motherhood. However, few see them as unqualified goods. Most are well aware of the coercive effects of such options on women; some are also concerned with the instrumentalization of embryos, fetuses, or children, and an increasing number are alarmed at the social cost of new technologies and their potential to exacerbate natural and social inequities of birth. With the newest innovations of cloning and stem cell research, concerns about reproduction and the embryo take a different turn, as questions of distributive justice in the allocation of research funds and access to promised therapies become predominant.

Maura Ryan has developed the economic criterion from a feminist and theological standpoint and pressed the larger question of whether and when the intensive use of technology serves the real interests of women.[118] Weaving in resources from law, medicine, theology, and first-person infertility accounts (including her own), Ryan skillfully nuances a judicious argument that infertility therapies should be viewed as reasonable medical remedies. Yet they can also reinforce women's "desperation" in the face of coercive social constructions of motherhood and can embody or exacerbate inequities in access to health care. From the standpoint of relief of suffering as a goal of medicine, the suffering caused by illness goes beyond the physical to include psychosocial dimensions, and these are particularly acute for the infertile. Both men and women see themselves "not as having imperfect or malfunctioning bodies, but as having spoiled identities."[119] Although medical treatment can play into the very ideologies that cause such reactions, bioethics must be realistic about "the ends of medicine." Medicine can primarily address only the physical causes of infertility; in cases in which those cannot be removed, the person will need to rely on other personal and social resources to resolve the suffering of infertility. And although medicine as such cannot resolve every social issue, it is still part of a social climate that may need transformation so that infertility may be more adequately "defined, lived, ministered to, and potentially transcended."[120]

One useful part of Ryan's study is her discussion of the relative weight of the biologically based aspects of parenthood and those aspects that involve affective and emotional ties and social and personal commitment. Although the latter are more definitive of human relationships in general, Ryan recognizes that the former are also relevant, though not decisive (e.g., in cases of adoption). Rather than trying to minimize either side of parenthood, she acknowledges that a right balance is important but not easy to find, and must be tailored to different kinds of circumstances.

Ryan pursues the justice aspects of reproductive technologies in the context of the common good by first defining parenthood as a form of social participation, the basic conditions of which society has some duty to provide. Health is a "capacity for acting in the world, for pursuing vital goals."[121] Even though women's life goals cannot be reduced to motherhood, bearing children may still be considered as a basic human capacity that some legitimately desire to realize and that can integrate those engaging in it into important social relationships.[122] However, the right to advanced infertility services is not defensible if it compromises the access of others to basic health needs or if it maintains the privilege of some by disadvantaging others.

Theologian Deborah Blake agrees and states even more strongly, "A fundamental moral concern surrounding the use of complex reproductive technologies is the lack of solidarity with the poor and personal complicity with an unjust structure." The use of such technologies cannot be exempted from their "social, economic, and political context" or from "responsibility for the common good."[123] In Ryan's view, infertility treatment ought to be funded on an equitable basis, which will require placing some limits on the types of treatments available by combining considerations of cost and likely effectiveness in view of the particular circumstances of the patient. For example, patients could be required to try less costly measures first, and limits could be placed on the number of times certain treatments should be used.

Finally, Ryan reflects the orientation of participatory theological bioethics when she turns to the resources of faith communities for a spirituality that can contend constructively with the problem of infertility, at both an individual and communal level. The inability to bear children is not a problem with which most religious traditions have dealt well, instead portraying barrenness as a curse and fertility as a blessing from God. More recognition could be given to adopting parents and infertile "hopeful parents" in community liturgies, while special liturgies could be developed to mourn both infertility and pregnancy loss, as well as to mark the end of "aggressive infertility treatment."[124] A "transformative spirituality" will not be built on "the expectation of miracles," but on "the constant companionship of God in the experience of infirmity, disappointment, or despair." Communities of faith need not deny reality, but can become sites where "transcendent hope" can be witnessed, and "the capacity to trust that all things, even our present sufferings, are working to good can be learned."[125]

Elisabeth Brinkmann probes similar possibilities by reaching into the Christian past for creative alternatives to liberal, radical, and care-based feminist approaches to reproductive technologies. Brinkmann draws parallels between medieval women who suffered because the birthing female body was construed as deficient by their culture, and modern women who suffer because infertility is construed as a deficiency from the womanly norm of motherhood. Just as medieval women overcame the idea they were "defective and misbegotten" by identifying with the suffering, bleeding, and "feeding" body of the crucified Christ, contemporary women can avoid the unsatisfying ethic of control proposed by modern infertility medicine and integrate their suffering "into a life of generativity" and "loving service to others," whether family building through adoption or other social commitments.[126]

The use of ARTs is not limited to creating pregnancy. They also enable unprecedented control over the health of the child to be born. In vitro fertilization, combined with advances in genetic analysis, has made it possible (whether in the context of infertility or not) to select embryos with certain characteristics. Originally performed to avoid gene-based diseases and abnormalities, PIGD can also be used to further preferences for identifiable "normal" traits. The inequitable social implications of this prospect are only too evident, as those with more income have access to greater levels both of "medically indicated" and of elective genetic intervention. Nevertheless, these technologies are promoted as expanding reproductive choice, even though they can also create stress for pregnant women and create a social bias against the birth of children that are predicted to suffer "abnormalities."

As the authors of an annotated bibliography note, many feminists resist the subtle control of procreation through criteria that are formulated in terms of genetic health, but are more defined by social than scientific norms. They also connect international population control with the medicalization of procreation.[127] Europeans, perhaps more than North Americans, are concerned with the social and medical ideologies that predetermine "free choice."[128] Genetic technologies are loaded with symbolic meanings. In the process of "individualization" that has occurred in postindustrial societies since World War II, individuals leave traditional belief systems and structures of power and support. Yet, rather than being "autonomous," the individual experiences "new forms of social entrenchment and control," exerted not by external authorities but by internalized norms that predetermine "free and autonomous" decisions.[129]

People in western societies perceive themselves to have a high degree of control over their personal lives, but this also heightens the expectation of greater individual accountability and responsibility.[130] Social pressure to become parents, but to avoid giving birth to "defective" and "burdensome" children; the belief of individuals and couples that they can and should have control over procreative abilities and outcomes; and the rapid development of sophisticated and profitable medical technology that offers such control are forces that converge to create an unbridled demand for ARTs and plentiful opportunities for those who furnish them to exploit individual desires while ignoring the common good. Regulation of ARTs in light of the restraining, educative, and enabling functions of the law is clearly long overdue.

Toward Regulation

The need for some form of improved social control over ARTs motivates the 1994 report of the President's Council on Bioethics, *Reproduction and Responsibility*,[131] as well as a comprehensive analysis published by the Hastings Center.[132] Both address problematic social trends. *Reproduction and Responsibility* concentrates its attention on technologies that involve manipulation of the embryo outside the human body, especially in ARTs. It identifies lack of information about the long-term health effects of these interventions on women and children and recommends a federally funded study of risks and benefits.[133] The PCB report frames its discussion in terms of substantive human goods, two of which are the "liberal" values of reproductive freedom and privacy. Others are relief of the suffering of infertility, confidentiality, compassion for children with genetic diseases, "human dignity" including the dignity of the body, parental and intergenerational relationships, justice in access, and "the fundamental value of human life and the respect owed to it in its various stages."[134] Ultimately the report acknowledges the need for greater public discussion, with the immediate need to prohibit "boundary-crossing" innovations such as reproductive cloning, the sale of embryos, and research on embryos after fourteen days of development. Although the report grants that the embryo deserves "special respect," it does not define this precisely. The report does reflect a development away from a single focus on federal legislation, discussing the possibility of a new regulatory agency, the use of government funds, and increased self-regulation by professional organizations as part of a multipronged strategy of governance.

The Hastings Center report by Erik Parens and Lori Knowles also highlights substantive as well as procedural issues, asking, "Are we in danger of allowing the market mentality to colonize childbearing, as it has already colonized much of our lives?"[135] "Liberty, equality, solidarity and justice" should all be determinants of policy on ARTs, as should "safety" and the more complex and difficult-to-define good of "well-being."[136] One threat to well-being is the tendency to view children in terms of characteristics rather than as valued persons, a concern that converges with many theological critiques. Parens and Knowles also realize that using genetics to give children social advantages potentially increases "the gap between the haves and have nots" and could underwrite stereotypes and biases embodied in dominant ideals of "human excellence."[137] (Genetic enhancement techniques will be addressed in the next chapter.)

Parens and Knowles warn that, even though controversial, human well-being should be a part of the public discussion and should even motivate regulation, rather than being dismissed as "speculative" or even "religious."[138] Like the PCB report, Parens and Knowles urge that embryos be respected. They believe that respect should increase with development and conclude that more public debate is needed on what types of manipulation or research on embryos are appropriate or tend to instrumentalize, with dangerous implications for the ways we view other life.[139] Like the PCB, they explore a variety of means and levels of oversight and observe that regulation will have to be pluralistic and incremental.[140] They review policies of the United Kingdom and Canada,[141] though they tend to lose sight of the justice concerns in moving to the international level.

The President's Council on Bioethics and Parens and Knowles provide approaches to a social bioethics that not only could accommodate religious participation but actually invites it. They represent the edge of a discourse about early life and reproduction that is no longer focused exclusively on the rights of the unborn versus reproductive rights, nor do they exalt privacy and autonomy or favor autonomy to the virtual exclusion of consideration of substantive goods and values. Regarding the latter, public debate is called for, paralleling the "deliberative democracy" model in which value traditions contribute substantively, yet in a mode that is respectful and reciprocal. Participatory democracy and faith-based activism also offer resources for understanding how theological bioethics could be influential in the future of debates about and controls on ARTs. Even more strikingly, these models help account for the possibility that the "public" perspectives represented in these two reports may already have been influenced by ethical concerns that have characterized the contributions of religious communities and theological bioethics for three to four decades.

A Global Perspective

Although these two reports concentrate on the North American scene, the same concerns and issues, especially justice and regulation, are even more acute internationally. When one puts ARTs in a global context, one realizes that their pervasiveness and popularity depend largely on their profitability and marketability to "first world" consumers. In other parts of the world, overpopulation is a greater problem than infertility, and family planning, prenatal care, maternal and infant mortality in childbirth, and deaths from early childhood diseases are much more urgent issues than new techniques to replace natural conception. One exception, or perhaps an illustration, is sex selection, which is used in many traditional societies to eliminate female fetuses or to select sperm or embryos that will result in the births of boys. In these cultures, women's status and sometimes lives are dependent on their ability to bear male heirs.[142]

Sex selection—which western feminists disapprove of with virtual unanimity[143]—nicely illustrates the tension between respect for cultural pluralism and a perceived need to draw at least some moral lines. Many or most geneticists and counselors around the world (trained largely in liberal traditions of respect for informed consent) in fact permit women to choose sex selection. Yet sex selection invariably perpetuates sexist attitudes toward and social denigration of women.[144] Take even a relatively innocuous case of preconceptual sex selection, the choice of a girl in a fairly gender-equal society, when a mother deeply wants to raise a daughter in addition to several sons. At the very least, sex selection promotes gender stereotyping and encourages parents to invest heavily in and try to control for having a child with specific types of characteristics.[145]

Yet, especially in the gender-unequal societies in which sex selection is most in demand, laws against sex selection are often ineffectual in the face of strong social pressures to bear a child of a given sex, usually male. The best approach to the problem is not to focus on the enactment of absolute prohibitions, but gradually to establish a "moral climate" in which girls and women are valued. The key is "to promote education for women and equality in the workforce," because societies place higher value on women when they engage in "productive" work outside the home. In developing nations, the ratio of women to men and women's longevity "directly parallel women's participation in the workforce." Therefore the solution to sex selection in nations such as India, Pakistan, and Bangladesh lies in the education and employment of women.[146]

Participatory Theological Bioethics: Infertility and Adoption

Illustrating the practical side of theological bioethics with regard to the issue of infertility in an ethos of individualism and consumerism, adoption can be seen as an important alternative practice. From a theological perspective, not only does adoption offer an option to women facing problem pregnancy, but also it witnesses to the Christian idea that "family" is inclusive and expansive, across lines of religion, race, and culture.[147] By offering adoption as one way to resolve infertility and create families, faith communities and theological leadership can counter the pressure toward expensive and stressful technological "solutions" to the inability of a couple to bear children.

John Paul II encouraged adoption as a means, not just of fulfilling parental desires but of contributing to the common good. Although natural kinship bonds are important to families and parenthood, they are not all-determinative. In adoption, children who are not able to remain with their birth families (obviously the ideal) are incorporated into new families in a compensatory way. "Christian parents will thus be able to spread their love beyond the bonds of flesh and blood, nourishing the links that are rooted in the spirit and develop through concrete service to the children of other families, who are often without even the barest necessities."[148] In his view, the very existence of so many children without families "suggests adoption as a concrete way of love."[149] Adoptive families testify that "this is a possible and beautiful way, despite its difficulties; a way, moreover, which is even more feasible than in the past in this era of globalization which shortens all distances."[150] Adoption is "a form of 'procreation' which occurs through acceptance, concern, and devotion. The resulting relationship is so intimate and enduring that it is in no way inferior to one based on a biological connection."[151] Maura Ryan places adoption under the virtue of "hospitality" and within a social justice framework. She points out, however, that not only infertile couples have a responsibility to care for the welfare of children in need of families.[152] In fact, Stephen Post sees adoption as a way that any Christian family can model in its own relationships of love the covenantal inclusiveness of Christian community.[153]

Adoption is a remedial measure, necessary in many cases and certainly of great promise for both adoptive parents and children. Yet it is important to remember that the need for adoption often or even usually is due to forms of social injustice. Adoption is a commendable choice for women or couples who want to avoid abortion but are unable to raise a child themselves or for families whose resources are stretched beyond the breaking point. Forms of open adoption, allowing for continuing contact between birth mothers and children, help alleviate some of the pain of loss for both, providing children with a sense of history and connection to their biological families. However, adoption is not the line of first defense against family disruption due to poverty and other types of social exclusion. Ensuring that children have families is always a greater priority than ensuring that childless couples have children; social support to keep children in their families or extended families of birth should be the first priority, with adoption in their countries or cultures of origin the preferred backup measure.

If none of these options are possible for a given child, international adoption holds great promise. Every effort must be made to ensure that children are released for adoption under ethical and noncoercive conditions and that they are not treated as marketable goods by for-profit, freelance "adoption facilitators" or privileged couples. In fact, reliable and ethical adoption services are best provided by reputable agencies, with licensed and salaried social workers, cooperating with similar counterparts representing U.S. birth mothers, or child service providers in international countries of origin. Couples, agencies, and countries accepting such children and placing them with families should always be attentive to and devote resources to alleviating the social conditions leading to family disruption in the first place. For example, Catholic Charities, historically a leader in adoption services in the United States, now places much more emphasis on measures to support poor families and children than on adoption services per se; it advocates for services that can help keep families together and welcome new children, such as housing and health care. Holt International Children's Services, a Protestant evangelical agency that began international adoptions in the United States after the Korean War, devotes a significant portion of its resources to in-country family reunification, family and unwed mother support services, and foster care programs, educational sponsorship, and adoption in the children's countries of origin.[154]

Conclusion

The bioethics of reproduction has been one of the most troubled spheres of cultural and policy debate in the United States in the past half-century. It is also an area in which theological participation has been constant, passionate, and divisive. Participatory theological bioethics today has the opportunity to help overcome cultural rifts over reproduction, embryos, and abortion. Theologians can and should continue to bring substantive values to the table, such as the value of early life, gender equality that has practical meaning in terms of education and employment, and social investment in the material needs of women, children, and families. Theological bioethicists should devote more attention in reproductive ethics than they have in the past to social justice and the common good, as indispensable to the exercise of reproductive freedom and responsibility. While abortion and reproductive technologies are promoted as free choices, a theological worldview can do much to uncover the ways in which patterns of access to social resources often force women into abortion or induce individuals and couples to "choose" means of reproduction that do more to support the infertility industry than to relieve infertility. The desires to procreate with one's spouse or to experience pregnancy, childbirth, and a biological connection to one's child are natural and good; infertility caused by physical dysfunction is a medical problem that deserves a medical response. Low success rates, disproportionate expense, the priority of other medical needs, and the availability of other solutions should, however, be part of public deliberation about the ethics and practice of assisted reproduction. Theological bioethics should participate in democratic social processes of dialogue toward regulation of ARTs and toward alternatives to abortion. Adoption is one alternative to abortion that can also offer those desiring to become parents the opportunity to build a family and to alleviate the consequences of negative factors that cause the disruption of birth families.

CHAPTER

7

BIOTECHNOLOGY, GENES, AND JUSTICE

The Human Genome Project (HGP) began in 1990 as an international consortium of scientific teams. It planned to map the entire human genome by 2005, on a budget of $3 billion. The major supporters of the HGP are the United Kingdom's Wellcome Trust, a large medical charity, and the U.S. federal government's National Institutes of Health (NIH). International collaborators include Germany, France, Japan, and China.

In 1998, about midway through the fifteen-year research process, the HGP received a surprise challenge from a private, for-profit corporation, Celera Genomics, headed by J. Craig Venter, a former NIH researcher. Intent on getting immediate practical results from genetic knowledge and on patenting and using that knowledge not only to address medical needs but also to make profits by selling subscriptions to Celera's database, Venter proposed to sequence the human genome by 2003. He built on information that had been made public by the HGP, but denied public access to Celera's results. In response, the public consortium moved its projected completion date to 2003 as well. In June 2000, the two teams announced a rough draft of about 90 percent of the genome, with the remainder to be filled in later. The fact that the rivals made their discoveries public jointly at the White House, and in the presence of U.S. President Bill Clinton and British Prime Minister Tony Blair (by satellite), signaled mutual accommodation among academic, political, and business interests in genetics and a seeming commitment to place American research in the context of international cooperation. However, the next several years of genetics research only intensified ethical debates about genes, patents, profits, and the common good.

The Genome: Metaphors and Politics

The 1997 United Nations Educational, Scientific, and Cultural Organization (UNESCO) *Universal Declaration on the Human Genome and Human Rights* refers to the human genome as underlying "the fundamental unity of all members of the human family" and as belonging to "the common heritage of humanity," the benefits of which belong to all.[1] At stake here is the public or private character of knowledge about genes and the patentability of life-forms and of genetic knowledge. A patent confers the right to retain control over "intellectual property" so as to protect profits. Critics of patents on genes or life-forms say there is a duty to make knowledge and beneficial applications available to a wide circle of potential beneficiaries. Genetic knowledge should not be owned by individuals and corporations. The rhetoric used to present the decoding of the human genome is both a shaper and an indicator of the climate of public debate about genetics and biotechnology. It reveals many of the complexities, even contradictions, of cultural attitudes toward the ethical and social questions they pose.

Finding the right image to express excitement and capture the public imagination seems to evoke almost as much competitive spirit as the scientific race. It is also an exercise in metaphor making as political act. Among the images for the genome or its sequencing, the more overused ones come from the technical world of construction, machinery, and computers. Some that appeared in *The New York Times* on the day of the announcement include the following: set of instructions, instruction manual, manual of the human machine, blueprint, programming code, master parts list, and model of high performance.[2] These metaphors connote a strong, even deterministic, correlation between genetics and human function, downplaying the role of environmental and social factors. Other metaphors are textual and seem to suggest a more complex and culturally mediated relation between genetics and the person: human genetic library, book of life, booklet of life, code to life on Earth, working draft, and atlas. Another high-profile category of imagery alludes to pioneering, voyages of discovery, and the conquest of frontiers. This category works to place genetic science in a noble social context. It easily invokes the honor and idealism that U.S. audiences willingly attach to their national history and the supposed moral mandate that lies behind American claims to international precedence. Other metaphors are religious and refer to creation, divine knowledge, and divine control over nature. Generally used to evoke awe at genetic discovery, they can also be used by critics to suggest the hubris involved in intruding on divine sovereignty.

What might be gained by those who promote genetic discoveries or control the results? Basic knowledge about human biology, and about processes, conditions, and even behaviors and mental states linked to biology, is promised by this advance. Beyond this, it opens up multiple avenues to the prevention or treatment of disease and the improvement of human health and capabilities. The new genomics (a half-century after the discovery of DNA) is emerging under the morally attractive aegis of health benefits for "humanity." Genetics research might alleviate causes of suffering and death such as cancer, cardiovascular disease, dementia, and diseases with a clear link to specific genes (such as Huntington's disease and cystic fibrosis). Opportunities to find cures for disease, to avoid passing on genetic difficulties to children, and even to enhance our characteristics or those of future generations seem to open new vistas for human enterprise, freedom, and happiness. Already genetic information is being put to use to carry out genetic tests on humans, to improve drugs' performance by tailoring them to varieties of diseases, and to splice genes across species of plants and bacteria. All of these techniques are ostensibly aimed at great benefit for humans and relief of suffering, and all have potential to be highly profitable. While some caution that clinical applications will come slowly, others predict that genomics will soon revolutionize the practice of medicine and extend the average human lifespan beyond ninety years within the next half-century.

For instance, the new science of regenerative medicine exploits the body's internal communications system to get it to respond to damage and disease by repairing tissue and bolstering the immune system. Personalized medicine is also on the horizon, offering drugs tailored to the individual genetic makeup of the patient, thus enhancing the effectiveness of treatments for ailments such as cancer, heart disease, and some forms of mental illness. To the extent that diseases may be linked to specific genes, genetic testing will be able to identify who has a proclivity toward a certain affliction, allowing preventative measures to be taken. Diagnostic testing raises the possibility of detecting genetic liabilities *in utero,* or even at the embryonic stage. Medical science may be able to intervene in germ cells or embryos to remove or change a gene, so that its effects not only would be prevented in one individual but also would not be passed on to the next generation. Such possibilities raise the questions of what is to count as a defect, how to gauge the seriousness of a genetic threat, and how to evaluate the appropriate course of action given its presence. Yet attempts to avoid illness may cause unexpected harms, because genes are complex and their functions not fully understood. Moreover, the genome of every individual is sure to contain "errors" whose actual results will depend on many factors, including interaction with other genes, the environment, medical care, lifestyle, and even culture.

Ethical Questions

The HGP has spurred almost as many ethical and social questions as it has biotech start-up companies. Is genetic information completely private, or should access be given to family members, insurers, employers, or public health agencies? What about screening, counseling, and treatment programs? Should they be mandatory or optional, publicly or privately funded, universal or targeted at suspect populations? If screening and treatment are available, will that result in less tolerance for persons with genetic disabilities? Alternatively, genetic science will be able to identify links to positive traits such as intelligence, memory, or socially desirable details of appearance. Is it just as valid to enhance the genetic code as to remove or cure pathologies? What is to count as a genuine improvement, and who will be able to obtain one?

One of the most pressing and perplexing ethical dimensions of the new genomics research is the just use of genetic knowledge in an era of economic globalization. U.S. law, policy, and even philosophy tend to frame social justice questions in terms of individual rights, civil liberties, procedural solutions to conflict, and equality of opportunity. U.S. individuals and organizations frequently approach the social aspects of genetics by prioritizing freedom and self-determination—of scientists, businesses, consumers, and even the nation as an international actor with particular "values" and "interests." This focus on rights can neglect the social and economic bases of health and disease and the effect on social institutions and patterns of individual choices and enterprise.[3] African, Asian, Latin American, and, to an extent, European cultures put a higher priority on social and economic rights within a community than they do on individual privacy and choice.

The furor about the genome goes beyond medical implications. It represents the confluence in the modern age of science as the most respected mode of knowledge, medicine as a new priesthood whose altruism is assumed, and the economy as the most important social institution for defining power and control over social resources (more on economics to follow). Scientists who can promise health benefits come across as the saviors of humanity and as our redeemers from human suffering. Profits and acclaim may encourage researchers to welcome this role, but the public is also responsible for entrusting to, even demanding of, science and technology the alleviation of social and personal problems that deserve a more holistic and realistic response. Religious traditions warn us not to place too much trust in even the most worthy human solutions to suffering, even though any humane solution should be earnestly pursued. Like technologies once harnessed to military and territorial conquest (in the last century, building the atomic bomb or putting a man on the moon), technology in medical guise may turn out to be another means of power-seeking, and its consequences should be predicted with moral and social circumspection.

Those who herald genomics' success hold up the alleviation of disease and the prerogative of the scientist or corporation to capitalize on genetic knowledge. Often hidden from view is the fact that neither medical nor commercial benefits are going to be universally shared. While North Americans and Europeans seek answers to cancer and other enigmatic diseases, millions die around the world from treatable causes such as malaria, anemia, and tuberculosis. Does it serve the common good, even in the United States, to provide new genetic treatments for the privileged, while so many go uninsured? Does it serve the global common good to devote billions to new genetic inventions while more basic health needs are so dire and while great gaps in other basic needs such as food, housing, education, and clean water bring early death to many?

Some years ago, Paul H. Silverman already noted a transfer of knowledge from "academic medical centers" to "the private enterprise arena" through the formation of new companies, in-house research, and alliances and acquisitions. The for-profit mode of the market influences the shape research takes. "The increase in research and development activity by these firms is designed to position them competitively for what is expected to be a major diagnostic market potential."[4] Biotech corporations do not promote research for its own sake or promote healing as an end in itself. Rather, they seek to identify and fill a market niche, then advertise aggressively both to providers and to prospective consumers. Successful marketing will make the first product out difficult to displace even when improvements come along and will encourage the production of "me too" drugs, that is, pharmaceuticals that are only marginally different from the original, but different enough to escape its patent protections. Financial considerations play a huge role in the development of new research into therapeutic applications and in availability to consumers.

In her scathing attack on drug industry practices, former *New England Journal of Medicine* editor Marcia Angell accuses companies of abandoning unprofitable products despite medical need, which results in shortages of drugs and vaccines for conditions such as prematurity, hemophilia, cardiac arrest, flu, pneumonia, diphtheria, tetanus, whooping cough, measles, mumps, and chicken pox.[5] Even in the faltering economy of 2002, the ten drug companies in the Fortune 500 were more profitable than the other 490 businesses together.[6] According to Angell, "big pharma" markets aggressively and misleadingly hires researchers whose results it controls, bribes doctors, and spends huge sums lobbying Congress and supporting the political campaigns of supporters. For example, in the 1999–2000 election season, pharmaceutical corporations gave $20 million in direct contributions and $65 million in "soft" money to candidates they wanted to influence.[7]

The drug industry's sphere of influence extends to academic medical centers and universities, eroding their objectivity, independence, and commitment to the common good. Drug companies are major benefactors to medical schools.[8] Universities and their faculty conduct paid trials for industry, receive a cut of the profits, and may even hold stock in the company. Yet they are often denied information about similar trials in other institutions and about the overall results, so that the manufacturer's interpretation of the outcomes will be incontestable. Sheldon Krimsky claims that the "unholy alliance" between pharmaceutical companies and scientists has led to the demise of public interest science.[9] Rather than pursuing solutions to social problems and honestly evaluating the effects of new technologies, research scientists allow their priorities to be dictated by commercial interests and their personal or institutional stake in the profits.[10]

The individual rights of investigators, investors, and companies to sell biomedical tools enjoy a priority in our legal and political system that is unmatched by the right of other members of society to a "decent minimum" of health care, much less by practical means of structuring behavior patterns so that they contribute to the common good and further a humane, holistic approach to health, illness, suffering, finitude, scarcity, and social interdependence. How the rights of investors and researchers ought to be exercised and limited presents a challenge to state, national, and now international regulatory agencies and lawmakers.

I would certainly not rule out market investment and entrepreneurial biomedical research as ethical means of making a living, enhancing one's scientific reputation, staking out a share in the key social institutions of twenty-first-century North American society, or exploiting the opportunities of globalization. All of the above, however, are subject to moral restraints. They should come under legal and regulatory limits that help societies, international bodies and alliances, and transnational institutions (including markets and corporations) to retain, or if necessary reinvent, the legal and ethical standards of behavior that safeguarded individual rights and the common good in what may have been a simpler biomedical age.

Benefits, Access, and Justice

Though at the present time the health benefits of genetics research are more prospective than real, the directions in which they are developing are largely determined by perceived "need," that is, market demand. People who already have access to basic nutrition, hygiene, and health care and who do not run a high risk of early death from communicable diseases such as malaria and tuberculosis are most likely to be interested in genetic diagnosis and treatment for less common or less severe diseases. Treatments for diseases that affect the most people in the most developed parts of the world will be created first by pharmaceutical companies. The WHO estimates that pneumonia, diarrhea, tuberculosis, and malaria, which account for over 20 percent of the world's disease burden, receive less than 1 percent of the total public and private health research funds. Of the 1,233 new drugs marketed between 1975 and 1999, only 13 were approved specifically for tropical diseases, and 6 of these were developed under special grants from the WHO and the United Nations Development Program.[11]

In the case of diseases that strike both rich and poor and for which genetic diagnosis or treatments are available or in the process of development—such as thalassemia and diabetes—access to genetic interventions is dependent upon ability to pay. Thalassemia is under control in the United States and Europe, but in most other countries of the world thousands of children a year die of this condition. Diabetes is on the rise globally, and genomic research is moving toward therapy, but there is no more reason to expect that the benefits will be any more available to impoverished families than are tests for thalassemia or AIDS drugs. Meanwhile, evidence mounts that knowledge of the genomics of pathogens could lead to much more effective prevention and treatment of communicable diseases such as malaria, tuberculosis, dengue fever, meningitis B, hepatitis B, and even African AIDS.[12] Yet funding for the necessary research is not plentiful, and access to benefits is very constrained for the majority of the world's population. This will be even more true of "luxury" or "discretionary" genetic services, such as enhancement of "normal" traits.

Right now, clean water, food, basic health care, perinatal care, and the AIDS pandemic are of mightier concern in most cultures than genomics. Questions of justice in the development of genetic medicine thus arise in at least the following areas: more equitable health resource allocation in general, nationally and globally; shaping the future applications of genetic medicine so that both rich and poor are served; and possibly redistributing or "sharing" profits from genetic biotechnologies so that "advances" aimed at a "first world" market will contribute to a rise in health in the developing world.

Although there has been some discussion of global justice in the philosophical and theological literature on genetics,[13] such analysis has not trickled down much to the scientific and business communities or to the public debate, nor has it taken hold in the policy arena in this country. For example, an overview of the implications of the HGP by Francis Collins and Victor McKusick, U.S. leaders of the project, focuses its ethical concerns on misuses of genetic information in light of health insurance and employment law in the United States.[14] A 2001 report of the National Bioethics Advisory Commission (NBAC) on ethics in international research demands, rightly enough, that U.S. researchers abroad adhere to informed consent standards similar to those required at home, but does not envision a larger policy community in which U.S. standards might come under scrutiny or in which international standards would be cooperatively developed.[15]

Although 5 percent of the HGP budget is devoted to study of and education about Ethical, Legal, and Social Issues (ELSI), much of the work funded has concentrated on concerns about privacy and autonomy, tacitly or explicitly framed against U.S. constitutional, legal, and judicial traditions. An agenda-setting conference held in the United States in 1991 by the ELSI program of the HGP highlighted insurance, employment, and the civil liberties of suspected criminals subjected to genetic testing as key moral topics. Reproductive medicine, the area in which much genetic research and intervention are carried out, is governed almost exclusively by the principle of informed choice. In contrast, the international organization of scientists collaborating in the Human Genome Project refers to the human genome as "part of the common heritage of humankind" and recommends that research follow "principles of justice and solidarity" applied internationally.[16] The HGP itself is an international endeavor, interweaving the interests and expertise of several cultures. The discovery of a common genetic code confirms that human beings across cultures share basic physical characteristics, needs, and vulnerabilities. This suggests the need for a global approach to genomic ethics and policy and the restraint of some types of investigation and application for the sake of the general welfare.

Patents

The gateway to profit is the patent. A patent gives its holder the right to exclusive use of an invention for twenty years, during which time royalties are charged for licenses to use the patented information, either for a marketable application or for further research. Researchers want to patent any potentially useful knowledge about genes as fast as possible (even before they have figured out a specific use) so that that knowledge can be sold to drug companies. One justification for patents is that they provide incentive for investment and work in areas that are potentially of benefit to many. But the downside is that they channel resources toward only the most profitable research and help limit accessibility to those who can pay.

U.S. business interests have thus far had a disproportionate influence on the development and coordination of international patent law. The Brazilian theologian Marcio Fabri mentions a case in which a U.S. corporation claimed to have found a cure for asthma in an African coastal tribe. It then sold DNA samples from tribe members to a German pharmaceutical company for $70 million without any remuneration whatsoever to the DNA donors. "This little example shows that genetics has become a field of economic and political endeavor that national and international policies cannot ignore."[17]

Although patent laws vary nationally or regionally, an international regime of patent law has been established by means of the World Trade Organization's requirement that member nations respect intellectual property rights as defined by North American and European standards. Adherence to the 1995 TRIPS agreement (Trade Related Aspects of Intellectual Property Rights) is part of the price of entry into the global economic market, and noncompliant members will be placed on trade "watch lists" that threaten eventual trade sanctions and discourage investment even in the short term. At least in theory, patents can only be obtained for inventions, not discoveries in nature, and patentable inventions must have clear and specific utility. Enforcement of these criteria has been questionable in practice. Patent applications have been filed for genes and segments of genes, even though these are not inventions, and no useful process or product based on them has yet been proposed in any detail. According to a U.S. Department of Energy report, more than 3 million gene-related patent applications have been filed, mostly in the United States, Europe, and Japan.[18]

In the emergent global market, patented drugs are big international business. The announcement in February 2001 by Celera Corporation and the HGP that the number of functional human genes may be much smaller than anticipated may mean that pharmaceutical companies will be able to produce genetically engineered drugs more quickly, even though there may turn out to be fewer of them to produce, and production may depend on further study of the proteins genes code for, not just knowledge of the genes themselves. Drug development is expected to customize drugs both to the genetic causes of particular diseases and to the genetic profiles of individuals. Among the early targets for new gene-based drug products are asthma and Alzheimer's.

But what kind of social implications will the manufacture of genetically engineered drugs have? International control of currently available drugs through patent laws gives us a preview of a likely scenario. The ongoing controversy over AIDS drugs, involving developing countries, transnational pharmaceutical companies, and the World Trade Organization, illustrates the future of control over other genomics based tests, treatments, and "improvements." According to international trade agreements, companies can "segment" the market for their products, meaning that they can charge different prices for the same product in different countries. Although TRIPS provides that countries can set intellectual property rights aside in the case of a "national emergency," efforts of the South African government to pass and act on a law permitting parallel importing to help address its AIDS crisis were fought tooth and nail by a coalition of big pharmaceutical companies. It was not until the World Trade Organization Ministerial Conference in Doha, Qatar, in 2001, after a prolonged battle, that its rules were renegotiated to permit the importing of generic drugs or their components from foreign countries where prices may be lower. And the specific arrangements under which this could be accomplished were still in contention until August 2003, when an agreement was finally reached to allow generics manufacturers to produce enough drugs to supply foreign markets.[19]

Bioethical policy, especially in the United States, and perhaps most crucially in the area of genetics, has not caught up with the emerging, inequitable, and confounding world order in which transnational corporations seek profits around the world, unaccountable to any one governing authority. It has barely begun to deal with the fact that genomics research and development are driven largely by the market and that the market for genetic tests and, in the future, for the benefits of stem cell research and pharmacogenomics is or will be international. The development of these techniques "by the private sector on a for-profit basis means that they will be beyond the means of many citizens, making them available only to a narrow, wealthy segment of society."[20] The flip side of the global marketing of genetic therapies (and, eventually, enhancements) is that a great deal of investment will go into the most profitable applications and not necessarily into those that affect the most people or cause the most suffering.

Genes, Justice, and Theology

A common good framework defines justice in terms of the good of a whole society and all its members, with "society" being given an increasingly global range. Justice is an objective criterion of moral relationships that sees persons, groups, and communities as interdependent and as having an equal right to share in the material and social conditions of human well-being. No one has a right to private property gained at the expense of the basic human needs of other persons or groups. Active efforts must be made to include those who have previously been excluded from participation in the common good (the preferential option for the poor). According to the principle of subsidiarity, neither should government control activities that can be successfully carried out at the local level, nor should it neglect to direct and coordinate such enterprises to the extent necessary to serve justice. Justice goes beyond individuals to consider the common good and any particular social development by its effects on the interdependent welfare of all. Today, in the era of transnational corporations, joint international efforts to contain violence and alleviate natural disasters, and a growing sense of shared responsibility for the environment, the common good has an ever more global meaning.

Religious traditions and theologians are not generally opposed to the promise of genetic science in alleviating human suffering caused by disease, disability, and early death. Religious traditions offer few if any absolute definitions of human "nature" that specify clearly what is and is not a transgression, in the sense of a breach or change of "the natural" that upsets divinely ordained limits. Citing various popes and teaching bodies, the CHA surmises that "the church is not opposed to genetic research that respects personal dignity, supports human life, and upholds the common good. When it is aimed at the prevention, treatment, and elimination of disease, genetic research can be morally good."[21]

But many worry about the cumulative social effects of certain attitudes of control over the human species, such as extending the lifespan indefinitely or selecting characteristics of children by design and passing them on to future generations through germ line modification. Increasingly, these social concerns are taking the shape of a justice agenda framed by the common good and backed by religious symbols and theological warrants. In 1997, John Paul II urged "the responsible international bodies to commit themselves to drawing up effective legal guarantees to ensure that the health of those who do not have a voice will also be promoted in its entirety and that the world of health care will be imbued with the logic of solidarity and charity rather than with the dynamics of profit."[22]

Feminist theologians in particular have brought their social concerns to this area. The exclusionary tendencies of genetics research are given poignant testimony in the silence on the wonders of the HGP by those whose health care concerns are more basic. African American theologian Emilie Townes weaves a "womanist ethic of care" around urgent needs of black Americans.[23] Foremost among these are a very inadequate health care delivery system for basic needs and the lack of an integrated approach to health that includes spiritual and psychological dimensions. Genetics comes up in the context of diseases that particularly afflict African Americans, including low birth weights, hypertension, obesity, diabetes, breast cancer, asthma, and HIV/AIDS. Townes realizes that, though genes can predispose to certain conditions, multiple environmental factors come into play in causing disease. These include cultural determinants of diet and the symbolism of food, environmental risks, social constraints or influences on behavior, and lack of access to early diagnosis and treatment.[24] Genetic "miracles" will never resolve the health problems of people who continue to subsist under multiple conditions of deprivation. From the womanist theologian's perspective, genetic interventions do not offer hope for the future, because "the careless drive toward entitlement without responsibility" has resulted in an extremely unhealthy atmosphere for women and men unable to purchase health care.[25]

Breast cancer is a good example, one noted frequently by feminist bioethicists. In some cases, breast cancer risk is increased by genetic factors. However, the fact that black women are hit by this disease less frequently than white women, yet die of it in greater numbers, is not due to genetics. Black women have less access than white women to mammograms, early intervention, and treatment. Theologian Susanne DeCrane insists "the reality of the survival rate of black women from breast cancer demands a commitment from the community to pursue *aggressively* the underlying causes of the disparity."[26] These causes are more social than genetic. Genetic tests for susceptibility are emerging. But for those with no access to basic care, or who face bias in seeking treatment, just how relevant is genetic testing to their own heath status and future? African Americans and others who have suffered racial or ethnic discrimination are wary of the idea that genetic tests and treatments will serve their welfare rather than creating new bases for racist and exclusionary policies and institutions. As one scholar worries, "Without some of the critical questions raised by the African and African American encounter with scientific racism, how can we be sure that the good of this research will be appreciated, and how will we build effective safeguards against exploitation?"[27]

Many theologians respond in the narrative and prophetic modes of discourse in order to reinvigorate the commitment of religious communities to approach genomics with a sense of humility and to apply genomics with a commitment to fairness. The narrative approach does not necessarily exclude ethical and policy discourse, but serves more generally to reaffirm communal values within an expansive, normative worldview. Narrative and prophetic discourse can even serve as a vehicle to introduce associated values into the public sphere. For instance, Laurie Zoloth reaches into the Jewish "world of the Talmud" to find metaphors that set human creativity under God and allow for instances in which human activity justifiably transgresses the "natural." She takes stories of magic, sorcery, and alchemy to provide metaphors for research in genetics. While the rabbis permit some instances of magic, limits are set against worshipping a thing made or hawking the "elixir of life" in the marketplace, thus recommending a "duty of justice."[28] Zoloth's reflections are not meant only for Jews, but for Christians and others who are seeking novel insight into the human problems of genetic identity and intervention.

Similarly, Sondra Ely Wheeler believes that all theistic traditions talk about material reality as creation and engage in discernment in view of the creative intention of God.[29] Making the point that critical selection of metaphors within traditions is important, Therese Lysaught points out that metaphors drawn from accepted practices of killing, such as self-defense and just war, slant discourse toward justification of new practices under discussion. Alternative metaphorical strands, focused on values of peace, compassion, and healing, might lead to greater caution.[30] Andrea Vicini, noting the prevalence of metaphors of discovery and conquest that are applied to the HGP, suggests that biblical metaphors of healing would help reconnect genetic knowledge to the holistic good of persons in their relationships.[31] Brent Waters suggests that the best way to approach the value of embryonic life is under the rubric of love of neighbor. This metaphor can encourage dispositions of care and caution, even though there are "no easy or obvious choices to be made when the needs, obligations, and limitations of *all* the neighbors involved are taken into account."[32]

Some religious advocates of human genetic intervention have used the metaphor of the human person as "co-creator" or "created co-creator" with God to advance a benign picture of human genetic opportunities and freedoms.[33] The "co-creator" metaphor serves largely to license human genetic intervention and to frame it with an optimistic attitude toward the potential benefits of scientific advances. The driving concern behind the metaphor seems to be throwing off irrational restraints of tradition and allowing religion to endorse those aspects of scientific investigation that promise significant benefits for human health and happiness. Others object that metaphors of divinely aligned creativity seem to legitimate much while offering few criteria for the responsibility and proper ends of scientists.[34] Bart Hansen and Paul Schotsmans point out that a *created* co-creator may have a responsibility to develop creation in line with the divine intention, but that the process of doing so will be marked by the limits and moral failure that characterize the human condition.[35]

Perhaps it is not surprising that some consider religious value systems subjective, vague, or unrealistic. Who is to judge whether their narratives are truly prophetic, and how are they to be connected to ethics and policies that are public? Audrey Chapman takes issue with the seeming reluctance of many religious critics to enter into the kind of precise ethical analysis necessary to advance toward clear and feasible policy recommendations. She believes that "it is not enough for them to stimulate the moral imagination" if they "do not illuminate where to draw the precise boundary between genetic interventions representing responsible expressions of human stewardship, co-creation, or partnership with the divine and those that are extensions of human hubris or pride."[36]

In reality, some theologians and churches are quite prepared to move toward such recommendations; they tend to be those with a more conservative stance toward the value of the embryo. Their policy recommendations tend toward prohibiting or limiting embryo research.[37] However, the move from narrative to policy is not always laid out in the clear ethical terms and arguments that might make sense to those who do not share the narrative. An uncertain connection between narrative discourse and policy also arises when socially progressive theological bioethicists want to send up warning signals and influence social priorities without necessarily proposing that restrictive legislation is a possible or productive route toward better policy.

Clear ethical thinking is always to be desired. The rhetorical use of narratives and symbols cannot simply be substituted for ethical argument, especially when the aim is to specify provisions of public policy. Yet it is not always possible to draw precise ethical or policy lines on social justice requirements. Nevertheless, even when ethical argumentation is tentative or incomplete, it can still be possible for theological bioethics to operate at the participatory level. It can begin to initiate more just practices or practices in which contentious points can be "backgrounded" in favor of ways of going forward on agreed aims. Further treatment of the links between theological discourse and policy will appear in the following discussion on stem cell therapy. A concluding discussion of examples of participatory theological bioethics addressing genetics and ethics through practices will take up examples of local action in the United States, then turn to genetically modified foods for global parallels and precedents for human genetics.

Stem Cell Research

Some day, medical science may be able to heal or alleviate ailments such as Alzheimer's, Parkinson's, diabetes, spinal cord injuries, heart disease, and cancer by giving patients new cells that have been guided to act as replacements for their own damaged tissue. Sometimes the starting "stem cells" could be culled from organs and tissue in the recipient's own body, such as bone marrow, ensuring a perfect match. But many scientists argue that more promising research is being conducted on even less specialized and hence more versatile stem cells taken not from adults but from very early embryos, about a week after fertilization. At that point the embryo is a sphere whose inner cell mass contains many as yet undifferentiated cells. They can still form any tissue of the body, or even a new embryo. In 1998, scientists began culturing these cells to develop new therapies for disease. But harvesting stem cells means destruction of the embryo.

Research on embryonic stem cells thus presents bioethics with a classic moral dilemma: Is it ever right to cause some evil to achieve a greater good? Does the end justify the means? Those who put a priority on advancing medical relief for physical suffering focus attention on the good to be gained and minimize or negate the value of the embryo lost. Others, who see the embryo as having value in its own right, and who put a priority on protecting "the unborn," believe saving lives through medical advances cannot justify the direct taking of other lives. To the means/end conflict must be added still another complication. Neither the means nor the end can be looked at in isolation from their contexts and all the ramifications any attempt to balance the two would have for the welfare and moral fabric of society. Does sacrificing embryos lead to a general disrespect for life and even its commercialization? Would prohibition of such research constitute dangerous restriction of scientific inquiry and signify callousness toward those who suffer serious illness? What do we have to say to the justice question of who will get to use these new therapies if produced?

From 1996 until 2000, the United States banned the use of federal money for embryo experimentation, including stem cell research. This restriction did not apply to privately funded research. The NIH interpreted the law to mean that federally funded researchers could use stem cells if they were derived from embryos by private companies. In 2000, the NIH issued revised guidelines, permitting scientists using public grants to use stem cells derived by others. Publicly funded scientists could use cells from frozen human embryos, originally created as part of infertility treatment.

When George W. Bush took office as U.S. president in 2001, he reconsidered this policy. He decided to permit federal funding of stem cell research only on cell lines that had been derived before August 9, 2001, the day of the announcement of the new policy. Originally the number of such lines was estimated to be about sixty, but eventually the number of usable lines was pared down to about twenty.[38] Bush assigned the task of further study and the submission of an advisory report to the President's Council on Bioethics (PCB).

The PCB did not reach a unanimous position on the matter and included alternative evaluations of stem cell research in its report.[39] These represent prevalent viewpoints in American society, including positions taken by theologians and religious denominations. Although the latter tend to have a protective view of early life, not all have defined the embryo as having full moral status, and not all preclude any research use.[40] Some PCB members favored the funding of stem cell research and even the creation of embryos for research, provided that they were destroyed within fourteen days. In the view of these members, embryos up until that point have "a developing and intermediate moral worth that commands our special respect," but experimentation is not inconsistent with respect, as long as it is regulated. "These embryos would not be 'created for destruction,' they would be destroyed in the service of a great good."[41] Other members felt that there was no special respect due the early embryo and that the only moral requirement was the consent of the donors. However, a third position represented a more "mainstream" balance to the first position (held by many, even a majority in U.S. society). This is the position that "it is morally wrong to exploit and destroy developing human life, even for good reasons, and that it is unwise to open the door to the many undesirable consequences that are likely to result from the research."[42] The report did not prompt any immediate change in federal policy, though it did illustrate contrary ways of thinking about stem cells that enjoy currency in cultural and political debates.

The proponents of moral arguments about embryos, especially arguments aimed at public policy outcomes, do well to recognize that they "are reasoning about something that is by nature mysterious, something conceived in darkness, something whose presence in cases of natural conception cannot be known until after the fact."[43] Even though now the embryo can be observed as "a life-in-process in the laboratory," the microscopic view exposes something whose "meaning seems inadequately explained by what we see; its significance seems hidden from sight."[44] Policy dilemmas may require compromise; they may also require reliance on factors beyond the status of the embryo in itself. Justice in relation to health care is just as important a determinant of moral public policy on stem cells and other aspects of embryo research as the status of the research subject.

Even within the limits stipulated by Bush, the federal government spent $25 million in 2003 to fund studies involving human embryonic stem cells. Meanwhile, many stem cell investigators turned to private groups for funding. Some funds came from interest groups such as the Juvenile Diabetes Foundation; others came from investors hoping to gain control over therapeutic inventions and make a profit. In 2004, researchers at Harvard began raising millions for a stem cell institute. The governor of New Jersey signed legislation establishing a state-supported stem cell research facility, and voters in California went to the polls to vote on a referendum to permit the state to spend $300 million on stem cell research. The ballot measure, which was approved by voters, had support from a variety of sources, including scientists, investors, patient advocacy groups, and the Bill and Melinda Gates Foundation.[45] Advocates of the measure recruited wealthy supporters, celebrity disease victims, and Nobel laureates as spokespersons, not to mention the advocacy of film star and state governor Arnold Schwarzenegger. The promotion campaign included the promise of more than 100 million lives saved, financial benefits for all, and the threat of a competitive loss to other countries if this opportunity to create embryos for stem cell research did not materialize.[46] In 2005 the Massachusetts state legislature approved a bill endorsing the creation of embryos for stem cell research, as long as they are not allowed to develop beyond fourteen days.

On the one hand, such initiatives embody subsidiarity and allow public participation. On the other hand, they reveal how public opinion makers can influence the outcome with inflated claims that conceal private interests. They also raise the question of whether it is a good thing to have embryo research proceed without uniform federal regulation. Public-private entrepreneurship can commit public money without requiring public accountability and gives the biotechnology industry a major role in determining the use of public funds. It may threaten other state-funded social programs, which ultimately could undermine equity in other areas, including those related to health.[47] Stem cell research in the United States has become an area of public participation and even "participatory democracy," but it also endangers the appropriate role of government in making sure that "democratic" social movements do not confer greater advantages on those already possessing the power and resources to influence the direction of the movement.

In April 2005, the prestigious National Academies, a self-elected group of scientists that advises government, issued a set of guidelines intended to provide ethical standards for private stem cell research by universities and companies.[48] These guidelines recommended the creation of embryos for research, within a fourteen-day limit on development; limitation of payment to egg donors to direct costs, such as travel; and permission to place human embryonic stem cells in animals, as long as they are not primates. The National Academies' report reflects the interest of scientists and corporations in facilitating the acceptance of so-called therapeutic cloning, as the limits do not exceed what is now common practice in private stem cell research. The report does not address questions of justice in access to benefits in relation to the common good. It does, however, recommend that an oversight body be established that would include ethicists and public representatives.

Theology, Justice, and Stem Cell Research

Theologians and religious communities have a role to play in bringing research expenditures under the umbrella of the common good. Research on and use of embryos are intended to relieve suffering, but are also driven by gains for researchers, clinics, and pharmaceutical companies. There is no guarantee that stem cell-derived therapies will be shared with the least advantaged or that the least advantaged would identify these therapies as their first health care priority. Hence policies that encourage research on embryos deserve intense scrutiny.

In 2001, a conference sponsored by Marquette University, the Catholic Archdiocese of Milwaukee, and the Wisconsin Catholic Conference brought together stem cell research scientists, public policy experts, and theological ethicists to discuss the ethics of stem cell research.[49] This project, spearheaded by Marquette University philosopher Nancy Snow, was already itself an exercise in participatory theological bioethics in that it convened discussion partners and an audience of different viewpoints and areas of expertise for a couple of days of exchange, argument, and socializing. The conference papers primarily employed the mode of ethical discourse, but the analyses offered were "expansively" grounded in theological premises and narrative references. They also indicated policy outcomes that would be consistent with the authors' theological commitments and explicitly defined the relationship of theological ethics to policies.

Scientists presented the prospects of both adult and embryonic stem cell investigations. Among the theologians, one presented a defense of stem cell research, premised on the rudimentary moral status of the embryo and the acceptability of the creation of spare embryos from in vitro fertilization.[50] Six theologians, all Catholic, expressed varying levels of hesitation about such research, with two condemning it completely as an unacceptable instrumentalization of human life.[51] The remaining four did not take absolute positions on the status of the embryo, but discouraged embryo research, taking into consideration both respect for developing human life and social justice in access to potential benefits.[52]

Attention to the common good as including the welfare of those who do not now have the means to obtain even basic health care has generally been lacking in the debates about stem cells. Given that this is a crucial dimension of stem cell ethics and policy, theological bioethicists should make a special investment in broadening the usual analysis beyond the embryo to justice and access.[53] Feminist theologians Karen Lebacqz, Laurie Zoloth, and Suzanne Holland note that among the aspects of stem cell research needing more consideration are "profit and commodification of important parts of human living" and "the perennial and intractable issue of social justice and how to distribute the benefits and burdens that will inevitably be associated with this research."[54] Justice in health care has been a concern for both Zoloth and Lebacqz in previous works, and Lebacqz has raised important questions about the inequitable social ramifications of the funding and exploitation of the HGP. Both use biblical stories to indicate that a fair and righteous community is an inclusive one.[55]

Margaret McLean represents a pervasive concern in feminist theological analysis of genetics as a whole when she voices concern that,

> given our country's growing economic divide and the fact that private companies are funding the leading edge of biotechnology, it seems likely that, left undisturbed, stem cell technology will be available to some but not all. This portends further stratification of human health and well-being within the richest country in the world.

She proposes an ethic based on "fairness of access" to new technologies, taking into account the "social lottery" that affects "the weaker members of society, especially children and those left poor in money, health, and access."[56] Her language reflects a Christian "preferential option for the poor." Her words recall those of the parable of judgment in Matthew 25, where Jesus rewards with eternal life those who have served him in the person of the hungry, thirsty, imprisoned, and sick. McLean sees it as imperative in the age of biotechnology that "we expand our moral imaginations to account for and be accountable to marginalized persons and concern ourselves with the shaping of a just future. Power is to be exercised on behalf of the least of us today and for the seven generations to come."[57] As Holland points out, new technologies on sale to elites will further limit women's decision-making capacity and exploit their bodies, as ova are commercialized, and the poor—largely female and people of color—are excluded from therapeutic benefits.[58]

Clearly, there are many unresolved issues related to the ethics of stem cell research. Yet, as in the case of many social issues, "inaction" is not an option. This type of research is already well under way. The task is therefore not to decide "prospectively" whether it is a good idea, but to subject it to moral guidance and restraints, acknowledging its potential for beneficial outcomes while limiting the social damage and moral compromises it involves. Theologian Paul Lauritzen draws an analogy to moral thinking about war; criteria of "just war" present a theologically backed and publicly meaningful framework with which to assess moral possibilities and obligations in the midst of circumstances that are already problematic, are ambiguous, and in which social decision making cannot be avoided. In Christian tradition, "just war" thinking can be used to discourage and restrain a practice without necessarily drawing an incontrovertible line against it. Lauritzen wields just war theory with the expectation that it can exclude an activity as well as defend it.

Although Lauritzen does not see the embryo as having the full value of an infant, he sees as "equally implausible" the idea that it is "merely cellular material."[59] Therefore destroying it is morally problematic and should be avoided. From just war tradition, Lauritzen mentions the criteria of just cause, proportion, and last resort. In particular, he argues that stem cell research fails last resort, as it has not yet been demonstrated that there are benefits to be gained from the use of embryo cells that could not also be gained by the use of adult stem cells. Scientists seem to want to ensure that research can proceed on both fronts. Yet no concrete therapies have yet been developed from embryonic stem cells. On the side of embryonic cells, there may be greater pliability and ability to develop into a number of different types. However, adult stem cells have already been used in successful though still experimental treatments for some otherwise fatal ailments such as leukemia and heart disease.

Other just war criteria can also be applied to this problem, expanding Lauritzen's analysis. The just cause test could certainly be met by the aim to find cures for disease. But what about proportion? The proportionality of destroying embryos to gaining results must be partly determined by the status of the embryo and partly by the significance of the benefits—both uncertain matters. The criterion of proportion leaves stem cell research in a dubious position at best.

Another standard just war criterion also brings uncertainty—reasonable hope of success. Promises of success are motivated by the optimism and hope of researchers and the demands of disease constituencies. By the same token, these promises may be exaggerated. So reasonable hope of success is in doubt as well. A further criterion of just war is right intention. This moral concern likewise casts a shadow over stem cell research. Is the ultimate intention the relief of suffering or financial gain and prestige? Commercial interest in the embryo and its cells tends to vitiate the integrity of the arguments of those who want to use it. Private companies supplying stem cells must be remunerated for their services. There are tremendous financial incentives for researchers to investigate medical uses of stem cells so as to sell their knowledge to for-profit pharmaceutical companies or to work directly for those companies. At the very least, we must acknowledge the reality of mixed motives.

Even in a just war, there are limits that must be observed. The limit of means in war is another relevant criterion. Would limits be maintained in stem cell research? Indications are not promising, as stem cell research seems to expand readily in response to demand from investing corporations. An indispensable guide to the conduct of war is noncombatant immunity. In the research arena, a parallel standard is the protection of human subjects. Virtually every analyst of stem cell research and other genetic research stipulates that safety to consumers or patients is a key criterion, as well as the informed consent of research subjects. In the case of the embryo research, the "subject" will be destroyed, and no consent is possible. There is no consensus that an embryo is a "human subject" in the conventional sense of the term. However, "respect" does demand certain limits on its use.

Under U.S. law, the only blanket protection the embryo is afforded is immunity to being bought or sold. This limit is only partly observed in practice, because products derived from embryos, like stem cells, can be sold. Other suggested limits are that embryos not be preserved longer than fourteen days (the approximate time of individuation, and hence, in the view of some, personhood) and that embryos not be created expressly for the purpose of research. Whether these limits are adequate is debatable, and the incremental relaxation of limits is a likely prospect—similar to the inevitable death and destruction that accrue to noncombatants in war and make the morality of war ambiguous to most theological critics.

It seems unlikely that philosophers and embryologists will agree on some all-or-nothing developmental line of demarcation, after which an embryo must be treated with all the dignity of a person and before which its value is negligible. Practically, the search for such a line seems to result more in denial of status before the "magic moment" than in enhanced protection after, and this is surely a major motivation of the repeated insistence of various religious groups that the early embryo be given the benefit of the doubt. I find it difficult to reconcile respect for the embryo as even a rudimentary member of the human species with any practices or policies that would permit its creation for purely instrumental purposes.

Although it is true that couples undertaking infertility treatments permit the creation of "spare" embryos, this is done within a context in which the aim is to bring some or most of those embryos to life; in which those seeking therapy fear that they will have too few viable embryos, not too many; and in which their appreciation of the likelihood that they will have to freeze or destroy embryos is clouded by their single focus on pregnancy and what it requires. The hesitancy of many to actually dispose of unused embryos is evidence of their progenitors' ambivalence in regarding them simply as a means to an end. As a matter of fact, there are hundreds of thousands of embryos cryopreserved around the world. Though this number is excessive, and though the numbers of spare embryos should in principle be severely reduced or even eliminated, current supplies should furnish adequate resources for at least the immediate future of stem cell research. Even if many frozen embryos turn out to be unusable, work with the pool of those available should be attempted before the creation of new embryos is declared medically necessary. Meanwhile, continuing research on adult stem cells may bring positive results.

The goods to be weighed in stem cell research are not limited to the safety of embryos or to the development of medical science or even to cures for devastating disease. They include a commitment to all those who are marginalized in the present health care access system, as well as a commitment to improve the moral quality of relationships in the social body. The just war criterion of proportion comes into play here again. It is not just a matter of proportion between the value of the embryo, the harm done to it, and the good that may come to those who benefit from therapies down the road. There is also the matter of the general use of research funds and the need for money devoted to medical care and its development to be equitably or "proportionately" shared. On this score, the incremental public and private financing of stem cell research is a step in the wrong direction.

Finally, justifying a war requires the engagement and consent of a legitimate authority. Who is that authority in the case of genetics research? Federal and state governments are involved; so are national advisory bodies. Research done with federal funds must also pass the scrutiny of institutional review boards in the host institution. However, funding that comes from private sources is subject to little or no formal restraint or scrutiny, other than, perhaps, accountability to the boards of directors and shareholders that monitor corporate business and profits. Therefore the discrepancy of funding sources and types and levels of regulation is a moral issue in stem cell research, as well as in other types of genomics. Even if stem cell research ought not to be banned, it could be situated and controlled on a spectrum of other health care needs through cautious funding policies; aggressive peer review; regulatory and legal oversight applying to all research, however funded; and stringent limits on patent grants, devised in view of collaborative international policy.

A compromise policy might respect the dignity of the embryo—a dignity whose exact nature and extent are in doubt, at least for the general public—by permitting research only on those embryos destined to be destroyed or allowed to die in any event, that is, "excess" embryos that remain after infertility therapy. Such a policy would expand the number of embryos available for research, thus also respecting the potential alleviation of human suffering that stem cell research offers. A national policy on embryo research should apply to both privately and publicly funded research. A policy of greater restriction of researchers receiving federal dollars simply encourages the for-profit pharmaceutical industry to proceed with the creation of embryos for research alone, with tacit social approbation that is parasitic on the widespread (though inaccurate) public perception that embryo research is generally restricted or even forbidden by "national" policy. In fact, a uniform national policy or legislation on the use of embryos for research could do more than restrict such research to leftover IVF embryos; it could prohibit the patenting of information obtained by research on embryos. This would help ensure that those advocating such research are truly dedicated to its disease-alleviating potential and are undertaking the destruction of embryos in the pursuit of the public interest. Such a policy would prioritize the common good rather than private profits in defining the limits of stem cell research. While not necessarily conforming in every respect to Christian principles or ideal practices, a policy of significant limitation (such as uniform public-private regulation, no creation of research embryos, and no patent profits from embryo research) would represent a "middle axioms" approach. To achieve such an outcome, theological bioethicists should cooperate with others to seek a net increase in social welfare, while enacting moral constraints to the extent concretely possible within current political conditions.

In summary, theological bioethicists are drawing on distinctive narratives to take a prophetic stance against uncritical acceptance of stem cell research as a scientific and research imperative. Using theologically informed language about solidarity, power, and justice, they are expanding the horizon of value and meaning within which the benefits of stem cell research are evaluated. Even without universal agreement on the status of the embryo, the justice concerns of theological bioethics may sound a chord with others critical of the patterns of health care access in the United States and abroad, and reservations about stem cell technologies may increase. European societies are more cautious than the United States about permitting embryo research, and in 2005, the UN General Assembly approved a declaration urging all nations to prohibit all forms of human cloning, including the "therapeutic cloning" of embryos for research on stem cells.[60]

Genetic Enhancement

Whereas stem cell research is widely practiced and has been the subject of much debate, genetic enhancement is still largely prospective and has not received as much public or theological attention. Yet it is an equally momentous and perplexing issue, and one that is sure to have even greater implications for social justice. Up until now, manipulation of human genes has been justified mainly in terms of relieving or curing pathologies. To the extent that diseases have genetic causes, genetic engineering may be able to treat them by somatic cell therapy, that is, by introducing healthy genes into a patient in order to counter his or her condition. Somatic cell therapy is generally regarded as a good, and ethical questions have been directed at safety and risk. The means by which new genes can be introduced and controlled, without causing new and perhaps greater problems for the recipient, are highly imperfect. Recipients of experimental gene therapies have died as a result; hence somatic cell therapy is reserved for the most desperate cases, in which no other alternatives are available.

Germ-line therapy is even more controversial. In germ-line therapy, genetic changes in an embryo are made to allow a child to develop without an inherited anomaly. He or she would carry copies of the corrected gene in every cell and would pass them on to offspring. On the one hand, germ-line therapy promises not only to correct but to eradicate inherited genetic disease from a reproductive line. On the other, the same risks that accompany somatic cell therapy arise here, and any deficiencies or "mistakes" in the result will be passed on as well. In fact, germ-line therapy in embryos is unlikely to become a common means of avoiding inherited disease, because in vitro fertilization and preimplantation diagnosis make it possible in most cases to simply select embryos without a defect. Thus germ-line intervention is more likely to be a conduit for adding "beneficial" genes than for correcting dysfunctional ones. Because of the risky and unpredictable nature of germ-line therapy, and because it is a type of control over future generations in the face of extreme uncertainty about outcomes, many ethical analysts have concluded that germ-line therapy should be excluded completely. In 2000, the American Association for the Advancement of Science adopted the position that there should be a ban on all inheritable genetic modification until questions of safety and efficacy have been resolved and until a public oversight process is in place.[61] This conclusion is not an absolute judgment based on the nature of the therapy or of the human genetic code, but a prudential judgment based on likely outcomes and risks.

Genetic enhancement carries the ethical questions about somatic and germ-line gene therapy a step further, adding a new dimension. In gene "therapy," a disease or dysfunction is in play, a genetic event that interferes with human health and functioning. In enhancement techniques, a normally constituted or functioning individual would be the recipient of an intervention to "improve" his or her characteristics and capabilities. The point would not be to relieve suffering but to confer advantage. Enhancement might be aimed at a trait with a fairly clear genetic basis, such as muscular strength or height, or it might attempt to modify complex traits that are highly interdependent with environmental factors, such as intelligence or musical ability.

There are multiple areas of unclarity in the ethical analysis of enhancement. The most obvious is that it is much easier to define "disease" than it is to define "normal" functioning, and thus to define what "enhances" it. A second, related source of ambiguity is that the same techniques that are already used to remedy "disorders" could be employed to increase characteristics or abilities of those who do not suffer from deficiencies. A parallel from traditional medicine is the use of human growth hormone to increase the height of children of abnormally short stature. Not only is it hard to define what is normal height, but normal height could also be increased by the same means. In the area of genetics, gene-based therapies to increase muscle strength in children who suffer from Duchenne muscular dystrophy are already in development. These same "therapies" could be employed to increase normal muscle mass, conferring, for example, an advantage in athletic competition, or to overcome the "normal" effects of aging. The negative policies on the use of performance-enhancing drugs by professional or Olympic athletes indicate that enhancement engineering might be met with resistance as "unfair." Organizations such as the International Olympic Committee, UNESCO, and the World Anti-Doping Agency are already investigating these potential uses of genomics.[62] At the same time, the use of such drugs—or other means of enhancement—is not always easy to define, detect, and control.

For example, aging is a normal and universal process, yet its effects are debilitating. Would drugs or genetic interventions to treat, delay, or eliminate aspects of the aging process count as therapy or enhancement? What would such interventions mean for cultural attitudes toward aging and decline and support for the debilitated elderly? What if wealthier segments of society were able to access interventions against aging, hence losing personal investment in social institutions of support for the aged? Or life might be prolonged, and with it the period of time of increasing debilitation, leading to a burden on social resources to the disadvantage of younger generations.[63]

What if individuals could purchase genetic enhancements for themselves or their children, or even have their embryos modified so that their entire genetic line would inherit a change "for the better"? Such choices would no doubt be influenced by cultural paradigms of excellence, whether in regard to appearance, talent, personality, or intelligence. The prevalence of cultural norms would be "selected for" by those with the purchasing power to realize their ambitions. Even more certain is the fact that those ambitions would involve a desire for competitive "superiority." One group of scholars draws a conclusion from aging research that applies more widely: "The first lesson that has emerged from the biogerontologists' experience is simple: while fighting disease always garners more public funding than health promotion, new biomedical enhancements will always have a bigger private market than new disease cures."[64] On the market, unsafe and ineffective means to promised benefits will be a problem, along with the actual advantages that will accrue to more lucky or prudent consumers. According to another scholar, the greatest social danger from enhancement genetics is

> a highly individualized marketplace funneled by an entrepreneurial spirit and the free choice of large numbers of parents that could lead us down a path, albeit incrementally, toward a society that abandons the lottery of

> evolution in favor of intentional genetic modification. The discoveries of genetics will not be imposed upon us. Rather, they will be sold to us by the market as something we cannot live without.[65]

It is difficult to argue or demonstrate that genetic enhancement involves a violation of human nature or human dignity, especially if the measure is the individual human being and his or her "natural" or "created" assets and abilities.[66] It would also be difficult to "outlaw" enhancement techniques by such standards, because the line between therapy and enhancement is gray. Treatments developed for therapeutic ends can and will generate enhancement opportunities. The major objection to the introduction of genetic enhancements is not that they are unnatural but that they are unfair. The availability of enhancement would confer even greater advantages on people who already control a disproportionate amount of resources and, furthermore, would permit users to shape future generations according to their standards of beauty and success.

One rejoinder might be that the wealthy and powerful already have the ability to pass on favored characteristics and abilities to their children by means of selective and expensive educational and cultural opportunities and that genetic means to the same ends would not represent a significant adjustment in the ways human societies work already. There is some truth to this reply. The "lottery of evolution" is already not so random. People select mates partly on the basis of qualities that can be inherited. Yet there is a difference between genetic and cultural enhancement techniques. The difference is that "cultural" means allow a much greater equalizing role for human freedom and for circumstantial risk or contingency.

Social opportunities afforded by wealthy or powerful families to their children require more voluntary response by the children in order to be effective and to be communicated further down the family line than would genetic changes. Circumstantial factors also have more opportunity to encourage or interfere with the transmission of values and assets, creating more diversity and flexibility in inheritance patterns than would be the case with genetically based individual traits. This is true even though most genetic "abilities" are to a greater or lesser extent interdependent with environmental factors. The passing on of genetic characteristics to children is still less dependent on confirmatory social conditions than is the passing on of cultural identity. Conversely, in the social transmission of goods and capabilities, new generations of families without unusual social assets are able to manipulate their individual circumstances to maximize their chances to gain goods or position. Freedom and contingency in the transmission of social assets tend to level or at least reconfigure the social playing field more regularly than would likely be the case if assets (or preferences) were genetically inscribed.

It might be that genetic treatments for cosmetic problems such as wrinkles or baldness, or enhancement of some abilities, such as disease resistance, could be accepted without dire effects on social relationships or the common good. However, these "highly seductive" technologies should not be accepted merely because there are "gaps in public policy or an aggressive marketplace." Extensive public discourse is necessary to achieve the scrutiny these inventions deserve and the regulation they require.[67] Theology can participate in this process, utilizing all its modes of discourse and focusing especially on considerations of equity and the common good.

Participatory Strategies for Theological Bioethics

A premise of this book is that religious groups and theological bioethicists often seem to lack access to policy-forming bodies at the national level; their testimony to national advisory bodies may serve as a "token" of respect for the variety of moral beliefs within the culture but is not very important in defining final reports. Theological bioethicists themselves admit an appreciable degree of uncertainty in establishing the practical policy "payoff" of their values and commitments. They are often better at narrative and prophetic discourse than at ethical and policy analysis.

Religious thinkers often seem unable to draw specific and well-warranted policy conclusions about genetics from their background narratives and general beliefs.[68] Perhaps if their contributions were more ethically coherent, they would be more influential on policy at the national level. It may be the case, however, that the role of a theological worldview is at least as much to challenge a social ethos as it is to specify policy outcomes that are required by the worldview. The challenge can be mediated into the social world at multiple levels and in multiple communities of discourse and practice, as well as through many institutions, beyond federal policy. Many different policy initiatives could address health inequities; it may be difficult or impossible to show conclusively that any one is the inevitable outcome demanded by theological ethics.

The debate about gene patenting is a good example. Patents are not objectionable in principle but should be subject to what John Paul II has referred to as a "social mortgage on property." Before the 1999 annual general meetings of the World Bank and International Monetary Fund, John

Paul II stated that "the Church has consistently taught that there is a 'social mortgage' on all private property, a concept which today must also be applied to 'intellectual property' and to 'knowledge.' The law of profit alone cannot be applied to that which is essential for the fight against hunger, disease and poverty."[69] He did not draw specific policy conclusions. The "social mortgage" metaphor advances the ethos of solidarity in both ethical and socially prophetic terms, without specifying exactly what policy is necessary to guarantee that the mortgage will be paid. Investors and inventors have a right to profit from their work and are entitled to exclude others from appropriating it for their own profit. However, this right and this entitlement have limits. The use of legal patent rights is morally problematic when it becomes a means to protect disproportionate financial gain for some while preventing others from gaining access to lifesaving medicines or treatments. The views of John Paul II and other religious and moral leaders were influential in relaxing patent controls on AIDS drugs for the poor.

Another line of critique adopted by religious bodies and theologians has to do with respect for human nature and the integrity of human and nonhuman life forms. This critique of patenting holds that no one should be able to assert rights over any class of components of the human body, such as genetic sequences, or over species of plants or animals, even if they have been created by genetic engineering. This type of thinking is not against all technology, but reflects a religiously grounded conviction that "biological patents constitute a threat to the dignity and sanctity of life."[70] An example of this second critique is the 1995 Joint Appeal against Human and Animal Patenting issued by representatives of several Christian, Buddhist, Jewish, Muslim, and Hindu religious denominations.[71] The issuing of the appeal was "participatory" in that it gathered interreligious participants in a common action and received significant public attention in the press and from scientists and churches. In contrast to John Paul II's use of the "social mortgage" metaphor, the content moved from religious symbols to a policy conclusion. There was not much ethical analysis in between.

The signatories all agree that "humans and animals are creations of God, not humans, and as such should not be patented in human inventions."[72] It is difficult to move from this general affirmation to specific ethical reasons that show that patenting genes is a violation of human nature or that patented life-forms demeans dignity. In fact, the Joint Appeal represents the views of many religious bodies but by no means a consensus; not all can agree that the symbol of "creation" requires one and the same policy outcome. Differences persist even in churches whose representatives signed the statement. According to Chapman, "the Joint Appeal can be characterized as more of a public policy declaration than a work of ethical or theological analysis."[73]

Another way to put the point is to say that the Joint Appeal, in a move not uncharacteristic of religious critiques of genetics, moves from narrative discourse directly to a stance on policy that is "prophetic" rather than ethically warranted. In fact, it is not clear why patenting would always be a violation of human, animal, or plant "nature" or of "creation." The driving concern seems instead to be that ceding control over life-forms to profit-making enterprises is likely to have bad consequences for future social attitudes and practices and, hence, to harm the common good. Social justice is a primary concern, perhaps the main concern, behind religious resistance to patenting of life-forms, even if not the only concern. The same is true of the fear of commercialization in genetics in general, or in the use of new reproductive technologies. It is hard to "prove" that payments to egg donors or the purchase of genetic tests to diagnose abnormalities in gametes or embryos violates some inherent quality of reproduction or of early life that should be protected absolutely. What is more clear is that distribution of medical resources by ability to pay results in very inequitable access, as well as the gearing of services offered to the needs or preferences of those best placed to purchase them.

These consequences should be contested by theological bioethics, but drawing policy conclusions that are inadequately defended is counterproductive because it undermines the credibility of religious voices. Sometimes it is better to express moral concerns and the religious values behind them, then join with others in seeking to establish better alternative practices that address those concerns, even if some moral issues remain unresolved. Within religious communities or in activities by which churches and theologians engage with the larger community, distinctive values such as justice, respect for life, and the healing of illness receive practical expression. For instance, the *Ethical and Religious Directives* for Catholic institutions state that no one is to be the subject of either therapeutic or nontherapeutic genetic experimentation unless that person or a surrogate has given consent. Although the solution of abortion is excluded, genetic counseling and prenatal testing "may be provided in order to promote responsible parenthood and to prepare for the proper treatment and care of children with genetic defects."[74] Catholic health facilities and clinics value freedom from genetic disease but also avoid the destruction of early life. The Catholic voice in bioethics gains credibility to the extent that it actually succeeds in establishing inclusive practices of healing and care, rather than just insisting that social policy conform to the specific morality derived within the religious tradition.

Moral directives regarding genetics and counseling are placed within an overall Catholic health care mission in which more equitable access and service to the poor are higher values. Within the larger picture, genetic services (or infertility services) are a secondary priority compared to basic health care for the underserved. The CHA, for example, spends its public advocacy resources primarily on health care reform and basic needs such as housing, rather than on debating new reproductive technologies and stem cell research. This in effect makes a practical "statement" about distributive justice in relation to biotechnology. It contributes to a reshaping of social priorities away from funding for profitable genomics and toward funding for those who are presently uninsured or who cannot get humane care when suffering terminal illness or debilitating old age.

In 2004, the CHA, using member consultation and work by a committee of experts, prepared a "toolkit" to address the practical and pastoral implications of, and the moral problems associated with, new "advances" in genetics.[75] The materials include a CD-ROM, with a scientific overview, theological framework, and outline of ethical issues, and three documents presenting selections from church teachings on genetics, a case book, and a constructive statement toward a "Catholic vision" of genomics. Acknowledging that genomics presents boundless opportunities for the improvement of human well-being, the vision statement also invokes Jesus' healing in the context of human wholeness, spiritual values, and ultimate finitude. The statement stresses the importance of allocating research and clinical resources in light of the common good and of a just distribution of benefits.

> Our enduring commitment to the disadvantaged and our option for the poor requires a careful and delicate balancing with regard to the pursuit of genomics—for example, balancing the pursuit of the goods of genomics with efforts to ensure that the basic human needs of all our citizens are adequately met; balancing the pursuit of genomics with meeting the health needs of the poor and effecting reform of a health care system with so many injustices.[76]

The document goes on to acknowledge the benefits that genomics may bring and attends to generally recognized moral problems such as informed consent and confidentiality. Yet it also raises for Catholic health care questions such as whether trust in genetic testing and treatments exceed the benefits realistically to be delivered, and whether the implementation of gene-based diagnostic and treatment programs in Catholic facilities is the best way to meet the commitment to serve the poor and disadvantaged. The intended audience is executives, boards, and sponsors of Catholic hospitals, as well as ethics committees, direct care leaders, and educators.

Protestant theologians similarly place genetic counseling within a value perspective that relativizes biotechnology as a solution to human problems and stresses values of respect and compassion. There may be a greater tendency than in recent Catholic bioethics to focus attention on the individual counseling relationship. A fairly lengthy report on genetic counseling from the Lutheran bioethics institute, the Park Ridge Center (Chicago), stresses the need for expertise in scientific information related to genetics and for pastoral sensitivity in dealing with clients. Religious values and narratives are important in counseling about genetic disease, as this issue engages persons in the limit experiences of birth and death; giving a religious dimension to genetic decision-making is important to help persons cope with suffering and healing.[77]

As theological bioethicists engage policymakers and scientists with more frequency about genetics-related practices that are quickly becoming institutionalized, the moral color of the structures channeling costs and benefits is receiving a higher profile. In the participatory as well as analytical and policy modes, a 2003 conference at St. Louis University (a Jesuit institution) drew together interests and expertise from the medical, legal, business, and theological realms and repeatedly surfaced the theme of social justice. A Catholic moral theologian and health care administrator makes a plea to limit advocacy for individual needs, in view of attention to the good for many and to public health ethics, and sounds a note that rings through most of the other essays.[78] The message is brought toward the realm of practice by experts from different disciplines, suggesting how ideals might be reflected in concrete structures or policies regarding, for example, corporate behavior, patent law, pediatric medical standards, genetic screening programs, health insurance, and "informed consent" in different social and political contexts.

Genomics and Global Participatory Bioethics

Although genomics is not yet perceived to have enough impact on basic health needs to mobilize constituencies whose levels of deprivation across the board are dire, that could change as awareness increases in developing countries and specific gene-based vaccines and drugs to target AIDS, malaria, hepatitis, and diabetes grow closer to reality. A model for activism on human genetics already exists in the form of international mobilization against genetically modified foods, in which religious participation is high.[79] Similar forms of "participatory democracy" for genetics and human health could be extended or developed from existing advocacy networks for justice in national and worldwide health care.

Promoters of genetically modified crops maintain that they will help feed the poor. Opponents contend that there is no evidence that such crops are cheaper or more nutritious. Moreover, European activism against "Frankenfoods" has raised levels of resistance in the European Union, if not in the United States, and seed manufacturers like Monsanto need new outlets for an increasingly unpopular product. Under the guise of humanitarian aid, U.S. corporations and government are trying to force acceptance in other nations in the form of food donations. However, the introduction of such crops risks displacing local varieties, creating dependence on imported products (especially when the imported seeds are "designed" to be difficult to make or reproduce), putting subsistence farmers out of business and raising levels of poverty throughout Asia and Africa.

There is still some argument (especially in Africa) that genetically modified foods could someday benefit the poor by enhancing nutrients or resistance to adverse environmental conditions. Yet, a growing international advocacy network, making extensive use of the Internet, is working hard to solidify local opposition and reveal the corporate profits that an altruistic façade protects. In 2000, an international organization of fifteen Catholic NGOs published a study calling for affected nations to resist patent law by making as wide a use as possible of the discretionary power allowed them under World Trade Organization regulations and to seek the moral high ground with Catholic social teaching, especially the pope's declaration that there is "a social mortgage on property" requiring the rich to fulfill obligations to the developing world.[80]

In February 2003, a consultation on "Biotechnology and Agriculture—a Faith-Based Perspective" was held in Chicago. Many of the sponsoring or cooperating organizations already had strong relationships and had participated in a conference in September 2002. They included but were not limited to Agricultural Missions in New York,[81] the National Council of Churches of Christ in the U.S.A., the National Catholic Rural Life Conference, the Evangelical Lutheran Church in America, Lutheran World Relief, the Presbyterian Hunger Program, the Episcopal Church of the United States, the South African Catholic Bishops Conference, the Catholic Bishops' Conference of the Philippines, Catholic Relief Services, Bread for the World, the Maryknoll Office for Global Concerns, and the Adrian Dominicans (a Catholic women's religious order). In addition, individual representatives also arrived from El Salvador, Nicaragua, Haiti, and Ghana. A 2002 report was circulated from the Church and Society Commission of the Conference of European Churches, Bioethics Working Group.

The Chicago meeting resulted in a position paper available for individuals and groups to sign or to publicize, declaring that agricultural genetic engineering has not been demonstrated to safeguard "the common good, human dignity, the sacredness of life and stewardship." The paper calls into question the marketing of crops by large private companies for profit, equating private control by patent law under current global trade policies with a threat to local food systems. The church has a responsibility "to monitor developments and educate its membership" according to principles of accountability and social justice. In order to further these aims, the conference participants use an e-mail list to circulate information, news, and opportunities for cooperation, mobilization, and protest. One item within the first three months after Chicago was a report on "Principles for Global Corporate Responsibility: Bench Marks for Measuring Business Performances," the work of a coalition of religious organizations and advocacy groups from twenty-two countries.[82] Another was an invitation to participate in a four-week United Nations Food and Agriculture Organization Internet conference on "regulating GMOs in developing and transition countries."[83] Statements were also circulated from the Catholic bishops in the Philippines and Brazil and from African organizations; reports and news items were submitted on regulation or boycotts of genetically modified foods in the European Union, the United States, and Asia.

Religious and theological analysis continues to be controversial in the area of plant genetics, as in that of human genetics, and for the same reason: promises of "benefits" and "relief of human suffering" meet with skepticism and counterevidence about implementations that further disadvantage the poor. In 2004, the National Academy of Sciences (U.S.) issued a report asserting that genetically engineered crops pose no unique health risks, but it called for further long-term study and for tightening of scrutiny of individual products before they go to market, measures that underscored the uncertainty of the health risk finding.[84] A couple of months later, the Vatican and the United States cosponsored a conference in Rome on genetically modified foods and world hunger that critics saw as a lobbying effort by commercial interests hoping to expand the market and to displace competition from traditional farming methods. The event, held at the Gregorian University, was prejudicially entitled "Feeding a Hungry World: The Moral Imperative of Biotechnology."[85] The U.S. ambassador to the Holy See defended promotion of genetically modified crops, asserting that "the worst form of cultural imperialism is to deny others the opportunities we have to take advantage of new technologies to raise up our human condition." But adversaries rejoined that world hunger is not a problem of production but of distribution, and that genetically modified crops serve mostly U.S. multinational biotechnology corporations. The "opportunities" available to the wealthy and well-fed include the right to own land, sell its products at a fair price (or receive subsidies), buy the expensive pesticides necessary to maintain genetically modified crops, choose between farming and other types of education and employment, and even hire workers by whose labor they profit.[86]

At the Vatican meeting, International Cooperation for Development and Solidarity (CIDSE) and Caritas Internationalis circulated a joint statement representing "international networks of Catholic non-governmental agencies with longstanding experience in the fight against hunger and for food security."[87] Together, CIDSE and Caritas represent 177 relief, development, and social service organizations in more than two hundred states and territories throughout the world. They conclude,

> GM crops do not address the root causes of hunger, including lack of access to land, water, energy, affordable credit, local markets and infrastructures. Greater investment in agriculture and rural development, true commitment to land reform, more participatory decision-making within institutions and fairer rules governing international agricultural trade and regulations on corporations are some of the key changes needed in order to address these complex causes of hunger.[88]

Much the same could be said about disease and human genetics. Pharmacogenomics and gene therapy are not needed to address the causes of most diseases and premature deaths of the poor. Adequate food, clean water, and basic health care would reduce maternal and infant mortality, cut deaths in early childhood, and curtail the ravages of malaria, tuberculosis, and sleeping sickness. These and other diseases, such as AIDS, have roots in social causes such as lack of employment opportunity and denial of social resources to women. Although there is a possibility of genetic means of combating these diseases, for example, by enhancing immunity or disabling malaria-spreading mosquitoes, these research avenues are not pursued as avidly by those in possession of capital as those that connect the profit motive with the demands of the rich: cures for cancer, heart disease, obesity, and Alzheimer's.

There are other justice-oriented moral and social analyses of disease, genomics, and access whose explanatory language and agenda converges with that of theological bioethicists. The WHO has recommended focused action in local communities to reduce disparities in poor health and life expectancy, with help from investments by donor organizations and nations. Locally based and internationally enabled measures have shown their potential for success in the SARS epidemic, and in advances in the campaign to eradicate polio.[89] A list of biotechnologies that could help improve health in developing countries was drawn up by a research team of experts from twenty-eight countries and published in 2002. Their ten recommendations are more affordable diagnoses of infectious diseases, vaccines against infectious diseases, more efficient drug delivery systems, environmental improvement, sequencing pathogen genomes, female controlled contraceptives and barriers against sexually transmitted disease, bioinformatics to identify drug targets and pathogen-host interactions, crops with enhanced nutrients to counter specific deficiencies, and more affordable therapeutic products, such as insulin, made using recombinant technologies.

The authors urge individual countries to assess the usefulness of these technologies in their local contexts and to focus on those promising the most benefit. Associations of developing countries are encouraged to pool collective efforts and resources. Pharmaceutical and biotechnology industry associations are urged to work with members to determine the status of work on these and similar technologies in their research and development plans and to form partnerships with WHO and developing countries to create and distribute these products. The results of the study are also proposed as guides for policies of major international donors and bilateral aid agencies, such as the U.S. NIH, the Rockefeller Foundation, the Gates Foundation, and the Wellcome Trust.[90]

It is true that advances in genomics will probably not mean very much to the third of the world population that lives on less than $2 a day.[91] Genomics may simply be diverting resources away from efforts toward adequate food, water, sewage disposal, and other global public health needs. Nonetheless, recommendations like those above may have beneficial effect if they are accompanied by a greater willingness on the part of rich countries and drug and biotech companies to share knowledge and increase investments. The ultimate goal must be for developing countries to achieve a position where their access to health resources is under their own control and sustainable. Partnerships could be formed with regional groupings, such as the Asia-Pacific Health Research Forum and the African Health Research Forum, and should involve scientists and institutions from developing countries that have already made some advances in genomics, such as Brazil, India, China, Malaysia, and Thailand, as well as the Third World Academy of Science.[92]

At both the theoretical and practical levels, it appears that there is some agreement of theological, philosophical, and policy bioethics on the importance of solidarity, participation, and a preferential option for the poor. A remaining challenge is for this convergence of viewpoints to make a practical difference large enough to contest in any significant way the control that economic interests have over access to health care resources. Bioethical discourse about access and justice tends to concentrate on conversionary rhetoric and arguments, aiming moral persuasion at the "haves" and moral encouragement at the "have nots." A major asset of theological discourse is that it can explicitly name personal and structural resistance to change as sin, not only placing it under a judgment but defining it in relation to a normative order as nonnormative and unacceptable. The sinful intransigency of inequitable social structures and their beneficiaries is something to be actively resisted. Participatory theological bioethics has a special obligation to go beyond exhortation. It should help identify and act upon "pressure points" in the "webs of transformation" around genomics and other biotechnologies, points at which pressure can be applied to "the powers" to bring about change even without or before conversion. Advocacy for AIDS drugs has provided one example.

In the same vein, theological bioethicists should urge that steps be taken by philanthropists and other funders to devise means of forceful intervention in the business practices of biotech companies. Michael Kremer, an expert in development economics, estimates that about half of all global health research and development in recent years was undertaken by private industry, with less than 5 percent going to diseases specific to poor countries.[93] Doctors Without Borders recognizes that international research in the private sector is driven by financial returns rather than public health needs (just as is private research in the United States). Sixty percent of all profits from international pharmaceutical sales are made in the United States, whereas Africa represents only 1 percent of worldwide sales. Firms have limited incentives to invest in such diseases, because the market is poor and profits are sure to be low.[94]

Kremer makes the case that foreign-aid donors should issue advance contracts for purchase of needed products such as malaria vaccines, thus stimulating research and guaranteeing that development would serve those in dire need. "Push" programs could subsidize research in desirable areas. "Pull" programs would reward research outputs by committing in advance to buy a product as a specified price. Both are important, but the latter have a special advantage in situations in which research is funded for a product that may not bring the greatest reward in money or prestige. The actual uses of grant money and their outcomes are hard to monitor in push programs, and funding can get diverted to more financially or professionally profitable purposes. In pull programs, money does not change hands until the desired outcome is produced. Another advantage of pull programs is that investors can promise to pay for a drug or vaccine, no matter who develops it. Thus, the danger of preferential treatment of certain countries or teams in awarding grants is avoided.

Push and pull programs enhance or reinforce the work of moral persuasion by offering practical incentives based on self-interest to accomplish good deeds. These incentives are coercive, or a counter-use of power, to the extent that they employ tacit threats to change behavior. The threat is of lost productivity and earnings and of slippage relative to the positions of market competitors. These programs would make the development of biotechnology for the poor seem more attractive even to those corporations whose agents are not motivated by altruism or for whom the "preferential option for the poor" is not important. "A price of $15 for the first 200 million people immunized, plus revenues from modest sales outside the program, would give a potential vaccine developer a net present value of revenues that would be comparable to the revenues from products developed for commercial purposes." Yet the program would cost investors nothing if a viable product were not developed.[95] Corporations such as GlaxoSmithKline have been working on projects such as a malaria vaccine over a period of many years in order to serve the developing world. These projects do represent a commitment to use scientific knowledge to serve the public good. Yet they are slow to reach fruition because they have a low institutional priority compared to financial accountability to shareholders. International public interest and service organizations and donors should do more not only to encourage but to pressure corporations toward responsibility for global health needs.

A number of organizations, including national governments, the World Bank, and private foundations like the Gates Foundation, have the resources to enter into pull contracts. In addition, the concept of purchase commitments has been endorsed by elements within the Clinton and Bush administrations, the United Kingdom, the WHO, the World Bank, and the Gates Foundation, with a few initiatives proposed or in progress.[96] As in other aspects of global security, the cooperative international control of biotechnology and the turning of new developments to the common good rather than to destructive or divisive ends (such as bioterrorism) requires "wisdom and courage," but is also an exercise in prudence and self-protection.[97] To be effective, it will require persuasive appeals to altruism and justice, quasi-coercive appeals to self-interest, appropriate manipulation of market incentives, and public participation.

Representative processes of judgment are important both for credibility and for competence and effectiveness, especially when global matters are at stake. While those in whom power is vested are invariably reluctant to give it up, experience shows that participatory processes are necessary to accomplish goals that are beneficial to all. In fact, without participation, not even the interests of the more powerful can be made secure. Global oversight of biotechnology is necessary not only to distribute benefits equitably and to avoid destructive applications but also to monitor against inadvertent biotechnological or genomic catastrophes. The National Academy of Sciences recently recommended that the national oversight system be strengthened and that an international regulatory process be adopted.[98]

Conclusion

Genetic science and its applications constitute a realm in which the nature, tasks, and tools of participatory theological bioethics are superbly demonstrated. As participatory, a theological bioethics defined by an "option for the poor" joins its narrative, prophetic, ethical, and policy discourses to participatory intervention in social structures that govern human relationships. Using theological symbols and claims such as creation, image of God, love of neighbor, and care for the poor, theological bioethics relates these to mediating concepts such as solidarity, common good, and distributive justice. It develops and learns by means of practices in which Christians join with members of other faith traditions and with institutions and organizations focused around other types of identity, many of which intersect with religious communities and membership. For example, persons of differing moral commitments are concerned about the personal and social implications of patenting genes or funding stem cell research. Exploiting the resources of multileveled subsidiary sites of collective agency, theological bioethics brings an expansive religious worldview to bear on practices shared with or interacting with "the public sphere," dialectically understood.

FINAL REFLECTIONS

Theology is the "critical thinking" of religion, and the practices that make religion and theology concrete not only express theologies and their differences but help generate the theological expressions. According to Edward Schillebeeckx, Christian identity is actualized in new experiences and practices, and these practices have "a hermeneutical, critical and productive power" with respect to Christian theology.[1] For example, Christian medical providers who give care to the poor gain new insight into the social conditions and policies that do or do not support health. Theological bioethics can gain insight and change direction as a result of the liberative practices in which it engages. Yet this also means that, within a religious tradition, the same sort of interactive comparing, testing, criticizing, sorting, and converting or consensus-building must go on as goes on when religion or theology engages in the "public" sphere with nonreligious value traditions, theories, and practices. Theological bioethicists need to defend theoretically and display politically the values they believe to be key to their religious identities and those of their traditions.

The present work in theological bioethics endorses and promotes health care reform guided by the priority of the preferential option for the poor, within an ethics of the common good. With Robert Schreiter, I see as normative and even as pervasive in Christian ethics today the "global theological flow" that reflects "'the irruption of the poor'" (in the phrase of Gustavo Gutierrez).[2] The bioethical practice entailed by this theology is a new or renewed Christian social engagement for health care justice. This theological orientation challenges the control of market values in virtually every sphere of contemporary life, including health care, and especially their effect on the poor.

It is difficult if not impossible to accomplish goals of distributive justice by means of blanket characterizations, prescriptions, and prohibitions. Rather, justice in access to resources must be approached in different social sectors and arenas by means of appropriate interventions, directives, legislation, regulation, and policies that make particular practice areas and spheres of relationship more inclusive. The goal of humane health care for all is undermined by the regulatory or legal "normalization" of activities like physician-facilitated killing, the creation of research embryos, and the development of genetically tailored drugs that will be available to only a few. Participatory theological bioethics holds up democratically developed regulation as a current available means to exert control over liberalism, technology, and the market and to advance the cause of health care equity.

Religious congregations and educational institutions constitute a major potential forum in which to encourage and shape public deliberation on important public issues such as physician-assisted suicide, health care reform, patenting, germ-line engineering, stem cell research, and the responsibilities of privileged societies for global health. Religious traditions can resist the trend toward funding and development of every new and potentially profitable innovation, which is often virtually "pre-programmed once a new technique appears on the market."[3] They do this not only through various modes of "verbal" discourse (narrative, prophetic, ethical, and policy) but also through action (participatory). Theology and religious traditions can function as subversive authorities in reshaping cultural assumptions, values, norms, and institutions.[4] Beyond narratives, symbols, and ethical arguments, theologians within religious traditions and churches can be part of the reflective, critical instantiation of a different set of values in their own practices. They can also explore and introduce new models of political participation that engage religious communities with others in fostering broad-based and more democratic resolution of quandaries about the uses of health resources.

National policy is important but not the only route, or necessarily the most accessible route, for the contribution of religion and theology. In many dimensions of local, national, and global civil society, and in partnership with different levels of government and a variety of government agencies, theological bioethics can forward social practices that represent its values and expand their sphere of influence. Middle axioms are the instruments by which religious values and theological interpretation seek common ground with companion moral traditions and practices, yet also press along that ground toward a deeper or higher level.

The public sphere of arguments interlocking with practices is a realm of "criss-crossing communities" that can become a "web of transformation."[5] The liberal, scientistic, and market environments that presently control medicine and biotechnology can be subjected to critique and modified. This can happen only if and when resistant practices, as well as their narrative and argumentative languages, challenge the status quo. Theological bioethicists, feminist ethicists, liberation theologians, and all those interested in global health equity bring challenges from different directions, share agenda items, and discover points of mutual symbolic and argumentative intelligibility. Together they can roll back the technologization of the dying process, the commercialization of reproduction, the control of genetic information by for-profit corporations, and the exclusion of the majority of the world's population from health needs much more fundamental than ICU treatment, in vitro fertilization, stem cell therapies, and pharmacogenomics. The large and small successes of collective action against exclusionary pricing of AIDS drugs and against the corporate promotion of genetically modified plants and animals create the possibility of an analogous response to the global proliferation of biotechnology and indicate a new direction for theological analysis.

A conception of theological bioethics as participatory captures the influence theologians can have in the spheres of common life where they join with others in the search for the common good. This search is never concluded, satisfied, or even balanced; in fact, engagement rather than completion fulfills the meaning of the common good, as a network of historical relationships in which everyone continually participates in the practices relevant to their well-being. Theological bioethics in the twenty-first century must make a new commitment to public participation. It must work hard to transform local and global access to the basic goods of health care, so that justice, equity, and the common good move much further from utopia toward reality. Christian practices and theologies—bioethical or otherwise—will never completely change personal relationships or social institutions so that injustice is eradicated and suffering abolished. Total practical success has never been the measure or the expectation of Christian political action. Sin is a sorry fact of life in which religious traditions and theologians themselves are implicated, even as they protest the evil in the world.

Yet neither the reoccurrence of defeat nor the resistance of hostile ideologies can excuse the retreat of theological bioethics from the public and political realms. The stakes are too high for those who suffer in the present worldwide "system" of health injustice. The distinctively religious contribution of theological bioethics is to set courageous transformative practices against the horizon of an ultimate, personal power that both judges and sustains human efforts. It is in actions that Christian practice renews and makes good on its hope for change. Collaborative, participatory social action can and must bring more just and compassionate sharing of global health resources.

ACKNOWLEDGMENTS

I AM GRATEFUL for the generous support and encouragement of Georgetown University Press director Richard Brown, and of my friend and Boston College colleague Jim Keenan, the editor of the Moral Traditions series. They always had time to give advice, make sure this project moved ahead expeditiously, and give me confidence that what was once a series of disconnected essays in bioethics could turn into an integral work with a new thesis, focus, and relevance.

Two colleagues in theological bioethics, Karen Lebacqz and Paul Lauritzen, read the entire manuscript for Georgetown University Press and gave many invaluable suggestions, big and small. The most important of these—a point on which they agreed—was the recommendation to situate my own proposal against other religious attempts to intervene politically in the practices of medicine and research, especially in light of the 2004 national elections.

My research assistant, Sarah Moses, a Boston College Ph.D. candidate in ethics, located and conveyed to my office an astounding amount of research materials, some requiring a considerable amount of ingenuity to produce. As a member of the Community of Sant'Egidio, Sarah provided me with illustrations of their work among the elderly and AIDS patients internationally, which were woven into the project.

The Rev. Michael Place, until recently president of the Catholic Health Association, is also an advocate of health care justice. He graciously complied with my many requests for more access, information, and resources, supporting my use of the CHA along with Sant'Edigio as examples of a socially engaged and participatory theological bioethics.

Parts of the following chapters and articles served as a basis for the book; all have been revised and recombined into different chapters. Substantial new material has been added.

"Abortion, Sex, and Gender: The Church's Public Voice," The John Courtney Murray Forum Lecture 1993, *America* (May 22, 1993).

"Euthanasia: The Practical and Social Significance of Double Effect," in Todd A. Salzman, ed., *Method and Catholic Moral Theology: The Ongoing Reconstruction* (Fordham University Press, 1999).

"The Genome Project: More Than a Medical Milestone," *America* 183, no. 4 (August 12, 2000).

"Social Ethics of Embryo and Stem Cell Research," *Women's Health Issues* 10, no. 3 (May–June 2000).

"Stem Cells: A Bioethical Balancing Act," *America* 184, no. 10 (2001).

"Religion, Theology and Bioethics," in J. Sugarman and D. Sulmasy, eds., *Methods in Medical Ethics* (Georgetown University Press, 2001).

"Genetics, Ethics and Feminist Theology: Some Recent Directions," *Journal of Feminist Studies in Religion* 18, no. 2 (fall 2002).

"Bioethics, Theology, and Social Change," *Journal of Religious Ethics* 31, no. 3 (2003).

"Nature, Sin, and Society," in Harold Baillie and Timothy Casey, eds., *Genetic Engineering and the Future of Human Nature* (MIT Press, 2004).

"How Theology Moves into Public Bioethics," in David E. Guinn, ed., *Faith at the Frontiers: A Reader in Religion and Public Bioethics* (Oxford, forthcoming).

"Genetics, Theology, Common Good," in Lisa Sowle Cahill, ed., *Genetics, Theology, Ethics: An Interdisciplinary Conversation* (New York: Crossroad, 2005).

NOTES

Unless indicated, websites were accessed between July and October 2004.

Introduction

1. Edward Schillebeeckx, "The Religious and the Human Ecumene," in *The Language of Faith: Essays on Jesus, Theology, and the Church* (Maryknoll, NY: Orbis Books and SCM Press, 1995), 262. On the biblical basis of concern for the poor in health care, see Scott E. Daniels, "Biomedical Ethics and U.S. Health Policy," and John F. Kilner, "A Biblical Mandate for Cultural Engagement," in *BioEngagement: Making a Christian Difference through Bioethics,* ed. Nigel M. de S. Cameron, Scott E. Daniels, and Barbara J. White (Grand Rapids, MI: Eerdmans, 2000), 142 and 23, respectively. See also my essay "The Bible and Christian Moral Practices," in *Christian Ethics: Problems and Prospects,* ed. Lisa Sowle Cahill and James F. Childress (Cleveland, OH: Pilgrim Press, 1996), 3–17.

2. Schillebeeckx, "Religious and the Human Ecumene," 261.

3. Jim Wallis, "Neither Republicans nor Democrats Have a Clue," *Boston Theological Institute Newsletter* 24, no. 19 (2005): 2. See also Jim Wallis, *God's Politics: Why the Right Gets It Wrong and the Left Doesn't Get It* (San Francisco, CA: HarperSanFrancisco, 2005).

4. Terms such as "right," "left," "liberal," "conservative," "neoconservative," and "progressive" are frequently used in public debates but are hard to define. In fact, they do not denote hard and unitary positions or viewpoints. "Right" and ""conservative" are usually associated with pro-life, pro-family, and anti-gay causes. However, it is certainly possible to be feminist and pro-life or to support the sanctity of marriage and want to extend marriage to gays. Even more difficult to line up than stances on sex and gender are those on economics and political participation. People on either the "right" or the "left" can support individual autonomy and privacy in the economic sphere and think of civil and political rights primarily in terms of "civil liberties." This is true of both "neoconservatives" and "liberals," who often do not agree on sex and gender ethics. The term "progressive" is thus sometimes used to refer to a politics that aims for a political process that is more inclusive along the socioeconomic and racial-ethnic spectrum and that also puts more emphasis on socioeconomic and material rights such as housing, education, employment, and health care. This brief discussion is meant more to indicate the complexity of these distinctions, rather than to define terms precisely. I identify more with "progressive" politics, thought of as a commitment to social justice, the common good, sex and gender equality, ethnic-racial inclusion, and a critical attitude toward state-

sanctioned killing, such as capital punishment, war, physician-assisted suicide, and abortion. I also see "progressive politics" as a big umbrella, under which a variety of groups could come together, even if not always in agreement on every issue.

5. As a work in bioethics, this project does not include the display or defense of a complete constructive theological ethics. I treat the relation of bioethics to Catholic moral theology and Catholic social ethics in *Bioethics and the Common Good* (Milwaukee, WI: Marquette University Press, 2004). Works in theological ethics that define the essential meaning of Christian ethics in ways similar to my own project, combining a biblical "option for the poor" with a commitment to public discourse about solidarity and the common good, include Cristina Traina, *Feminist Ethics and Natural Law: The End of the Anathemas* (Washington, DC: Georgetown University Press, 1999), and David Hollenbach, *The Common Good and Christian Ethics* (Cambridge: Cambridge University Press, 2002). The social encyclicals of John Paul II sound similar themes, e.g., *Sollicitudo Rei Socialis* (1988), as do many varieties of liberation and political theology.

6. Edward Schillebeeckx, *The Schillebeeckx Reader*, ed. Robert Schreiter (Edinburgh, UK: T&T Clark, 1984), 118. This passage was originally published in 1971.

7. Robert Schreiter, *The New Catholicity: Between the Local and the Global* (Maryknoll, NY: Orbis, 1997).

8. The preferential option for the poor is a term developed by liberation theology to denote a solidarity with the poor that motivates affirmative action by the more privileged, with the aim of changing social structures. The concept derives from Jesus' commands to serve one's neighbors, especially those most in need. It has been adopted by John Paul II to express the mandate of Catholic social teaching (see the encyclical *Gospel of Life* [*Evangelium vitae*], 1995, nos. 18, 40–41).

Chapter 1

1. These are infamous research projects, in which African American men were left untreated for syphilis even after treatments had been shown effective (Tuskegee syphilis study), and in which mentally retarded children were exposed to hepatitis (Willowbrook State School). See Jeffrey P. Kahn, Anna C. Mastroianni, and Jeffrey Sugarman, *Beyond Consent: Seeking Justice in Research* (New York: Oxford University Press, 1998) 3–4; and Warren T. Reich, "Bioethics in the United States," in *Bioethics: A History*, ed. Corrado Viafora (Bethesda, MD: International Scholars Publications, 1996) 83–87. The Nuremburg code may be found in Tom L. Beauchamp and LeRoy Walters, *Contemporary Issues in Bioethics* (Belmont, CA: Wadsworth, 1978), 404–5.

2. Reich, "Bioethics," 88.

3. Students of Gustafson who entered the field early on included James Childress (a Quaker, who usually writes from a philosophical perspective), Allen Verhey (developing biblical ethics within the Reformed tradition), Stanley Hauerwas (a Methodist, whose proposal of a communitarian, narrative ethics has been immensely influential), and Margaret Farley (a Roman Catholic and major contributor to feminist bioethics). David Smith (an Episcopalian) has worked at the intersection of theology, philosophy, and policy; Warren Reich (a Catholic) edited the *Encyclopedia of Bioethics*. Charles E. Curran argued that Catholic moral theology in general should be more historical and applied this to norms in bioethics. William E. May (also a Catholic) defended Catholic Church teaching

on bioethics, while William F. May (a Methodist) turned his attention more to the social and professional roles and obligations of physicians than to practical problem solving. Robert Veatch has expanded the interreligious dialogue among many traditions. For further discussion, see LeRoy Walters, "Religion and the Renaissance of Medical Ethics in the United States," in *Theology and Bioethics: Exploring the Foundations and Frontiers,* ed. Earl E. Shelp (Dordrecht, Neth.: Kluwer, 1986), 3–16; Warren Thomas Reich, "Bioethics in the United States," in *History of Bioethics: International Perspectives,* ed. Roberto Dell'Oro and Corrado Viafora (San Francisco, CA: International Scholars Publications, 1996) 83–118; and James F. Childress, "Religion, Theology and Bioethics," in *The Nature and Prospects of Bioethics: Interdisciplinary Perspectives,* ed. Franklin G. Miller (Totowa, NJ: Humana Press, 2003), 43–67.

4. Warren T. Reich, *Encyclopedia of Bioethics* (New York: Macmillan, 1978).

5. The theologian on NBAC was James Childress; the theologian on the PCB is Gilbert Meilaender.

6. Richard A. McCormick, *Health and Medicine in the Catholic Tradition* (New York: Crossroad, 1984).

7. One of his more famous and influential pieces in this regard was "To Save or Let Die: The Dilemma of Modern Medicine," *Journal of the American Medical Association* 229 (1974): 172–76. The essay was published simultaneously in *America* 131 (July 1974).

8. See Walters, "Religion and the Renaissance," 3–16; and Warren T. Reich, with the assistance of Roberto Dell'Oro, "A New Era for Bioethics: The Search for Meaning in Moral Experience," in *Religion and Medical Ethics: Looking Back, Looking Forward,* ed. Allen Verhey (Grand Rapids, MI: Eerdmans, 1996) 96–115.

9. Thomas A. Shannon, "Bioethics and Religion: A Value-Added Discussion," in *Notes from a Narrow Ridge: Religion and Bioethics,* ed. Dena S. Davis and Laurie Zoloth (Hagerstown, MD: University Publishing Groups, 1999), 31.

10. See Philip Hefner, "The Evolution of the Created Co-Creator," in *Cosmos as Creation: Theology and Science in Consonance,* ed. Ted Peters (Nashville, TN: Abingdon, 1989), 211–33. For an example of this sort of argument about genetic technology, and a discussion of some alternatives, see Ted Peters, *For the Love of Children: Genetic Technology and the Future of the Family* (Louisville, KY: Westminster/John Knox Press, 1996).

11. For some grounds for this approach to theological ethics, see chapter 1, notes 1, 4, and 5.

12. Daniel Callahan, "Why America Accepted Bioethics," *The Hastings Center Report* 23, no. 6 (1993): S8.

13. Ibid.

14. Daniel Callahan, "Religion and the Secularization of Bioethics," *Hastings Center Report* 20 (July/August 1990): 2–10; Courtney Campbell, "Religion and Moral Meaning in Bioethics," *Hastings Center Report* 20 (July/August 1990): 4–10; Hauerwas, *Suffering Presence: Theological Reflections on Medicine, the Mentally Handicapped, and the Church* (Notre Dame, IN: University of Notre Dame, 1986); Hauerwas, "How Christian Ethics Became Medical Ethics: The Case of Paul Ramsey," in *Religion and Medical Ethics: Looking Back, Looking Forward,* ed. Allen Verhey (Grand Rapids, MI: Eerdmans, 1996), 61–80; Brent Waters, "What Is the Appropriate Contribution of Religious Communities in the Public Debate on Embryonic Stem Cell Research?" in *God and the Embryo: Religious Perspectives on Stem Cells and Cloning,* ed. Brent Waters and Ron Cole-Turner (Washington, DC: Georgetown University Press, 2003), 19–28.

15. See Tom L. Beauchamp and James F. Childress, *Principles of Biomedical Ethics,* 5th ed. (Oxford, UK: Oxford University Press, 2001). The first edition of this work appeared in 1979. (See n. 16.)

16. John H. Evans, *Playing God? Human Genetic Engineering and the Rationalization of Public Bioethical Debate* (Chicago: University of Chicago Press, 2002), 88. These four principles were first given a philosophical explanation and defense in Beauchamp's and Childress's *Principles of Biomedical Ethics* (1979), which has subsequently seen five editions. However, they had been earlier articulated as principles for public policy at a conference convened in 1974 by the National Commission for the Protection of Human Subjects of Behavioral and Biomedical Research (created by Congress in 1973). This conference or "retreat" issued recommendations in the form of the 1978 *Belmont Report,* named after the conference center, Belmont House. The report was submitted to the Department of Health, Education, and Welfare, which adopted it as public law governing federally funded research. (See Evans, *Playing God?,* 83–89; and Callahan, "Religion and the Secularization of Bioethics," S3.)

17. John Rawls, *A Theory of Justice* (Cambridge, MA: Harvard University Press, 1971), 395–99; see also Rawls, *Political Liberalism* (New York: Columbia University Press, 1993), 178–95.

18. Rawls, *Theory of Justice,* 396.

19. Evans, *Playing God?* 127–31.

20. Ibid., 158–65.

21. Jeffrey Stout, *Ethics after Babel: The Languages of Morals and Their Discontents* (Boston: Beacon Press, 1988), 282 and 283, respectively.

22. Ibid., 284 and 285, respectively.

23. David H. Smith, "Religion and the Roots of the Bioethics Revival," in Verhey, *Religion and Medical Ethics,* 2–18; Gustafson, *Intersections: Science, Theology, and Ethics;* Gustafson, "Styles of Religious Reflection in Medical Ethics," in *Religion and Medical Ethics,* ed. Verhey, 81–95; Reich, "New Era for Bioethics," 96–115; Richard A. McCormick, "Theology and Bioethics: Christian Foundations," in *Theology and Bioethics: Exploring the Foundations and Frontiers,* ed. Earl Shelp (Dordrecht, Neth.: Kluwer, 1986), 95–113; and Cahill, *Bioethics and the Common Good.*

24. Evans, *Playing God?* 197.

25. He cites the groundbreaking work of Amy Gutmann and Dennis Thompson, *Democracy and Disagreement* (Cambridge, MA: Harvard University Press, 1996).

26. Albert W. Dzur and Daniel Levin, "The 'Nation's Conscience': Assessing Bioethics Commissions as Public Forums," *Kennedy Institute of Ethics Journal* 14, no. 4 (2004): 351.

27. Mark Hanson concludes his Introduction to a set of Hastings Center papers on the engagement of religious groups and theologians with the ethics of gene patenting and cloning with the observation that "policy discourse was impoverished by an inability to accommodate religious insights in productive ways." Mark J. Hanson, ed., *Claiming Power over Life: Religion and Biotechnology Policy* (Washington, DC: Georgetown University Press, 2001), x. In the same volume Courtney Campbell rightly urges religious thinkers and communities to put up "meaningful resistance" to the dominant focus on autonomy, but envisions the audience of such appeals primarily as "public policy" and "the policy process." Campbell, "Meaningful Resistance: Religion and Biotechnology," in *Claiming Power over Life: Religion and Biotechnology Policy,* ed. Hanson, 26. The identification and development

of other avenues of religious and theological influence on social practices is important. In the same volume, Andrew Lustig and Audrey Chapman push further in this direction. Lustig, "Human Cloning and Liberal Neutrality: Why We Need to Broaden the Public Dialogue," in *Claiming Power over Life: Religion and Biotechnology Policy,* ed. Hanson, 30–52; Chapman, "Religious Perspectives on Biotechnology," in *Claiming Power over Life: Religion and Biotechnology Policy,* ed. Hanson, 112–43.

28. John H. Evans, "John H. Evans Responds," *Journal of the Society of Christian Ethics* 24, no. 1 (2004): 216.

29. Meilaender serves on the PCB. Childress has served on NBAC (1996–2001), as well as on the Human Fetal Transplantation Research panel, the National Organ Transplantation Task Force, and the Recombinant DNA Advisory Committee.

30. Gilbert Meilaender, "Comments of Gilbert Meilaender," *Journal of the Society of Christian Ethics* 24, no. 1 (2004): 192.

31. Jeffrey Stout, "Comments of Jeffrey Stout," *Journal of the Society of Christian Ethics* 24, no. 1 (2004): 190.

32. Ibid.

33. James Childress, "Comments of James Childress," *Journal of the Society of Christian Ethics* 24, no. 1 (2004): 200.

34. This is confirmed by the fact that Bush's reelection was perceived by Christian conservatives as vindication of their social goals and as an encouragement to push forward with state and local initiatives on same-sex marriage, public education, and abortion. See Neela Banarjee, "Christian Conservatives Press Issues in Statehouses," *New York Times,* December 13, 2004, A1, A18.

35. In 2005, the United States gave 15 hundredths of 1 percent to foreign aid, the smallest percentage among major donor countries. See Celia W. Dugger, "U.N. Proposes Doubling of Aid to Cut Poverty," *New York Times,* January 18, 2005, A6. See also a U.N. Millennium Project report on global poverty, *Investing in Development,* released in January 2005, at www.unmillenniumproject.org

36. Sarah Linn, "Gay-'marriage' foe takes petition to churches," *Washington Times,* June 19, 2004, C10.

37. Jim Wallis, "'After the Election . . .' Neither Republicans nor Democrats Have a Clue," *Boston Theological Institute Newsletter* 34, no. 19 (2005): 1–2. See also Jim Wallis, *God's Politics: Why the Right Gets It Wrong and the Left Doesn't Get It* (San Francisco, CA: HarperSanFrancisco, 2005).

38. Charles Taylor, "Politics and the Public Sphere," in *New Communitarian Thinking: Persons, Virtues, Institutions, and Communities,* ed. Amitai Etzioni (Charlottesville: University Press of Virginia, 1995), 185–86.

39. Ibid., 190–96.

40. William M. Sullivan, "Institutions as the Infrastructure of Democracy," in *New Communitarian Thinking,* ed. Etzioni, 175.

41. According to Nicholas Wolterstorff, a good number of citizens exercise their religious convictions and identities by basing their contributions to political issues on them, whether they are directly expressed or not. Hence the "liberal" idea of a religion-free zone is unworkable and unfair. Wolterstorff, "The Role of Religion in Political Issues," in *Religion in the Public Square: The Place of Religious Convictions in Political Debate,* Robert Audi and Nicholas Wolterstorff (Lanham, MD: Rowman & Littlefield, 1997), 77.

42. Carolyn Merchant, *The Death of Nature: Women, Ecology and the Scientific Revolution* (San Francisco, CA: Harper and Row, 1980), 164–71.

43. Dorothy Nelkin and M. Susan Lindee, *The DNA Mystique: The Gene as a Cultural Icon* (New York: W. H. Freeman and Co., 1995), 39, 198.

44. Lustig, "Human Cloning and Liberal Neutrality: Why We Need to Broaden the Public Dialogue," in *Claiming Power over Life: Religion and Biotechnology Policy,* ed. M. J. Hanson, 33–36.

45. Ronald Cole-Turner, *The New Genesis: Theology and the Genetic Revolution* (Louisville, KY: Westminster/John Knox Press, 1993), 54.

46. See the BIO website, www.bio.org

47. Statement by BIO president Carl B. Feldbaum, Washington, DC, April 14, 2003, PRNewswire, retrieved from www.bio.org

48. Dan Eramian, "Stem Cell Research: The Dialogue between Biotechnology and Religion," speech delivered during "Managing Controversy in Science and Health" at the Global Public Affairs Institute, Dublin, Ireland, May 7, 2002, retrieved from www.bio.news

49. David R. Loy, "The Religion of the Market," *Journal of the American Academy of Religion* 65, no. 2 (1997): 275.

50. Ibid., 276.

51. Cynthia Moe-Lobeda, *Healing a Broken World: Globalization and God* (Minneapolis, MN: Fortress Press, 2002), 48–65.

52. Ibid., 62.

53. John Gray, *Liberalism* (Minneapolis: University of Minnesota Press, 1986), 90–91.

54. See, e.g., Norman Daniels, *Just Health Care* (Cambridge: Cambridge University Press, 1985); and Richard B. Miller, *Children, Ethics and Modern Medicine* (Bloomington and Indianapolis: Indiana University Press, 2003).

55. Allen Buchanan, Dan W. Brock, Norman Daniels, and Daniel Winkler, *From Chance to Choice: Genetics and Justice* (Cambridge: Cambridge University Press, 2000), 80, 147, 314.

56. Ibid., 97–98.

57. Miller, *Children, Ethics, and Modern Medicine,* 123–25.

58. Ibid., 125.

59. Ibid., 269, 274.

60. Ibid., 254.

61. Brian Stiltner argues that liberalism, feminism, communitarianism, and other "philosophical schools," such as religion and theology, make "substantive" and not merely procedural arguments and that these imply "comprehensive accounts of human beings and what is of value to them." Hence, all can and should contribute to policy formation, as part of the common good. Brian Stiltner, "Morality, Religion, and Public Bioethics: Shifting the Paradigm for the Public Discussion of Embryo Research and Human Cloning," in *Cloning and the Future of Human Embryo Research,* ed. Paul Lauritzen (Oxford: Oxford University Press, 2001), 184. Stiltner is right, but the resemblances among these approaches go beyond the kinds of contributions they make to philosophical argument, and the sphere of their influence goes beyond public policy in the narrow sense.

62. Roger Lincoln Shinn, *The New Genetics; Challenges for Science, Faith, and Politics* (Wakefield, RI: Moyer Bell, 1996), 92.

63. James M. Gustafson, *Varieties of Moral Discourse: Prophetic, Narrative, Ethical, and Policy* (Grand Rapids, MI: Calvin College, 1988); and *Intersections.*

64. Gustafson, *Intersections,* 39.

65. Ibid., 54.

66. Ibid., 41.

67. Ibid., 19.

68. See Childress, "Religion, Theology, and Bioethics," 56–57.

69. Beverly Wildung Harrison, *Our Right to Choose: Toward a New Ethic of Abortion* (Boston: Beacon Press, 1989).

70. Janice Raymond, "Preface," in *Man-Made Women: How New Reproductive Technologies Affect Women,* Gena Corea et al. (Bloomington and Indianapolis: Indiana University Press, 1987), 12.

71. Karen Lebacqz, "Theology, Justice and Health Care: An International Conundrum" (paper presented at the University of Uppsala, Uppsala, Sweden, April 2002), 6.

72. Margaret A. Farley, "Feminist Theology and Bioethics," in *Theology and Bioethics,* ed Earl E. Shelp (Dordrecht, Neth.: D. Reidel Publishing Company, 1985), 163.

73. Ibid., 174.

74. Barbara Hilkert Andolsen, "Elements of a Feminist Approach to Bioethics," in *Feminist Ethics and the Catholic Moral Tradition: Readings in Moral Theology, No. 9,* ed. Charles E. Curran, Margaret A. Farley, and Richard A. McCormick (New York: Paulist Press, 1996), 342–43. This essay first appeared in *Religious Resources and Methods in Bioethics* in 1994.

75. Ibid., 378.

76. See Daniel P. Sulmasy, *The Healer's Calling: A Spirituality for Physicians and Other Health Care Professionals* (New York: Paulist, 1997); Benedict Ashley and Kevin O'Rourke *Health Care Ethics: A Theological Analysis,* 3rd ed. (St. Louis, MO: Catholic Health Association, 1978), 389–412; and Vigen Guroian, *Life's Living toward Dying* (Grand Rapids, MI: Eerdmans, 1996).

Chapter 2

1. Albert Jonsen and Stephen Toulmin, *The Abuse of Casuistry: A History of Moral Reasoning* (Berkeley: University of California Press, 1988); James F. Keenan, S. J. and Thomas A. Shannon, *The Context of Casuistry* (Washington, DC: Georgetown University Press, 1995).

2. Jonsen and Toulmin, *Abuse of Casuistry,* 19, 341.

3. James F. Keenan, "Proposing Cardinal Virtues," *Theological Studies* 56 (1995): 709–29; "Whose Perfection Is It Anyway?: A Virtuous Consideration of Enhancement," *Christian Bioethics* 5 (1999): 104–20; "Casuistry, Virtue and the Slippery Slope: Major Problems with Producing Human Embryonic Life for Research Purposes," in *Cloning and the Future of Human Embryo Research,* ed. Paul Lauritzen (Oxford: Oxford University Press, 2001); see also Keenan and Shannon, *Context of Casuistry,* 227–28.

4. Papal encyclicals will be cited in text with reference to numbered paragraphs.

5. Audrey Chapman, *Faith, Power and Politics: Political Ministry in Mainline Churches* (New York: Pilgrim Press, 2001), 124.

6. J. H. Oldham and W. A. Visser't Hooft, *Church, Community and State,* vol. 1, *The Church and Its Function in Society* (London: George Allen and Unwin, 1937), 210, 238.

7. Ronald Preston, "Middle Axioms," in *The Westminster Dictionary of Christian Ethics,* ed. James F. Childress and John Macquarrie (Philadelphia: Westminster Press, 1986), 382.

8. John C. Bennett, *Christian Ethics and Social Policy* (New York: Scribner's Sons, 1956), 77, 79.

9. Oldham and Visser't Hooft, *Church, Community and State,* 210.

10. Charles Villa-Vicencio, *A Theology of Reconstruction: Nation-Building and Human Rights* (Cambridge: Cambridge University Press, 1992), 9.

11. Ibid., 283, 276, 279.

12. Schreiter, *New Catholicity,* 111.

13. For a general discussion, see David Hollenbach, *Common Good and Christian Ethics.*

14. See Jean Porter, "The Virtue of Justice," in *The Ethics of Aquinas,* ed. Stephen J. Pope (Washington, DC: Georgetown University Press, 2002), 277–79.

15. Charles Curran, *Catholic Social Teaching, 1891–Present: A Historical, Theological and Ethical Analysis* (Washington, DC: Georgetown University Press, 2000), 189.

16. Ibid., 189–91.

17. Julie Clague, "Patently Unjust? International Efforts to Ensure Biotechnology Benefits All" (paper presented at "Transforming Unjust Structures: Capabilities and Justice," sponsored by the Von Hugel Institute, St. Edmund's College, Cambridge University, June 26–27, 2003). Also see Severine Deneulin, Mathias Nebel, and Nicholas Sagovsky, eds., *Capability and Justice; Towards Structural Transformation* (Dordrecht, Neth.: Kluwer Academic Press, forthcoming), in which Clague's paper will be published.

18. Francesca Polleta, *Freedom Is an Endless Meeting: Democracy in American Social Movements* (Chicago: University of Chicago Press, 2000), 125–26.

19. Ibid., 218–19.

20. Woodstock Theological Center, Ethics in Public Policy Program, *The Ethics of Lobbying: Organized Interests, Political Power, and the Common Good* (Washington, DC: Georgetown University Press, 2002), 64.

21. Ibid., 66.

22. Ibid., 83.

23. Ibid., 92–93.

24. Polleta, *Freedom Is an Endless Meeting,* 18.

25. Amy Gutmann and Dennis Thompson, *Democracy and Disagreement* (Cambridge, MA: Harvard University Press, 1996).

26. Ibid., 79, 84–85.

27. Ibid., 3, 91–92.

28. Ibid., 4–5.

29. Ibid., 129, 144–45, 148–49.

30. Ibid., 132–37.

31. Ibid., 92, 273, 301–6, 349.

32. Ibid., 273.

33. Daniel J. B. Hofrenning, *In Washington but Not of It: The Prophetic Politics of Religious Lobbyists* (Philadelphia: Temple University Press, 1995), 2.

34. Stephen Warner, "Changes in the Civic Role of Religion," in *Diversity and Its Discontents: Cultural Conflict and Common Ground in Contemporary American Society,* ed. Neil J. Smelser and Jeffrey C. Alexander (Princeton, NJ: Princeton University Press, 1999), 234.

35. Ibid., 237.

36. See Kenneth D. Wald, Lyman A. Kellstedt, and David C. Leege, "Church Involvement and Political Behavior"; and David C. Leege, Kenneth D. Wald, and Lyman A. Kellstedt, "The Public Dimensions of Private Devotionalism," in *Rediscovering the Religious Factor in American Politics,* ed. David C. Leege and Lyman A. Kellstedt (Armonk, NY: M. E. Sharpe, 1993), 121–38 and 139–56, respectively. On the positive connection between religious and political participation, see also Sidney Verba, Kay Lehman Schlozman, and Henry Brady, *Voice and Equality: Civic Voluntarism in America* (Cambridge, MA: Harvard University Press, 1995) and Robert Wuthnow, "Beyond Quiet Influence: Possibilities for the Protestant Mainline," in *The Quiet Hand of God: Faith-Based Activism and the Public Role of Mainline Protestantism,* ed. Robert Wuthnow and John H. Evans (Berkeley: University of California Press, 2002), 392.

37. Wald, Kellstedt, and Leege, "Church Involvement," 122.

38. Ibid., 4.

39. Ibid., 20.

40. Stephen Hart, *Cultural Dilemmas of Progressive Politics: Styles of Engagement among Grassroots Activists* (Chicago: University of Chicago Press, 2001), 119.

41. Ibid., 4.

42. Ibid., 28.

43. Ibid., 20, 223–24. See also Alan Wolfe, *One Nation, after All: What Middle-Class Americans Really Think about God, Country, Family, Racism, Welfare, Immigration, Homosexuality, Work, the Left, the Right, and Each Other* (New York: Viking Penguin, 1998).

44. Hart, *Cultural Dilemmas,* 4.

45. Reinhold Niebuhr, *The Nature and Destiny of Man,* vol. 1, *Human Nature* (New York: Charles Scribner's Sons, 1964), 88.

46. Hart, *Cultural Dilemmas,* 5.

47. Ibid., 8.

48. Ibid., 231.

49. Ibid., 46.

50. Ibid., 49–52.

51. Ibid., 190.

52. Ibid., 28.

53. Ibid., 89.

54. Ibid., 91.

55. Ibid., 95–96.

56. Paul Osterman, *Gathering Power: Re-building Progressive Politics in America* (Boston: Beacon Press, 2003).

57. Osterman, *Gathering Power,* 17.

58. Ibid, 206.

59. Ibid, 84–87.

60. Hart, *Cultural Dilemmas,* 205–6.

61. Amartya Sen, "What's the Point of Democracy?" *American Academy of Arts and Sciences Bulletin* 57, no. 3 (2004): 9.

62. Ibid., 10.

63. Richard Falk. "Religion and Globalization," *Bulletin of the Boston Theological Institute* 2 (2003): 2.

64. Abdullahi An-na'im, "Religion and Global Civil Society: Inherent Incompatibility or Synergy and Interdependence?" in *Global Civil Society 2002*, ed. Marlies Glasius, Mary Kalder, and Helmut Anheier (Oxford: Oxford University Press, 2002), 55.

65. Ibid., 57.

66. Ibid., 59.

67. Schreiter, *New Catholicity*, 16.

68. Mario Pianta, "Parallel Summits of Global Civil Society," in *Global Civil Society 2001*, ed. Helmut Anheier, Marlies Glasius, and Mary Kaldor (Oxford: Oxford University Press, 2001), 169.

69. Ibid.

70. J. S. Nye Jr. "Globalization's Democratic Deficit: How to Make International Institutions More Accountable," *Foreign Affairs* 80, no. 4 (2001): 3.

71. Anne-Marie Slaughter, "Everyday Global Governance," *Daedalus* 132 (2003): 83–90.

72. Ibid., 89.

73. Pianta, "Parallel Summits," 169.

74. Ibid., 171.

75. Robin Broad, ed., *Global Backlash: Citizen Initiatives for a Just World Economy* (Lanham, MD: Rowman and Littlefield, 2002).

76. Robin Broad, "Conclusion: What Does It All Add Up To?" in *Global Backlash*, 301.

77. Jerry Useem, "Globalization: Can Governments, Companies, and Yes the Protesters Ever Learn to Get Along?" *Fortune*, November 2001, 77–84. This article is discussed by Broad, *Global Backlash*, 303, and included in its entirety, 305–8.

78. Richard Falk, *Law in an Emerging Global Village: A Post-Westphalian Perspective* (Ardsley, NY: Transnational Publishers, 1998), 3–31.

79. Richard Falk, *Predatory Globalization: A Critique* (Malden, MA: Blackwell, 1999), 59.

80. Maura Ryan, "Beyond a Western Bioethics?" *Theological Studies* 65, no. 1 (2004): 174–76.

81. Lynn D. Robinson, "Doing Good and Doing Well: Shareholder Activism, Responsible Investment, and Mainline Protestantism," in *Quiet Hand of God*, ed. Wuthnow and Evans, 343.

82. Ibid., 352–53.

83. Ibid., 353–54.

84. Ibid., 355.

85. Information and the report, *God's Children Are Dying of AIDS* (July 12, 2004), can be accessed at the Christian Aid website: www.christianaid.org.uk

86. This statement, not directly attributed to Dr. Baggaley, was the conclusion of a Reuters online news report on Christian Aid efforts. "Christian Aid Calls on Religions to Work Together to Combat HIV/AIDS," July 12, 2004, retrieved from www.alertnet.org/thenews/fromthefield/108964031240

87. The conference was sponsored by the Wilstein Institute of Jewish Policy Studies and the Interreligious Center on Public Life, at Hebrew Union College and Andover Newton Theological School, Newton Centre, Massachusetts.

88. Vicki Brower, "Finding Biomedicines for Infectious Diseases," *Genetic Engineering News* 23, no. 2 (2003): 3. The article gives similar examples involving other companies as well.

Chapter 3

1. The Study to Understand Prognosis and Preferences for Outcomes and Risks of Treatment (SUPPORT) began in 1989, lasted four years, and was supported by a grant from the Robert Wood Johnson Foundation. For a discussion, see Ellen H. Moskowitz and James Lindemann Nelson, "The Best Laid Plans," special supplement, *Hastings Center Report* 25, no. 6 (1995): S3.

2. Timothy E. Quill, *Death and Dignity: Making Choices and Taking Charge* (New York: W. W. Norton, 1993), 49.

3. Ibid., 22.

4. Ibid., 52.

5. Daniel Callahan, "The Goals of Medicine: Setting New Priorities," special supplement, *Hastings Center Report* 26, no. 6 (1996): S20.

6. Institute of Medicine, *Approaching Death: Improving Care at the End of Life* (Washington, DC: National Academy Press, 1997), 260.

7. Ibid., 37.

8. Robert C. Atchley, *Social Forces and Aging: An Introduction to Social Gerontology* (Belmont, CA: Wadsworth Thomson Learning, 2000), 47.

9. Ibid., 50.

10. Ibid., 53–55.

11. Staff background paper for the President's Commission on Bioethics, "The Promise and the Challenge of Aging Research," December 2002, 2, retrieved from www.bioethics.gov/background/agingresearch.html

12. Ibid., 2–3.

13. Miguel A. De La Torre, *Doing Christian Ethics from the Margins* (Maryknoll, NY: Orbis Books, 2004), 193.

14. Institute of Medicine, *Approaching Death*, 57.

15. Emilie M. Townes, *Breaking the Fine Rain of Death: African American Health Issues and a Womanist Ethic of Care* (New York: Continuum, 1998), 61.

16. Atchley, *Social Forces*, 445.

17. Ibid., 448.

18. Ibid., 451.

19. See Albert I. Hermalin, ed., *The Well-Being of the Elderly in Asia: A Four-Country Comparative Study* (Ann Arbor: University of Michigan Press, 2002); Luise Hately and Gerald Tan, *The Greying of Asia: Causes and Consequences of Rapid Ageing in Asia* (London: Eastern Universities Press, 2003); Sinfree Makoni and Koen Stroeken, eds., *Ageing in Africa: Sociolinguistic and Anthropological Approaches* (Hampshire, England: Ashgate, 2002).

20. Albert I. Hermalin and Lora G. Myers, "Aging in Asia: Facing the Crossroads," in *Elderly in Asia*, ed. Hermalin, 4–5.

21. For some examples from the stories of old people in South Africa, see Els van Dongen, "Skeletons of the Past, Flesh and Blood of the Present: Remembrance and Older People in a South African Context," in *Ageing in Africa*, ed. Makoni and Stroeken, 257–76.

22. Jay Sokolovsky, "Starting Points: A Global, Cross-Cultural View of Aging," in *Cultural Context of Aging*, xvi–xxi.

23. Ann Biddlecom, Napaporn Chayovan, and Mary Beth Ofstedal, "Intergenerational Support and Transfers," in *Elderly in Asia*, ed. Hermalin, 209–10.

24. See, for example, Joan Weibel-Orlando, "Grandparenting Styles: The Contemporary American Indian Experience," in *Cultural Context of Aging,* 139–53.

25. Enee Devisch, Sinfree Makoni, and Koen Stroeken, "African Gerontology: Critical Models, Future Directions," in *Ageing in Africa,* ed. Makoni and Stroeken, 382.

26. Ibid., 280.

27. Harriet G. Rosenberg, "Complaint Discourse, Aging and Caregiving among the Ju/'hoansi of Botswana," in *Cultural Context of Aging,* 47–49.

28. Jane W. Peterson, "Age of Wisdom: Elderly Black Women in Family and Church," in *Cultural Context of Aging,* 276.

29. Ibid., 281.

30. Albert I. Hermalin, "Making the Choices: Policies and Research for the Coming Years," in *Elderly in Asia,* ed. Hermalin, 547.

31. Ibid., 551.

32. Ibid., 555.

33. Ibid., 572–73. See also Jay Sokolovsky, "Networks and Community: Environments for Aging," in *Cultural Context of Aging,* 317–29.

34. Sokolovsky, "Networks," 322–23. See also Yoko Tsuji, "An Organization for the Elderly, by the Elderly: A Senior Center in the United States," in *Cultural Context of Aging,* 350–63.

35. Sokolovsky, "Networks," 322.

36. Sokolovsky, "Starting Points," xxv.

37. See Clark E. Cochran and David Carroll Cochran, *Catholics, Politics & Public Policy: Beyond Left and Right* (Maryknoll, NY: Orbis, 2003), 92–112.

38. Joint International Research Group of the Institute for Bioethics, Maastricht, the Netherlands, and the Hastings Center, New York, "What Do We Owe the Elderly? Allocating Social and Health Care Resources," special supplement, *Hastings Center Report* 24, no. 2 (1994): S1–S12.

39. Ibid., S2.

40. Allen Verhey, *Reading the Bible in the Strange World of Medicine* (Grand Rapids, MI: Eerdmans, 2003), 11.

41. James F. Keenan, *The Works of Mercy: The Heart of Catholicism* (Lanham, MD: Rowman and Littlefield, 2005), 43.

42. See the Catholic Health Association report, *Catholic Health Care in the United States* (March 2004), at www.chausa.org

43. For more information, see the Catholic Health Initiatives website at www.catholichealthinit.org

44. www.gundluth.org

45. www.adventist.org/mission_and_service/health.html.en

46. www.santegidio.org/en/index.html

47. This and most of the information to follow is taken from the CHA website: www.chausa.org. This description is on the home page. An overview of the contents of the website may be found at www.chausa.org/CHASITE.ASP. The specific Web addresses of some of the more important sites and documents to be discussed will also be given. Others can be found through the sites mentioned.

48. The foregoing data and the identity statement are from a report called "Ministry Engaged: Catholic Health Care in the United States," March 2004, p. 1, retrieved through "About CHA" on the home page.

49. Ibid., 3.

50. Ibid., 4.

51. www.chausa.org/TRANSFORM/TRANSFORM.ASP

52. www.chausa.org/LONGTERM/LONGTERM.ASP

53. www.shausa.org/LONGTERM/HOUSING.ASP

54. John Paul II, "No Authority Can Justify Euthanasia," Address to the Thirteenth International Conference, "The Church and the Elderly," October 29–31, 1998, 3, retrieved from www.healthpastoral.org/wordsofpope/jpii07_en.htm. This link is available on the CHA website: www.chausa.org/LONGTERM/LONGTERM.ASP

55. Ibid., 4.

56. Families caring for elders with Alzheimer's face special burdens and are especially in need of a theological or religious self-understanding and community of support. One of the few to have addressed the burdens of family caregiving theologically is Stephen G. Post, *More Lasting Unions: Christianity, the Family and Society* (Grand Rapids, MI: Eerdmans, 2000), 151–76.

57. "Growing Old in America," retrieved from www.chausa.org/PUBS/PUBSART.ASP?ISSUE=HP0005. This also appeared in the CHA publication *Health Progress* (May–June 2000) in a feature "Special Section: Catholic Sponsored Housing."

58. Elderly Housing Coalition Committee on the Continuum of Care, "Providing an Affordable Continuum of Care for Low-Income Residents of Senior Housing," 1–2, retrieved from www.chausa.org/LONGTERM/PROVIDING_ER.ASP

59. www.chausa.org/PUBS/PUBSART.ASP?ISSUE=HP9903

60. www.chausa.org/chausa.org/LONGTERM/NURSIN.ASP

61. Chris Phillipson, "Ageism and Globalization: Citizenship and Social Rights in Transnational Settings," in *Cultural Gerontology*, ed. Lars Andersson (Westport, CT: Auburn House, 2002), 51.

62. Ibid., 52.

63. For discussions of religious practice and the elderly in several different cultures, see William M. Clements, ed., *Religion, Aging and Health: A Global Perspective*, comp. World Health Organization (New York: Haworth Press).

64. www.santegidio.org

65. See www.santegidio.org/en/solidarieta/anziani/autodet01.htm

66. *Come Rimanere a Casa Propria da Anziani* (Rome: Comunita da Sant'Egidio, 2003).

67. William E. May, *The Patient's Ordeal* (Bloomington: Indiana University Press, 1992), 120–41.

68. Sokolovsky, "Starting Points," xvii.

69. Jay Sokolovsky, "Culture, Aging and Context," in *Cultural Context of Aging*, 8.

70. Anthony P. Glascock, "When Is Killing Acceptable: The Moral Dilemma Surrounding Assisted Suicide in America and Other Societies," in *Cultural Context of Aging*, 62.

71. Ibid., 64.

72. Ibid., 62–63.

73. Ibid., 66–68.

74. For an argument that realistic limits should be set for medical care, in view of the inevitable facts of finitude, aging, and death, see Daniel Callahan, *What Kind of Life: The Limits of Medical Progress* (New York: Simon and Schuster, 1990), 151–57.

75. Congregation for the Doctrine of the Faith, *Declaration on Euthanasia*, May 5, 1980 (Boston: St. Paul Editions, 1980), 9. This document is also available in the *National Catholic Bioethics Quarterly* 1, no. 3 (2004): 431–47.

76. Congregation for the Doctrine of the Faith, *Declaration on Euthanasia,* 7.

77. Derek Humphry, *Final Exit: The Practicalities of Self-Deliverance and Assisted Suicide for the Dying,* 3d ed. (New York: Random House), 2002.

78. Quill, *Death and Dignity,* 125–129.

79. Betty Pelletz, "Suicide at 88 Ends 'Pointless Life,'" *Hemlock Quarterly,* April 1991, 6.

80. Quill, *Death and Dignity,* 124–25.

81. Anonymous, "It's Over, Debbie," *Journal of the American Medical Association* 259, no. 2 (1988): 272. For a discussion, see Quill, *Death and Dignity,* 123–24.

82. Quill, *Death and Dignity,* 9–16, 19–25. The story of Diane, "Death and Dignity: A Case of Individualized Decision-Making," was originally published in the *New England Journal of Medicine* 324 (March 1981): 691–94.For another viewpoint, see Rita Marker, "An Inside look at the Right-to-Die Movement," *National Catholic Bioethics Quarterly* 1, no. 3 (2002): 363–94.

83. For discussions of the Oregon law, see Katrina Hedberg and Susan W. Tolle "Physician-Assisted Suicide and Changes in Care of the Dying: The Oregon Perspective," in *Assisted Suicide: Finding Common Ground,* ed. Lois Snyder and Arthur L. Caplan (Bloomington: Indiana University Press, 2002), 7–16; and Kathleen Foley and Herbert Hendin "The Oregon Experiment," in *The Case Against Assisted Suicide: For the Right to End-of-Life Care,* ed. Kathleen Foley and Herbert Hendin (Baltimore: Johns Hopkins University Press, 2002), 144–74.

84. Hedberg and Tolle, "Changes," 9.

85. Statistics are available on the Oregon Health Division website, www.ohd.hr.state ,or.us/shc/pas/an-index.htm; and from the advocacy organization Compassion in Dying. Founded in 1993, Compassion in Dying supports patient choice, availability of adequate palliative care, especially pain relief, and assisted suicide. See www.compassionindying.org. Print literature is available from Compassion in Dying, Portland, Oregon (info@compas sionindying.org or 503–221–9556).

86. These statistics were taken from a Compassion in Dying brochure titled "Compassion in Dying Federation."

87. Foley and Hendin, "Oregon," 145.

88. Hedberg and Tolle, "Changes," 9–11.

89. "Compassion in Dying Federation."

90. Hedberg and Tolle, "Changes," 13–15.

91. Foley and Hendin, "Oregon," 145, 155.

92. Ibid., 168.

93. Ibid., 169.

94. Ellen Moskowitz, "The Consensus on Assisted Suicide," *Hastings Center Report* 33/ 4 (2003) 46–47.

95. A new collection focused on this experience appeared as this volume was going to press: Tom Meulenbergs and Paul Schotsmans, eds., *Euthanasia and Palliative Care in the Low Countries* (Leuven, Belg.: Peeters, 2005).

96. See P. J. van der Mass et al., "Euthanasia, Physician-Assisted Suicide, and Other Medical Practices Involving the End of Life in the Netherlands, 1990–95," *New England Journal of Medicine* 335, no. 22 (1996): 1699–1711; and Ezekiel Emanuel, "Whose Right to Die?" *The Atlantic Monthly* 279 (March 1997): 73–79.

97. Herbert Hendin, "The Dutch Experience," in *The Case Against Assisted Suicide,* ed. Foley and Hendin, 105.

98. Theo A. Boer, "After the Slippery Slope: Dutch Experiences on Regulating Active Euthanasia," *Journal of the Society of Christian Ethics* 23, no. 2 (2003): 226–27.

99. Zbigniew Zylicz, "Palliative Care and Euthanasia in the Netherlands: Observations of a Dutch Physician," in *The Case Against Assisted Suicide,* ed. Foley and Hendin, 122–43.

100. Boer, "Slippery Slope," 236.

101. Ibid., 238–39.

102. Zylicz, "Dutch Physician," 122.

103. Bruce Jennings, Daniel Callahan, and Arthur Caplan, "Ethical Challenges of Chronic Illness," special supplement, *Hastings Center Report* 18, no. 1 (1988): S12.

104. Ibid., S11.

105. Michael M. Mendiola, "Overworked, but Uncritically Tested: Human Dignity and the Aid-in-Dying Debate," in *Secular Bioethics in Theological Perspective,* ed. Earl E. Shelp (Dordrecht, Neth.: Kluwer, 1996), 138.

106. Gerald P. McKenny, *To Relieve the Human Condition: Bioethics, Technology and the Body* (Albany: SUNY Press, 1997), 31.

107. Stanley Hauerwas, *Truthfulness and Tragedy* (Notre Dame, IN: University of Notre Dame Press, 1977), 112.

108. Jennings et al., *Ethical Challenges,* S13.

109. See Daniel Callahan, "Bioethics: Private Choice and Common Good," and Thomas H. Murray et al., "Individualism and Community: The Contested Terrain of Autonomy," in *Hastings Center Report* 24, no. 3 (1994): 28–31 and 32–35, respectively.

110. Jennings et al., "Ethical Challenges," S14.

111. For overviews of various religious traditions on the problems of euthanasia and refusal of treatment, see Ron P. Hamel and Edwin R. DuBose, "Views of the Major Faith Traditions," in *Choosing Death: Active Euthanasia, Religion and the Public Debate,* ed. Ron Hamel (Philadelphia: Trinity Press International, 1991), 51–101.

112. Hauerwas, *Suffering Presence,* 75.

113. Ibid., 81.

114. Verhey, *Strange World,* 1. On the Christian tradition of care for the sick, see also Patrick Guinan, "Christianity and the Origin of the Hospital," *National Catholic Bioethics Quarterly* 4, no. 2 (2004): 257–63.

115. Verhey, *Strange World,* 94.

116. Christopher P. Vogt, *Patience, Compassion, Hope and the Christian Art of Dying Well* (Lanham, MD: Rowman and Littlefield, 2004), 139.

117. Ibid., 131–32; see chapter 3 on the *ars moriendi,* 15–51. *Ars moriendi* (the "art of dying") denotes a tradition of piety and literature that was particularly strong in the sixteenth and seventeenth centuries. Although it focuses on the individual, it also assumes that death is not an isolated event, that persons have multiple occasions to be present at the deathbeds of others, and that the church supports preparation for one's own death by means of instruction, prayer, and devotional reading. Vogt comments that this tradition has a bias toward the embrace of physical suffering that we would not regard as useful today.

118. See Carlos M. N. Eire, "Ars Moriendi," in *The Westminster Dictionary of Christian Spirituality,* ed. Gordon S. Wakefield (Philadelphia: Westminster, 1983), 21–22. Further resources on spirituality and death include Lucy Bregman, "Current Perspectives on

Death, Dying and Mourning," *Religious Studies Review* 25, no. 1 (1999): 29–34; Gerry R. Cox and Ronald J. Fundis, eds., *Spiritual, Ethical and Pastoral Aspects of Death and Bereavement* (Amityville, NY: Baywood, 1992); and Howard M. Spiro, Mary G. McCrea Curnen, and Lee Palmer Wandel, eds., *Facing Death: Where Culture, Religion, and Medicine Meet* (New Haven, CT: Yale University Press, 1996). The latter includes perspectives from Hinduism, Judaism, Chinese popular beliefs, Islam, and African American spirituality. The *ars moriendi* is a theme in several contributions.

119. Verhey, *Strange World*, 123. Verhey ends the sentence mentioning "complaint" with the words "and petition." Petitionary prayer certainly has a role in the Bible, but lament, as simply an agonized expression of human woe before a listening God, also has its place. The African American theologian Emilie Townes invokes the category of lament to communicate the emotions and spirituality of people deprived of adequate health care. Townes, *Breaking the Fine Rain of Death*, 9–16, 23–25.

120. Verhey, *Strange World*, 123.

121. Ibid., 305.

122. Ibid., 341.

Chapter 4

1. For the "classic" definition, see Gerald Kelly, *Medico-Moral Problems* (St. Louis, MO: Catholic Hospital Association, 1958), 128–35. For an overview and critical discussion, see Kevin W. Wildes, "Ordinary and Extraordinary Means and the Quality of Life," *Theological Studies* 57, no. 3 (1996): 500–512.

2. Pius XII, "Address to the Italian Anesthesiological Society," February 24, 1957, *Acta Apostolicae Sedis* 49 (1957): 146. Also available in *The National Catholic Bioethics Quarterly* 2, no. 2 (2002).

3. *Ethical and Religious Directives for Catholic Hospitals, Linacre Quarterly* (July–October 1949). Historical information on the *Directives* was provided by Ron Hamel, ethics director of the CHA, through the intermediary James Keenan.

4. For the early history of the CHA, see Christopher J. Kauffmann, *Ministry and Meaning: A Religious History of Catholic Health Care in the United States* (New York: Crossroad, 1995), 168–92.

5. See Kelly, *Medico-Moral Problems*, vii.

6. A notice inside the cover of the 1975 *Ethical and Religious Directives for Catholic Health Facilities* (Washington, DC: United States Catholic Conference, 1971) reads: "At the annual meeting of the National Conference of Catholic Bishops and the United States Catholic Conference, November, 1971, the Directives were approved as the national code, subject to the approval of the bishop for use in the diocese."

7. These are Kelly, *Medico-Moral Problems*; and McCormick, *Health and Medicine*.

8. The notes are mostly collected as Richard A. McCormick, *Notes on Moral Theology: 1965 through 1980* (Washington, DC: University Press of America, 1981).

9. Kelly, *Medico-Moral Problems*, 133–35. A large portion of David F. Kelly's *Contemporary Catholic Health Care Ethics* (Washington, DC: Georgetown University Press, 2004) is concerned with these issues and distinctions and provides a useful, critical overview (108–228). See also Richard A. McCormick, "Vive la Difference! Killing and Allowing to Die,"

America 177, no. 18 (1977): 6–12; and James F. Bresnahan, "Palliative Care or Assisted Suicide?" *America* 178, no. 8 (1998): 16–21.

10. Kelly, *Medico-Moral Problems*, 135.

11. Philip J. Boyle and Ellen Moskowitz, "Making Tough Resource Decisions: A Process for Considering Both Values and Costs," *Health Progress* 77, no. 6 (1996): 48.

12. Congregation for the Doctrine of the Faith, *Declaration on Euthanasia*, 8.

13. United States Conference of Catholic Bishops, *Ethical and Religious Directives for Catholic Health Care Services*, 4th ed. (Washington, DC: United States Conference of Catholic Bishops, 2001), no. 60. The 2001 version of the *Directives* is available at the USCCB website: www.nccbuscc.org/bishops/directives.htm

14. For several essays objecting to physician-assisted suicide on these grounds, see *The National Catholic Bioethics Quarterly* 1, no. 3 (2001); see also Michael Manning, *Euthanasia and Physician-Assisted Suicide: Killing or Caring?* (New York: Paulist Press, 1998); and Ashley and O'Rourke, *Health Care Ethics*, 3rd ed., 411–19.

15. *Declaration on Euthanasia*, 11–12.

16. National Conference of Catholic Bishops (NCCB), *Ethical and Religious Directives for Catholic Health Care Services* (Washington, DC: United States Catholic Conference, 1995). These guidelines were again revised, less extensively, in 2001 (cited in n. 13). The NCCB is now called the United States Conference of Catholic Bishops. The cited paragraph numbers and content of the 1995 *Directives* also apply to the 2001 version.

17. Ibid., no. 32. For discussion of shifts and nuances in the 1995 edition (e.g., more recognition of patient decision making), see James F. Keenan, "What's New in the Ethical and Religious Directives?" *Linacre Quarterly* 65, no. 1 (1998): 33–40.

18. Ibid., Introduction to part V (p. 13 of 20); and no. 61.

19. Ibid., nos. 21, 61.

20. Ibid., no. 58.

21. Ibid., Introduction to part V (p. 13 of 20).

22. John Paul II, "Address of John Paul II to the Participants in the International Congress on Life-Sustaining Treatments and Vegetative State: Scientific Advances And Ethical Dilemmas," March 20, 2004. An official Vatican English translation of the statement is available on the website of the National Catholic Bioethics Center: www.ncbcenter.org/press/04–03–20-LifeSustainingTreatments.html. It also appears in *The National Catholic Bioethics Quarterly* 4, no. 2 (2004): 367–70, titled "On Life-Sustaining Treatments and the Vegetative State: Scientific Advances and Ethical Dilemmas," 367–70; and again in *NCBQ* 4, no. 3 (2004), same title, 573–76. The Autumn 2004 issue of the *NCBQ* carries several articles on this speech, including Germain Kopaczynski, "Initial Reactions to the Pope's March 20, 2004, Allocution," *NCBQ* 4, no. 3 (2004): 473–82. The issue also contains eleven substantial letters commenting on the speech by moral theologians, Catholic physicians, and Michael Place, the president of the CHA. Like the development and revisions of the *Ethical and Religious Directives*, in concert with evolving medical, legal, and ecclesial perspectives and debates that bear on actual practices in health care, this exchange represents an expression of participatory theological bioethics. The CHA website provides to members "Resources for Understanding Pope's Allocution on Persons in a Persistent Vegetative State," including the pope's speech, a CHA statement referring readers to the *Ethical and Religious Directives*, an analysis of the speech in relation to past and other current teaching, and news articles for review: www.chausa.org/$MEMB/MISSSVCS/ETHICS/anh.ASP (Note: you must register before accessing this site.)

23. John Paul II, "Life Sustaining Treatments," no. 5.

24. Ibid., no. 3.

25. Ibid., no. 4

26. Ibid., no. 6.

27. Ibid., no. 4.

28. See Richard M. Doerflinger, "John Paul II on the 'Vegetative State': An Important Papal Speech," *Ethics and Medics* 29, no. 6 (2004): 2–4. See www.ncbcenter.org for the response of the National Catholic Bioethics Center to the speech; and *National Catholic Bioethics Quarterly* 4, no. 3 (2004) for several favorable responses. Peter Cataldo argues that the cessation of a person's conscious ability to seek the higher personal and spiritual goods of life is *not* a reason to cease preserving his or her biological life. Cataldo also provides a discussion of earlier figures in Catholic tradition who were influential in the development of the definition of "extraordinary" means. Peter J. Cataldo, "John Paul II on Nutrition and Hydration: A Change of Catholic Teaching?" *National Catholic Bioethics Quarterly* 4, no. 3 (2004): 513–39. See also William E. May et al., "Feeding and Hydrating the Permanently Unconscious and Other Vulnerable Persons," *Issues in Law and Medicine* 3, no. 3 (1987): 203–12.

29. Thomas A. Shannon and James J. Walter, "Implications of the Papal Allocution on Feeding Tubes," *Hastings Center Report* 34, no. 4 (2004): 18–20; Gerald Coleman, "Take and Eat: Morality and Medically Assisted Feeding," *America* (April 2004): 16–20; Ronald Hamel and Michael Panicola, "Must We Preserve Life?" *America* (April 2004): 6–13; John F. Tuohey, "The Pope on PVS: Does JP II's Statement Make the Grade?" *Commonweal* (June 2004): 10–12. Eileen P. Flynn, *Hard Decisions; Forgoing and Withdrawing Artificial Nutrition and Hydration* (Kansas City, KS: Sheed and Ward, 1990), provides an overview of the problem in relation to Catholic teaching. See also John J. Paris and Richard A. McCormick, "The Catholic Tradition on the Use of Nutrition and Fluids," *America*, May 2, 1987, 356–61.

30. Wildes, "Ordinary and Extraordinary Means"; McCormick, "To Save or Let Die," 172–76, also published in *America* 131 (1974); and James J. Walter and Thomas A. Shannon, eds., *Quality of Life: The New Medical Dilemma* (New York: Paulist Press, 1990). The latter includes a variety of positions on different sides of the issue.

31. Hamel and Panicola, "Must We," 13.

32. Thomas R. Kopfensteiner, "Death with Dignity: A Roman Catholic Perspective," *Linacre Quarterly* 63, no. 4 (1996): 73–74.

33. Ignatius Perkins criticizes contemporary culture because it "selectively affirms persons who matter and discriminates against others because of their socio-economic status, age, color, ethnicity, gender, or diagnoses as useless, burdensome." "The Dignity of the Person," *National Catholic Bioethics Quarterly* 4, no. 3 (2004): 456. See also Dan O'Brien, John Paul Slosar, and Anthony R. Tersigni, "Utilitarian Pessimism, Human Dignity, and the Vegetative State: A Practical Analysis of the Papal Allocution," *National Catholic Bioethics Quarterly* 4, no. 3 (2004): 497–512.

34. O'Brien, Slosar, and Tersigni, "Utilitarian Pessimism," 510.

35. Congregation for the Doctrine of the Faith, *Declaration on Euthanasia.*

36. Congregation for the Doctrine of the Faith, *Declaration on Euthanasia,* 12.

37. For an overview, including differing opinions of various Episcopal conferences, see Wildes, "Ordinary and Extraordinary Means," esp. 507–11.

38. Kelly, *Medico-Moral Problems,* 13–15. Richard McCormick lays out the conditions of double effect in *Ambiguity in Moral Choice* (Milwaukee, WI: Marquette University Theology Department, 1973), 7. For discussions, see Jorge Garcia, "Double Effect," in *Encyclopedia of Bioethics,* ed. Warren T. Reich, vol. 2, 2nd ed. (New York: Macmillan, 1995), 636–41; and Kelly, *Contemporary Catholic Health Care Ethics,* 108–23.

39. Many of the key contributions to this debate are included in Charles E. Curran and Richard A. McCormick, eds., *Readings in Moral Theology No. 1: Moral Norms and Catholic Tradition* (New York: Paulist Press, 1979). Some of the key names are Peter Knauer, Josef Fuchs, Louis Janssens, Bruno Schuller, and Richard McCormick. For further discussion, see Garcia, "Double Effect"; Bernard Hoose, *Proportionalism: The American Debate and Its European Roots* (Washington, DC: Georgetown University Press, 1987); and Cahill, *Bioethics and the Common Good,* 12–31.

40. McCormick, *Ambiguity in Moral Choice,* 50. See also Aline Kalbian, "Where Have All the Proportionalists Gone?" *Journal of Religious Ethics* 30 (2002): 7.

41. Margaret A. Farley, "Issues in Contemporary Christian Ethics: The Choice of Death in a Medical Context," *The Santa Clara Lectures* 1, no. 3 (Santa Clara, CA: Department of Religious Studies, Santa Clara University, 1995), 7–10.

42. Ibid., 11.

43. Ibid., 13.

44. Ibid., 13.

45. Timothy E. Quill, *A Midwife through the Dying Process* (Baltimore: John Hopkins, 1996).

46. Quill, *Death and Dignity,* 93–96.

47. Farley, "Choice of Death," 14.

48. See James J. Walter, "Terminal Sedation: A Catholic Perspective," *Update* 18, no. 2 (2002): 6–8.

49. Zylicz, "Dutch Physician," 138.

50. Quill, *Midwife,* 211.

51. Ibid., 210.

52. Timothy M. Quill, Rebecca Dresser, and Dan W. Brock, "The Rule of Double Effect—A Critique of Its Role in End-of-Life Decision Making," *New England Journal of Medicine* 337, no. 24 (1997): 1170.

53. Quill, *Midwife,* 210.

54. See John Keown, *Euthanasia, Ethics, and Public Policy: An Argument against Legalisation* (Cambridge: Cambridge University Press, 2002).

55. John J. Paris, "Active Euthanasia," *Theological Studies* 53 (1992): 25.

56. See Sidney Callahan, "A Feminist Case against Euthanasia: Women Should Be Especially Wary of Arguments for 'the Freedom to Die,'" *Health Progress* 77, no. 8 (1996): 21.

57. Frank Davidoff, "Lessons from the Dying," in *Assisted Suicide: Finding Common Ground,* ed. Lois Snyder and Arthur E. Caplan (Bloomington: Indiana University Press, 2002), 98.

58. Ibid., 104. Davidoff references Ezekiel J. Emanuel et al., "Attitudes and Practices of U.S. Oncologists Regarding Euthanasia and Physician-Assisted Suicide," *Annals of Internal Medicine* 133 (2000): 527–32.

59. See Kelly, *Contemporary Catholic Health Care Ethics,* 204.

60. Josephine M. Lumitao, "Death and Dying," in *Beyond a Western Bioethics: Voices from the Developing World,* ed. Angeles Tan Alora and Josephine M. Lumitao (Washington, DC: Georgetown University Press, 2002), 97.

61. Ibid., 99.

62. Ibid.

63. See Cardinal Joseph Bernardin, *The Consistent Ethic of Life* (Kansas City, MO: Sheed and Ward, 1988).

64. See M. Therese Lysaught, "Patient Suffering and the Anointing of the Sick," in *On Moral Medicine: Theological Perspective in Medical Ethics,* ed. Stephen E. Lammers and Allen Verhey (Grand Rapids, MI: Eerdmans, 1987), 356–63.

65. See Thomas A. Shannon and Charles N. Faso, *Let Them Go Free: A Family Prayer Service to Assist in the Withdrawal of Life Support Systems* (Kansas City, MO: Sheed and Ward, 1987); and Dolores L. Christie, *Last Rights: A Catholic Perspective on End-of-Life Decisions* (Lanham, MD: Rowman and Littlefield, 2003).

66. See an informational survey by the CHA, "Parish-Based Programs That Serve Aging and Chronically Ill Persons," *Health Progress* (March–April 1999), accessed from www.chausa.org/PUBS/PUBSART.ASP?ISSUE=HP9903&

67. Vogt, *Patience,* 136–38.

68. Cicely M. Saunders, Introduction, in *Oxford Textbook of Palliative Medicine* (Oxford: Oxford University Press, 1993), vi. See also Cicely M. Saunders, *Dying as They Live: St. Christopher's Hospice* (New York: McGraw-Hill, 1977), 153–79; Cicely M. Saunders, "Care of the Dying: The Last Refuge," *Nursing Times/Nursing Mirror* 82, no. 43 (1986): 28–30; and David A. Benahum, "The Historical Development of Hospice and Palliative Care," in *Hospice and Palliative Care: Concepts and Practice,* 2nd ed. (Boston: Jones and Bartlett, 2003), 3–5.

69. See Cicely M. Saunders, ed., *The Management of Terminal Disease* (London: Edward Arnold, 1978), a volume comprised of contributors all associated with St. Christopher's; and Cicely M. Saunders, "The Hospice: Its Meaning to Patients and Their Physicians," *Hospital Practice* 16, no. 6 (1981): 93–108.

70. Bruce Jennings, True Rynds, Carol D'Onofrio, and Mary Bailey, "Access to Hospice Care: Expanding Boundaries, Overcoming Barriers," special supplement, *Hastings Center Report* 33, no. 2 (2003): S6.

71. Ibid., S11.

72. Foley and Hendin, "Oregon," 303.

73. SUPPORT Principal Investigators, "Controlled Trial to Improve Care for Seriously Ill Hospitalized Patients," *Journal of the American Medical Association* 274 (1995): 1591–95.

74. For a discussion, see "Dying Well in the Hospital: The Lessons of SUPPORT," special supplement. *Hastings Center Report* 25, no. 6 (1995): S1–S36.

75. George Annas, "How We Die," *Hastings Center Report* 25, no. 6 (1995): S13.

76. Jennings et al., "Access," S3.

77. Ibid., S11.

78. Ibid., S4, S53–S54.

79. Ibid., S39.

80. Ibid., S5.

81. Daniel P. Sulmasy, "Health Care Justice and Hospice Care," special supplement, *Hastings Center Report* 33, no. 2 (2003): S14.

82. Ibid., S15.

83. Kathleen Foley, "Compassionate Care, Not Assisted Suicide," in *The Case Against Assisted Suicide,* ed. Foley and Hendin, 297.

84. True Ryndes and Linda Emanuel, "Is Discontinuity in Palliative Care a Culpable Act of Omission?" special supplement, *Hastings Center Report* (2003): S48.

85. Saunders, "Hospice Perspective," 285. See also C. Saunders and R. Kastenbaum, eds., *Hospice Care on the International Scene* (New York: Springer Verlag, 1997); Henk ten Have and David Clark, eds., *The Ethics of Palliative Care: European Perspectives* (Buckingham: Open University Press, 2002); and Kenji Eguchi, Jean Ikastersky, and Ronald Feld, eds., *Palliative Medicine: Current Perspectives and Future Directions* (Tokyo: Springer, 1998).

86. Robert Kastenbaum and Marilyn Wilson, "Hospice Care on the International Scene: Today and Tomorrow," in *Hospice Care,* ed. Saunders and Kastenbaum, 269–70.

87. For a more substantial discussion of the theological significance of Mother Teresa, see Lisa Sowle Cahill, "Mother Teresa: Postmodern Saint or Christian Classic?" *Criterion* 39, no. 3 (2000): 18–25, 37.

88. Michael Place resigned as head of CHA in 2005.

89. This is published as a large binder, with a book titled *Care of the Dying: A Catholic Perspective*; two monographs by theological bioethicist Richard Gula, *Euthanasia and Assisted Suicide: Positioning the Debate* and *Principled and Virtuous Care of the Dying: A Catholic Response to Euthanasia*; and four "modules" for implementing the perspective among health care governance leaders, administrators, physicians and nurses, and institutional mission leaders. It includes as appendices a bibliography and selected readings. The publication is available from the CHA, 4455 Woodson Road, St. Louis, MO, 63134–3797.

90. *Care of the Dying,* 45.

91. Ibid., 46.

92. Ibid., 47.

93. Ibid., 47–49.

94. Ibid., 63.

95. www.careofdying.org

96. International Colloquium of Catholic Bioethics Institutes, "Globalization and the Culture of Life Consensus Statement," *National Catholic Bioethics Quarterly* 4 (2004): 151–58.

97. Ibid., 157, nos. 11 and 12.

98. Ibid., 155.

99. For example, see of Christian Aid's website: www.christian-aid.org.uk/worship/group/chope/stories.htm

100. www.catholicrelief.org/our_work/where_we_work/overseas/africa/

101. www.catholicrelief.org/our_work/where_we_work/overseas/latin_america_and_the_caribbean/antilles/index.cfm

Chapter 5

1. Cynthia Smith, Cathy Cowan, Art Sensenig, Aaron Caitlin, and the Health Accounts Team, "Health Spending Growth Slows in 2003," *Health Affairs* 24, no. 1 (2005), accessed from http://content.healthaffairs.org/cgi/content/abstract/24/1/185?maxto

2. Institute of Medicine, *Insuring America's Health: Principles and Recommendations* (January 2004), retrieved from www.iom.edu/report.asp?id=17632. The entire report may also be accessed at the website of the National Academies Press: www.nap.edu/books/

0309091055/html. On data on the uninsured, see the August 2004 report of the U.S. Census Bureau, *Income, Poverty, and Health Insurance Coverage in the United States: 2003*, retrieved from www.censusgov/hhes/hlthins.html/

3. The United Nations General Assembly adopted the "United Nations Millennium Declaration" on September 18, 2000. The declaration is available at www.un.org/millenniumgoals

4. Dugger, "U.N. Proposes Doubling of Aid," A1, A6. See also UN Millennium Project, *Investing in Development: A Practical Plan to Achieve the Millennium Development Goals*, January 2005, retrieved June 2005 from www.millenniumproject.org,orunmp.forumone/eng_html_03.html

5. For overviews of some of these approaches, see Daniels, *Just Health Care*; Margaret Dahlgren, "The Concepts and Principles of Equity and Health," *International Journal of Health Services* 22 (1992): 429–45; Ezekiel Emanuel, "A Communitarian Health-Care Package," *The Responsive Community* (summer 1993): 49–55; Michael D. Reagan, *The Accidental System: Health Care Policy in America* (Boulder, CO: Westview Press, 1999), 12–15; Cochran and Cochran, *Catholics*, 6–12, 55–58.

6. Reagan, *Accidental System*, 3.

7. Institute of Medicine, *Insuring America's Health*, 7, retrieved from www.iom.edu/report.asp?id=17632

8. Mark V. Pauly, "Trading Cost, Quality, and Coverage of the Uninsured," in *The Future Healthcare System: Who Will Care for the Poor and Uninsured?* ed. Stewart H. Altman, Uwe E. Reinhardt, and Alexandra Shields (Chicago: Health Administration Press, 1998), 354.

9. Reagan, *Accidental System*, 20–21.

10. Laurene A. Graig, *Health of Nations: An International Perspective on U.S. Health Care Reform* (Washington, DC: CQ Press, 1999), 2. See also Paul Wallace, "The Health of Nations: A Survey of Health Care Finance," *The Economist*, July 17–23, 2004, 3.

11. Graig, *Health of Nations*, 182.

12. Martina Darragh and Pat Milmore McCarrick, "Managed Care: New Ethical Issues for All," *Kennedy Institute of Ethics Journal* 6 (1996): 189. This article is an extensive bibliographical overview of ethical analyses of managed care.

13. Wallace, "Health of Nations," 15.

14. Darragh and McCarrick, "Managed Care," 190.

15. Eduardo Porter, "Cost of Benefits Cited as Factor in Slump in Jobs," *New York Times*, August 19, 2004, A1.

16. Ibid., C2.

17. Institute of Medicine, *Insuring America's Health*, 1.

18. Ibid., 2.

19. Families USA, Special Report, "Working without a Net: The Health Care Safety Net Still Leaves Millions of Low-Income Workers Uninsured," April 2004, retrieved from www.familiesusa.org/site/PageServer?pagename=Uninsured_Index

20. National Governors Association, *Medicare Reform: A Preliminary Report* (June 2005), available from the website of the National Governors Association: www.nga.org

21. Robert Pear, "Drug Law Is Seen Leading to Cuts in Retiree Plans," *New York Times*, July 14, 2004, A1. The Medicare drug benefit bill, approved by Congress in 2004, was to take effect in 2006.

22. Families USA, "Working without a Net," 2.

23. Wallace, "Health of Nations," 6, 13.

24. Gina Kolata, "Health Plan That Cuts Costs Raises Doctors' Ire," *New York Times,* August 11, 2004, A1, A15.

25. For example, in 2004, General Electric, whose health care business was among its most profitable ($14 billion in sales), sought agreements with hospitals under which G.E. would offer technology, management and efficiency consulting, and options for financing as a package deal. Reed Abelson and Milt Freudenheim, "The Conglomerate Will See You Now: Is What's Good for G.E. Good for Health Care?" *New York Times,* July 18, 2004, Section 3, 1.

26. Interview, "Schroeder Reflects on the Uninsured," originally published by *American Health Line,* April 2, 2004; also available on the website of the Robert Wood Johnson Foundation: www.rwjf.org/news/featureDetail.jsp?id=25. The Robert Wood Johnson Foundation was begun in 1972 with the mission to improve health and health care in the United States. First concerned with access, it became focused in the 1980s on rising costs, and in the 1990s on reform of the health care system.

27. Institute of Medicine, *Unequal Treatment: Confronting Racial and Ethnic Disparities in Health Care,* retrieved from http://national-academies.org. See also a news release, "Minorities More Likely to Receive Lower-Quality Health Care, Regardless of Income and Insurance Coverage," at the same Web address.

28. See also Risa Lavizzo-Maurey, "Bias in Health Care," Newark, NJ, *Star-Ledger,* April 16, 2002, retrieved from www.rwjf.org/news/featureDetail.jsp?id=28. Dr. Lavizzo-Maurey is an African American physician and president of the Robert Woods Johnson Foundation.

29. Meredith Minkler, "Poverty Kills," *The Park Ridge Center Bulletin,* July/August 1999, 3–4.

30. Norman Daniels, Bruce P. Kennedy, and Ichiro Kawachi, "Why Justice Is Good for Our Health: The Social Determinants of Health Inequalities," *Daedalus* 128, no. 4 (1999): 215–51.

31. Reagan, *Accidental System,* 152–53.

32. Ibid., 153.

33. Interview, "Schroeder," 3.

34. Wallace, "Health of Nations," 17–18; Alain C. Enthoven, "Where Will Americans Obtain Their Health Insurance? The Job Link Revisited," in *Future Healthcare System,* ed. Altman, Reinhardt, and Shields, 319.

35. Uwe Reinhardt, "Employer-Based Health Insurance: R.I.P.," in *Future Healthcare System,* ed. Altman, Reinhardt, and Shields, 340.

36. Ibid., 347.

37. Pauly, "Trading Cost," 367, 369.

38. Reinhardt, "Employer-Based Health Insurance," 342.

39. Institute of Medicine, *Insuring America,* 5.

40. Ibid., 5–6.

41. Pauly, "Trading Cost," 364.

42. Ibid., 372.

43. News Release, "Survey: Uninsured Most Pressing Health Policy Concern," retrieved from the Robert Wood Johnson website: www.rwjf.org/news/features Detail.jsp?id=31

44. U.S. Bishops, "Resolution on Health Care Reform," *Origins* 23, no. 7 (1993): 97, 99–102. For a briefer updated statement, see "Health Care: The Uninsured," 2001, issued

by the Committee on Social Development and World Peace of the United States Conference of Catholic Bishops, available at www.usccb.org/sdwp/national/hlthcarebac.htm

45. Presbyterian Church (USA) [hereafter PCUSA], "An Affirmation on Advocacy on Behalf of the Uninsured" (2002), as part of its national health ministries, retrieved from www.pcusa.org/healthusa/policies/behalf-uninsured-htm

46. See Kauffman, *Ministry and Meaning.*

47. U.S. Bishops, "Resolution on Health Care Reform," 99, all from section IA.

48. Ibid., 100, section II.

49. Joseph Bernardin, "A Consistent Ethic of Life: An American-Catholic Dialogue," Gannon Lecture, Fordham University, 1983, in John P. Langan, ed., *Joseph Cardinal Bernardin: A Moral Vision for America* (Washington, DC: Georgetown University Press, 1998), 14.

50. Michael D. Place, "The Consistent Ethic of Life and Health Care Revisited," Second Annual Joseph Cardinal Bernardin Memorial Lecture, Catholic Theological Union, Chicago, 1999 (St. Louis, MO: Catholic Health Association, 1999), 2.

51. Ibid., 14.

52. Kauffman, *Ministry and Meaning,* 27.

53. See Suzy Farren, *A Call to Care: The Women Who Built Catholic Healthcare in America* (St. Louis, MO: Catholic Health Association, 1996).

54. CHA, *Advocacy Agenda: 2003 and 2004* (St. Louis, MO: Catholic Health Association, 2002); for further information, see www.chausa.org/CHASITE.ASP, where there are links to the updated advocacy agenda and advocacy resources.

55. Place, "Consistent Ethic Revisited," 26.

56. Larry S. Gage, "The Future of Safety-Net Hospitals;" and James Reuter and Darrell J. Gaskin, "The Role of Academic Health Centers and Teaching Hospitals in Providing Care for the Poor," both in *Future Healthcare System,* ed. Altman, Reinhardt, and Shields, 129–49 and 151–63, respectively.

57. Institute of Medicine, *America's Health Care Safety Net: Intact but Endangered* (Washington, DC: National Academies Press, 2000), 2.

58. Philip S. Keane, *Catholicism and Health-Care Justice: Problems, Potential and Solutions* (Mahwah, NJ: Paulist Press, 2002), 119.

59. Georgetown University Institute for Health Care Research and Policy, "Executive Summary," *A Commitment to Caring: The Role of Catholic Hospitals in the Health Care Safety Net* (St. Louis, MO: Catholic Health Association, 2002), iv. Also available at www.chausa.org/PUBLICPO/SAFTEYNET.ASP

60. Ibid., iii.

61. Ibid., ii.

62. Ibid., ii.

63. In 2004, Northridge Medical Center, Los Angeles, owned by Catholic Healthcare West, was forced to close, after having lost $1 million a month for a year. The hospital delivered 250 babies a month and had 26,000 emergency room visits a year. Some of its workload was to be transferred to Presbyterian Hospital, one mile away. California Healthcare West was to continue to operate a sister center, eight miles away. Nick Madigan, "Los Angeles Emergency Care Crisis Deepens," *New York Times,* August 21, 2004, retrieved from http://query.nytimes.com/search/query?srcht=s&srchst=&vendor=&query=%22Los+Angeles+Emergency+Care+Crisis+Deepens%22&date_select=site1week&submit.x=56&submit.y=10&submit=Search

64. Georgetown, *Commitment to Caring,* iv.

65. Townes, *Breaking the Fine Rain of Death,* 179.

66. Ibid., 180–81.

67. Place, "Consistent Ethic Revisited," 31.

68. B. Andrew Lustig, "Reform and Rationing: Reflections on Health Care in Light of Catholic Social Teaching," in *Secular Bioethics in Theological Perspective,* ed. Earl E. Shelp (Dordrecht, Neth.: Kluwer, 1996), 32. Lustig offers an overview of recent U.S. bishops' statements, in light of the common good tradition.

69. U.S. Conference of Catholic Bishops, *Directives,* 5, retrieved from www.usccb.org/bishops/directives.htm

70. Ibid., 12.

71. See a special issue of the *Journal of Medicine and Philosophy* 24, no. 3 (1999), edited by Kevin Wm. Wildes and M. Cathleen Kaveny, on the theme "Is Health Care A Commodity?"

72. Verhey, *Strange World,* 371–72.

73. CHA, *Continuing the Commitment: A Pathway to Health Care Reform* (St. Louis, MO: Catholic Health Association, 2000). Also available at www.chausa.org/PUBLICPO/PUBLICPO.asp

74. Ibid., "Foreword."

75. See Michael D. Place, "The Health Care Reform Equation," *America,* March 26, 2001, 8–13.

76. www.chausea.org/$memb/publicpo/ctuoverview.asp

77. See http://covertheuninsuredweek.org

78. www.chausa.org/PUBLICPO/PUBLICPO.ASP

79. CHA Staff, "Catholic Health Association Calls for Stronger National Will to Ensure Affordable and Accessible Health Care for All," citing a statement by President Michael Place, May 5, 2004, retrieved from www.chausa.org/newsrel/r04050a.asp

80. Michael D. Place, "The Health Care Crisis," *America,* December 13, 2004, 9.

81. Ibid.

82. CHA Staff, "Ministry Mobilized around the Uninsured," retrieved from www.chausea.org/$memb/publicpo/ctuoverview.asp

83. See several interfaith examples in PCUSA, "Affirmation on Behalf of the Uninsured," retrieved from www.apps.pcusa.org/health/usa/policies/behalf-uninsured.htm. See also the Christian Community Health Fellowship, at www.cchf.org; and the Interfaith health program, at www.ihpnet.org

84. CHA, Summary Report, "Catholic Ministries as Catalysts for Healthier Communities," retrieved from www.chausa.org/SAB/HEALTHIER_COMMUNITIES_ASP

85. CHA Staff, "Collaboration the Key to Providing Care for the Uninsured," retrieved from www.chausa.org/03ASSEMB/2003INSIDEM8.ASP

86. Debi Sampsel, "Community Networks: Partnerships between Catholic Charities and Catholic Healthcare Organizations," *Health Progress* 78, no. 1 (1997): 59–67.

87. Carter Center, *Strong Partners: A Report on Realigning Religious Health Assets for Community Health* (Atlanta: Carter Center, 1997), 75. This report resulted from a 1997 conference of the Carter Center's Interfaith Health Program, "Realigning Religious Health Assets," which it cosponsored with the Centers for Disease Control and Prevention. See also www.ihpnet.org/

88. William Foege, "The Value of Religious Health Assets," in *Strong Partners,* 4.

89. "Case History: Kansas Methodists Turn From Acute Care to Public Health," in *Strong Partners,* 74.

90. Gary Gunderson, "On Faith, Science, and Hope," in *Strong Partners,* 14.

91. Ibid., 20.

92. Gary Gunderson, *Boundary Leaders: Leadership Skills for People of Faith* (Minneapolis: Fortress Press, 2004), 58, 103.

93. Ibid., 127.

94. Ibid., 145.

95. Jon D. Fuller and James F. Keenan, "The Language of Human Rights and Social Justice in the Face of HIV/AIDS," *Budhi* (fall 2004): 211–31. Fuller and Keenan survey the contributions of theologians on the social ramifications of AIDS, citing many contributors to James F. Keenan, ed., with Jon D. Fuller, Lisa Sowle Cahill, and Kevin Kelly, *Catholic Ethicists on HIV/AIDS Prevention* (New York: Continuum, 2000).

96. Donald E. Messer, *Breaking the Conspiracy of Silence: Christian Churches and the Global AIDS Crisis* (Minneapolis: Fortress, 2004), 164.

97. Maria Cimperman, "Fundamental Ethics in an Age of AIDS" (Ph.D. diss., Boston College, 2003).

98. Edwin Vasquez, "The Brazilian Case: Applying a Catholic Understanding of the Common Good to Patent Law Regarding HIV/AIDS Drugs" (S.T.D. diss., Weston Jesuit School of Theology, 2005).

99. Tessa Marcus, *To Live a Decent Life: Bridging the Gaps* (Praetoria, South Africa: Southern African Catholic Bishops' Conference, 2004), 5.

100. Ibid., 41.

101. See Jon D. Fuller and James F. Keenan, "Church Politics and HIV Prevention: Why Is the Condom Question So Significant and So Neuralgic?" in *Between Poetry and Politics: Essays in Honor of Enda McDonagh,* ed. Linda Hogan and Barbara FitzGerald (Dublin: Columba Press, 2003), 158–81; James Olaitan Ajayi, *The HIV/AIDS Epidemic in Nigeria: Some Ethical Considerations* (Rome: Editrice Pontificia Universita Gregoriana, 2003), 153–69; Editorial, "When Dogma Costs Lives," *The Tablet,* June 2004; Eileen Flynn, *AIDS: A Catholic Call for Compassion* (Kansas City, MO: Sheed and Ward, 1985); Paul Farmer and David Walton, "Revealing and Critiquing Inequities: Condoms, Coups, and the Ideology of Prevention: Facing Failure in Rural Haiti," and Paulinus Ikechukwu Odozor, "Casuistry and AIDS: A Reflection on the Catholic Tradition," both in *Catholic Ethicists,* ed. Keenan, 108–19 and 294–302, respectively.

102. In early 2005, the Spanish Episcopal Conference briefly suggested that condom use against AIDS might be justifiable within limits, was rebuffed by Vatican officials, and precipitously made a retraction. Shortly thereafter, another Vatican official (Cardinal Georges Cottier, theologian to the pontifical household) advanced his own "strictly personal" opinion that the use of condoms by HIV-positive people was acceptable. The politics continue. See Julius Purcell, "Spain's Bishops Say Use of Condoms, Even to Prevent AIDS, Is Immoral," *Catholic News Service,* January 20, 2005, retrieved from www.catholicnews.com/data/stories/cns/0500360.htm; and "Papal Theologian Weighs Condom Use against AIDS," February 1, 2005, *Catholic World News,* retrieved from www.cwnews.com/news/viewstory.cfm?recnum=34990

103. BBC News, "Bush's AIDS Policy Faces Scrutiny," July 12, 2004, 1, retrieved from http://newsvote.bbc.co.uk/mpapps/pagetools/print/news.bbc.co,uk/2/

104. See Ajayi, *HIV/AIDS Epidemic,* 57–59.

105. For a more extensive discussion, see Lisa Sowle Cahill, "AIDS, Justice, and the Common Good," in *Catholic Ethicists,* ed. Keenan, 282–93.

106. Michael Wines, "Women in Lesotho Become Easy Prey for H.I.V.," *New York Times,* July 20, 2004, A1.

107. Ibid.

108. Gillian Patterson, "Braving Rows and Saving Lives," *The Tablet,* July 24, 2004, 8.

109. Ibid.

110. Southern African Catholic Bishops Conference, "A Message of Hope from the Catholic Bishops to the People of God in South Africa, Botswana and Swaziland," July 30, 2001, retrieved from the Bishops Conference website, www.sacbc.org.za/

111. Health News, "Continuing the Conversation," *Sunday Times* (South Africa), August 16, 2001, retrieved from www.suntimes.co.za/health/news/conversation.asp

112. Stuart C. Bate, ed., *Responsibility in a Time of AIDS: A Pastoral Response by Catholic Theologians and AIDS Activists in Southern Africa* (Pietermiaritzburg: St. Augustine College of South Africa, SACBC AIDS Office, and Catholic Theological Society of Southern Africa, in Association with Cluster Publications, 2003), ix.

113. Ajayi, *HIV/AIDS Epidemic,* 74–76.

114. Patterson, "Braving Rows," 8. At the 2004 Bangkok AIDS conference, reports were made of scientific work on vaginal microbiocides that women could use to block infectious agents. See Jon D. Fuller, "The XVth International AIDS Conference: A Scientific Perspective," *America,* August 30, 2004.

115. Mary-Jo DelVecchio Good, with Esther Mwaikambo, Erastus Amayo, and James M'Imunya Machoki, "Clinical Realities and Moral Dilemmas: Contrasting Perspectives from Academic Medicine in Kenya, Tanzania, and America," *Daedalus* 128, no. 4 (1999): 168–82.

116. Ajayi, *HIV/AIDS Epidemic,* 76–82; Wines, "Women in Lesotho," A1. In sub-Saharan Africa, 4 million children have lost one or both parents to AIDS; the number is expected to climb to 18 million by 2010. BBC News, "Annan Urges US to Fight Aids," July 13, 2004, retrieved from www.newsvote.bbc.co.ukmpapps/pagetools/print/news.bbc.co.uk/2/

117. United Nations Special Session on HIV/AIDS, "Declaration of Commitment on HIV/AIDS," August 2, 2001, retrieved from www.unaids.org/Declaration2706_en.htm.whatsnew/others/un_special/

118. For information about the fund, see www.theglobalfund.org/en/about/how. See also Deborah Sontag, "Early Tests for U.S. in Its Global Fight on AIDS," *New York Times,* July 14, 2004, A1, A10.

119. Fuller, "Scientific Perspective," 1.

120. Sontag, "Early Tests," A10.

121. Peter Piot, "Getting Ahead of the Epidemic," Bangkok, July 16, 2004, retrieved from the Kaiser Foundation website, at www.thebody.com/kaiser/piot_speech.html

122. For an extensive discussion of these developments, see Lisa Sowle Cahill, "Biotech and Justice: Catching Up with the Real World Order," *Hastings Center Report* 33, no. 5 (2003): 34–44.

123. Messer, *Breaking the Silence,* 102.

124. John Paul II, Tanzania, 1990, as cited in "Live and Let Live," the statement of CAFOD (Catholic Agency for Overseas Development, part of Caritas International) for

the World AIDS Campaign 2003–4, retrieved from www.cafod.org.uk/policy_and_analysis/policy_papers/hivaids/1

125. Archbishop Javier Lozano Barragan, "Holy See Delegation's Address to the UN General Assembly on HIV/AIDS," June 27, 2001, retrieved from the CAFOD website, at www.cafod.org/uk/resources/worship/church_statements/holy_

126. John Paul II, "Message for Lent 2004," December 8, 2003, retrieved from the Vatican website, at www.vatican.va/holy_father/john_paul_ii/messages/lent/docu

127. See www.nyumbani.org

128. "News Briefs," *America*, February 16, 2004, 5; BBC News, "Vatican Condemns AIDS Drug Firms," January 29, 2004, retrieved from httpc://news.bbc.co.uk/2/hi/Europe/3442217.stm

129. BBC News, "Kenyan Challenge to AIDS Drug Prices," February 21, 2001, retrieved from http://news.bbc.co.uk/2/hi/africa/1182633.stm

130. BBC News, "Vatican Condemns AIDS Drug Firms," January 29, 2004, retrieved from httpc://news.bbc.co.uk/2/hi/Europe/3442217.stm. The papal message presented at the press conference is the Lenten message cited in n. 125, above.

131. "News Briefs," *America*, 5.

132. www.caritas.org/, www.catholicrelief.org, www.jesuitaids.net, www.christian-aid.org, www.thegaia.org/

133. See the Sant'Egidio website, at www.santegidio.org/en/amicimondo/aids/notizie.htm

134. On the role of subsidiarity in the reform of access to health care, see Benedict M. Ashley and Kevin D. O'Rourke, eds., *Health Care Ethics*, 4th ed. (Washington, DC: Georgetown University Press, 1997), 114–16.

135. See, for example, the website of the South African Catholic Bishops Conference, for the "Message of Hope" on condom use, and for programs to provide treatment. www.sabc.org. See also SECAM (Symposium of Episcopal Conferences of Africa and Madagascar), *Our Prayer for You Is Always Full of Hope* (Accra, Ghana: SECAM Secretariat, 2003), 72–73, on condom use as a possible expression of love. Among the African bishops, Kevin Dowling of Rustenburg, North West, South Africa, has led the way in advocating for use of condoms as responsible. For a review of other international episcopal conferences and bishops who have taken a flexible approach to condoms, see Ajayi, *HIV/AIDS Epidemic*, 153–55. See also n. 100, above.

136. Messer, *Breaking the Silence*, 159–60.

137. See Margaret A. Farley, "Partnership in Hope: Gender, Faith, and Responses to HIV/AIDS in Africa," *Journal of Feminist Studies in Religion* 20, no. 1 (2004): 133–48; and George M. Anderson, "Sister-to-Sister: A New Approach to AIDS in Africa," *America*, August 4–11, 2003, 16–17.

Chapter 6

1. Editorial, "The Abortion Debate Today," *America*, February 16, 2004, 3.

2. According to the editorial cited in n. 1, a Gallup poll found in 2003 that 70 percent of respondents support a ban on partial-birth abortion. An earlier survey from the University of Michigan indicated that a ban was favored by 56 percent of the pro-choice respondents.

3. Kenneth L. Woodward, "Catholics, Politics & Abortion: My Argument with Mario Cuomo," *Commonweal,* September 24, 2004, 12.

4. Cochran and Cochran, *Catholics,* 183.

5. Statistics are available from the website of Planned Parenthood: www.planned parenthood.org/library/TEEN-PREGNANCY/teenpreg_fact.html

6. Cochran and Cochran, *Catholics,* 183.

7. Verhey, *Strange World,* 249–50.

8. Resources and a sense of the grassroots politics and ideological orientation of these approaches and of different expressions of the pro-life movement may be accessed at several websites. See Feminists for Life, www.feministsforlife.org; National Right to Life Committee, www.nrlc.org; and the USCCB Committee for Pro-Life Activities, www.usccb.org/prolife. The latter includes access to Catholic documents and teachings on a variety of pro-life issues.

9. Denise Lardner Carmody, *The Double Cross: Ordination, Abortion, and Catholic Feminism* (New York: Crossroad, 1986).

10. The encyclical, published in 1995, is available on the website of New Advent: www.newadvent.org/library/docs_jp02ev.htm. For a statement of the Catholic Church's position, see also *Declaration on Procured Abortion.*

11. Ibid., no. 3, citing *Gaudium et spes.*

12. Ibid., no. 5.

13. Ibid., no. 8.

14. Ibid., nos. 10, 12.

15. Contrast the penalty of excommunication for women who have abortions, in canon law. "A person who procures a completed abortion incurs a *latae sententiae* excommunication" (canon 1398), that is, an excommunication without an investigation or trial.

16. *Evangelium vitae,* no. 11.

17. Ibid., no. 12.

18. Ibid., no. 43. See also *Mulieris Dignitatem,* no. 14, and *Declaration on Procured Abortion,* no. 26.

19. Harrison, *Our Right to Choose,* 31.

20. John Paul II, "Letter to Women," *Origins* 25 (1995): 140, no. 6.

21. Ibid., no. 30.

22. See also Beverly Wildung Harrison, "Abortion: C. Protestant Perspectives," in *Encyclopedia of Bioethics,* ed. Reich, vol. 1, 34–38.

23. Margaret A. Farley, "Liberation, Abortion and Responsibility," in *On Moral Medicine,* ed. Lammers and Verhey, 434 (originally published in *Reflections* 71 [1974]).

24. Harry J. Byrne, "A Pro-Life Strategy of Persuasion," *America,* January 22, 2001, 15.

25. Among the many works on the abortion debate, four that provide a balance of perspectives of interest to theologians are Sidney Callahan and Daniel Callahan, eds., *Abortion: Understanding Differences* (New York: Plenum Press, 1984); Lammers and Verhey, eds., *On Moral Medicine;* Lloyd Steffen, ed., *Abortion: A Reader* (Cleveland, OH: Pilgrim Press, 1996); and Patricia Beattie Jung and Thomas A. Shannon, eds., *Abortion and Catholicism: The American Debate* (New York: Crossroad, 1988).

26. Lisa Sowle Cahill, "Abortion: B. Roman Catholic Perspectives," in *Encyclopedia of Bioethics,* ed. Warren Thomas Reich, vol. 1, rev. ed. (New York: Simon and Schuster Macmillan, 1995), 30–34.

27. Congregation of the Doctrine of the Faith, *Donum viate* (*Instruction on Respect for Human Life in Its Origin and on the Dignity of Procreation*), 1987, part I. The *Instruction* is published in *Origins* 16, no. 40 (1987): 697–711, and is reprinted in Thomas A. Shannon and Lisa Sowle Cahill, *Religion and Artificial Reproduction: An Inquiry into the Vatican Instruction on Respect for Human Life* (New York: Crossroad, 1988).

28. Kevin T. FitzGerald, "Human Embryonic Stem Cell Research: Ethics in the Face of Uncertainty," in *God and the Embryo: Religious Voices on Stem Cells and Cloning*, ed. Brent Waters and Ronald Cole-Turner (Washington, DC: Georgetown University Press, 2003), 131.

29. There are, of course, exceptions, and political tone is often in the eye of the beholder. In my view, among the exceptions are the pro-life feminism of Sidney Callahan, and the pro-choice feminism of Karen Lebacqz, both of whom seem to me to engage in an open and sympathetic way with the values and concerns of "the other side." See Sidney Callahan, "Abortion and the Sexual Agenda: A Case for Prolife Feminism," in *Abortion and Catholicism*, ed. Jung and Shannon, 128–40; and Karen Lebacqz, "Abortion: Getting the Ethics Straight," *Logos* 3 (1982): 47–60.

30. Lebacqz, "Abortion," 47.

31. Ibid., 50.

32. Discussions of the term "person" are myriad; for an introduction, see Mary B. Mahowald, "Person," in *Encyclopedia of Bioethics*, ed. Warren T. Reich, vol. 4, rev. ed. (New York: Macmillan, 1995), 1934–41.

33. For a philosophically precise overview and discussion, from contrasting yet mutually respectful perspectives, of the thesis that the embryo becomes a person after individuation, see Mark Johnson and Jean Porter, "Delayed Hominization," *Theological Studies* 56, no. 4 (1995): 743–70.

34. Sandra Harding, "Beneath the Surface of the Abortion Debate," in *Abortion: Understanding Differences*, ed. Callahan and Callahan, 208.

35. Mary Ann Glendon, *Abortion and Divorce in Western Law: American Failures, European Challenges* (Cambridge, MA: Harvard University Press, 1987), 53.

36. Ibid., 55.

37. Traci West, "The Policing of Poor Black Women's Sexual Reproduction," in *God Forbid: Religion and Sex in American Public Life*, ed. Kathleen M. Sands (Oxford: Oxford University Press, 2000), 135–54.

38. Frances Kissling, "Roe v. Wade, the Next Twenty-Five Years," *Conscience* 18/4 (1997/98) 3.

39. Woodward, "Catholics, Politics & Abortion," *Commonweal*, September 24, 2004, 13.

40. Germain Grisez, "Catholic Politicians and Abortion Funding," *America*, August 30–September 6, 2004, 19.

41. Mario M. Cuomo, "Persuade or Coerce? A Response to Kenneth Woodward," *Commonweal*, September 24, 2004, 15.

42. Mario Cuomo, "Religious Belief and Public Morality: A Catholic Governor's Perspective," in *Abortion & Catholicism*, ed. Jung and Shannon, 202–16.

43. U.S. Conference of Catholic Bishops, *Directives*, 4th ed., no. 45, retrieved from www.usccb.org/bishops/directives.htm. For an explanation of the analysis of abortion based on double effect, see Ashley and O'Rourke, *Health Care Ethics*, 4th ed., 252–70. While defending official Catholic teaching, Ashley and O'Rourke exemplify the strongly "partic-

ipatory" nature of most recent Catholic bioethics, in that they link their analysis to law, pro-choice and pro-life activism, health care institutions, and professional health education.

44. Christine E. Gudorf, "To Make a Seamless Garment, Use a Single Piece of Cloth," in *Abortion & Catholicism,* ed. Jung and Shannon, 284.

45. John Paul II, *Apostolic Exhortation on the Family (Familiaris Consortio)* (Washington, DC: United States Catholic Conference, 1982), 20–23, especially nos. 22–25.

46. Mary Jean Wolch, "An Open Letter from a Catholic Birth Mother," *Conscience* 17, no. 3 (1996): 25–28.

47. Angela Senander, "Standing with Pregnant Students," *America,* May 24, 2004, retrieved from www.americamagazine.org. The Jesuit statement to which Senander refers is "Standing for the Unborn: A Statement of the Society of Jesus in the United States on Abortion," reprinted in *America,* May 26, 2003.

48. Angela Senander, "Toward Liberation from Abortion: A Catholic Reflection on Abortion in the United States" (Ph.D. diss., Boston College, 2000).

49. Ibid., 16–20. See also Kathy Rudy, *Beyond Pro-Life and Pro-Choice: Moral Diversity in the Abortion Debate* (Boston: Beacon Press, 1996).

50. Mary C. Segers, "Reality Check," *Conscience* 18, no. 4 (1997–98): 38. See also Frances Kissling, "Is There Life after Roe? How to Think about the Fetus," in *Conscience* 25, no. 3 (2004–5): 11–20. Kissling, the president of Catholics for a Free Choice, argues that pro-choice advocates need to find better ways to recognize and articulate the value of the fetus and the difference that value makes in abortion decisions.

51. *Gaudium et spes,* no. 51.

52. Senander, *Liberation,* 103–5. Senander analyzes this and other documents in detail, tracing development since the 1960s.

53. Ibid., 108. She cites *Strengthening the Bonds of Peace,* the 1994 NCCB response to the papal encyclical against women's ordination, *Ordinatio Sacerdotalis.*

54. See the "Freedom to Serve" link on the CHA website, at www.chausa.org, as well as *The National Catholic Bioethics Quarterly* 4, no. 1 (2004), a thematic issue on "Conscience and Culture," which features articles on Catholic hospitals, pro-life nurses, contraceptive insurance mandates, mandated abortion coverage, and law and policy on "health-care conscience."

55. See Catholics for a Free Choice, *When Catholic and Non-Catholic Hospitals Merge: Reproductive Health Compromised* (Washington, DC: Catholics for a Free Choice, 1998); *Merger Trends: An Update to Reproductive Health Compromised* (Washington, DC: Catholics for a Free Choice, 1998); and Amy Nunn, Kate Miller, Hilary Alpert, and Charlotte Ellerton, "Contraceptive Emergency," *Conscience* 24, no. 2 (2003): 38–41.

56. Thomas Massaro, "United States Welfare Policy in the New Millennium: Catholic Perspectives on What American Society Has Learned about Low-Income Families," *Journal of the Society of Christian Ethics* 23, no. 2 (2003): 99.

57. Ibid., 110.

58. David W. Chen, "U.S. Seeking Cuts in Rent Subsidies for Poor Families," *New York Times,* September 22, 2004, A1, A21.

59. James R. Kelly, "Abortion Politics: The Last Decades, the Next Three Decades and the 1992 Elections," *America,* July 11, 1992, 8.

60. James R. Kelly, "A Dispatch from the Abortion Wars: Reflections on 'Common Ground,'" *America,* September 17, 1994, 8.

61. James R. Kelly, "Common Ground for Pro-Life and Pro-Choice," *America*, January 16, 1999, 13.

62. Ibid.

63. James R. Kelly, "A Catholic Votes for John Kerry," *America*, September 27, 2004, 17.

64. An example is the Public Conversations Project (PCP), which began in 1989 in Cambridge, Massachusetts, with the goal of promoting "constructive conversations and relationships among people who have differing values, world views, and perspectives about divisive public issues." Since its inception, dialogue about abortion has been one of PCP's major projects.

65. M. Cathleen Kaveny, "The Limits of Ordinary Virtue: The Limits of the Criminal Law in Implementing *Evangelium vitae*," in *Choosing Life: A Dialogue on Evangelium Vitae*, ed. Kevin Wm. Wildes and Alan C. Mitchell (Washington, DC: Georgetown University Press, 1997), 135.

66. John Courtney Murray, *The Problem of Religious Freedom* (New York: Missionary Society of St. Paul, 1965), 29–31.

67. David R. Obey, "My Conscience, My Vote," *America*, August 6–23, 2004, 12.

68. See Gregory A. Kalscheur, "John Paul II, John Courtney Murray, and the Relationship between Civil Law and Moral Law: A Constructive Proposal for Contemporary American Pluralism," *Journal of Catholic Social Thought* 1 (2004): 231–75, also available at www.bc.edu/schools/law/fac-staff/deans-faculty/kalscheurg/

69. M. Cathleen Kaveny, "Toward a Thomistic Perspective on Abortion and the Law in Contemporary America," *The Thomist* 55, no. 3 (1991): 358. Kaveny cites Thomas Aquinas, *Summa Theologiae*, I–II.97.2.

70. Kaveny, "Thomistic Perspective," 364–65; M. Cathleen Kaveny, "Autonomy, Solidarity, and Law's Pedagogy," *Louvain Studies* 27 (2002): 342, 349–53.

71. Kaveny, "Autonomy," 354.

72. For discussions of abortion internationally, see Rosemarie Tong, ed., *Globalizing Feminist Bioethics: Crosscultural Perspectives* (Boulder, CO: Westview Press, 2001); and *Reproductive Health Matters* 2 (1993), on the theme of abortion around the world.

73. For some of the divisive language in the coverage, see John Thavis, "U.N. Conference Struggles with Abortion Issue," *Arlington Catholic Herald*, September 15, 1994, 1, 12. For the official Vatican position, less divisively stated, see Archbishop Renato Martino, "Holy See: Partial Association with the Consensus," *Origins* 24, no. 15 (1994): 257, 259–64. For an adversarial pro-choice analysis, see Nafis Sadik, "Religion and Public Policy: Correcting the Balance: A Paper Presented in Stockholm and Madrid, October 2002," *Conscience* 23, no. 4 (2003): 37–39.

74. Bridget Burke Ravizza, "Human Rights Language and Liberation of Women" (Ph.D. diss., Boston College, 1999), 40.

75. Patrician Beattie Jung, "What Price Fertility?" in *Infertility: A Crossroad of Faith, Medicine, and Technology*, ed. Kevin Wm. Wildes (Dordrecht, Neth.: Kluwer, 1997), 174. For a more detailed treatment of these themes, see Lisa Sowle Cahill, *Sex, Gender and Christian Ethics* (Cambridge: Cambridge University Press, 1996), 243–46.

76. Miriam B. Rosenthal, "Therapy of Working with the Childless Woman: The Pathos of Unrealized Dreams, the Psychology of Female Infertility," in *Infertility: A Crossroad*, ed. Wildes, 39–40.

77. www.cdc.gov/reproductivehealth/art.htm

78. Eric Nagourney, "Condoms and Pelvic Inflammation," *New York Times,* August 17, 2004, D6.

79. Jane E. Brody, "The Risks and Demands of Pregnancy after 20," *New York Times,* May 11, 2004, D8.

80. See Robin Marantz Henig, *Pandora's Baby: How the First Test Tube Babies Sparked the Reproductive Revolution* (New York: Houghton Mifflin, 2003).

81. Assisted Reproductive Technology Surveillance—United States, 2001, retrieved from www.cdc.gov/mmwr/preview/mmwrhtml/ss5301a1.htm

82. Willy Lissens and Karen Sermon, "Preimplantation Genetic Diagnosis: Current Status and New Developments," *Human Reproduction* 12 (1997): 1759.

83. *2001 Assisted Reproductive Technology Success Rates: National Summary and Fertility Clinic Report,* retrieved from www.cdc.gov/reproductivehealth/ART01/section1.htm

84. Contribution of Assisted Reproductive Technology and Ovulation-Inducing Drugs to Triplet and Higher-Order Multiple Births—United States, 1980–97, retrieved from www.cdc.gov/mmwr/preview/mmwrhtml/mm4924a4.htm

85. Rhonda Shafner, "Egg Donation on the Rise as Alternative for Women in their 40s and 50s Seeking Pregnancy," Associated Press Newswires, February 10, 2002.

86. Gina Kolata, "A Record and Big Questions as Woman, 63, Gives Birth," *New York Times,* April 24, 1997, retrieved from www.nytimes.com/yr/mo/day/news/national/sci-older-mothers.hyml

87. Contribution of Assisted Reproductive Technology and Ovulation-Inducing Drugs to Triplet and Higher-Order Multiple Births—United States, 1980–97, retrieved from www.cdc.gov/mmwr/preview/mmwrhtml/mm4924a4.htm

88. Rebecca A. Jackson, Kimberly A. Gibson, Yvonne W. Wu, and Mary S. Croughan, "Perinatal Outcomes in Singletons Following In Vitro Fertilization: A Meta-Analysis," *Obstetrics and Gynecology* 103 (2004): 551–63. For another overview and sanguine assessment of trends in ART, see James P. Toner, "Progress We Can Be Proud Of: U.S. Trends in Assisted Reproduction over the First 20 Years," in *Reproductive Technologies: A Reader,* ed. Thomas A. Shannon (Lanham, MD: Rowman and Littlefield, 2004), 23–36.

89. American Society for Reproductive Medicine, *Guidelines on Number of Embryos Transferred,* revised and amended (Birmingham, AL: American Society for Reproductive Medicine, 1999).

90. See Thomas A. Shannon, "Human Cloning: Religious and Ethical Issues," in *The New Genetic Medicine: Theological and Ethical Reflections,* Thomas A. Shannon and James J. Walter (London: Rowman and Littlefield, 2003), 120–39. See also Glenn McGee, ed., *The Human Cloning Debate,* 2nd ed. (Berkeley Hills, CA: Berkeley Hills Books, 2000), for a variety of analyses, including Jewish, Protestant, Catholic, Buddhist, and Islamic, as well as the "Executive Summary" of the 1997 presidential advisory report, *Cloning Human Beings: Report and Recommendations of the National Bioethics Advisory Commission.*

91. Gina Kolata, "The Heart's Desire," *New York Times,* May 11, 2004, D1.

92. See www.ronsangels.com/auction.html and www.ronsangels.com/sperm.html

93. Deborah D. Blake, "Infertile Couples: Psychological Needs, Social Responsibilities," in *Infertility: A Crossroad,* ed. Wildes, 154–55, 158.

94. For example, see Bob Shacochis, "Missing Children: One Couple's Anguished Attempt to Conceive," *Harper's Magazine,* October 1996, 55–63.

95. G. Pennings, "Reproductive Tourism as Moral Pluralism in Motion," in *Reproductive Technologies,* ed. Shannon, 99.

96. Richard E. Blackwell et al., "Are We Exploiting the Infertile Couple?" *Fertility and Sterility* 48 (1997): 735.

97. Ibid., 737–38.

98. Ibid., 737.

99. Ibid.

100. One exception was Joseph Fletcher, prophet of "situation ethics" according to the norm of "love," who welcomed the separation of "babymaking from lovemaking" as an opportunity for the extension of human control over destiny. See Joseph F. Fletcher, "Ethical Aspects of Genetic Controls: Designed Genetic Changes in Man," *New England Journal of Medicine* 285 (1971): 781.

101. Paul Ramsey, *Fabricated Man: The Ethics of Genetic Control* (New Haven, CT: Yale University Press, 1970), 38. For an argument along similar lines, see Oliver O'Donovan, *Begotten or Made?* (Oxford: Clarendon Press, 1984). O'Donovan is especially concerned about the possibility that children may come to be viewed as "products."

102. Richard A. McCormick, *How Brave a New World?* (New York: Doubleday, 1981), 319. For a similar argument, see Eileen P. Flynn, *Human Fertilization in Vitro: A Catholic Moral Perspective* (Lanham, MD: University Press of America, 1984). Of special interest is Flynn's use of the moral theology of "probabilism" to handle complex cases for which different moral solutions can be plausibly derived.

103. McCormick, *How Brave a New World,* 326.

104. See, for example, Karen Lebacqz, ed., *Genetics, Ethics and Parenthood* (New York: Pilgrim Press, 1983).

105. See, for example, Flynn, *Human Fertilization in Vitro;* and Sidney Callahan, "The Ethical Challenge of the New Reproductive Technology," in *Medical Ethics: A Guide for Health Professionals,* ed. John F. Monagle and David C. Thomasma (Rockville, MD: Aspen Publishers, 1988), 26–37. For another view, that the "theology of the body" of John Paul II rightly cautions against technological intervention in reproduction, see Paula Jean Miller, "The Body: Science, Theology and Humanae Vitae," *Logos* 3, no. 3 (2000): 154–65.

106. Farley, "Feminist Theology and Bioethics," 182.

107. *Instruction,* II.B.5.

108. Ibid.

109. Ibid.

110. See the *Directives,* nos. 38 and 39.

111. For a discussion of the arguments, see Ashley and O'Rourke, *Health Care Ethics,* 3rd ed., 247.

112. A brief overview is provided by Shannon, *Reproductive Technologies.* Wildes, *Infertility: A Crossroad,* is a collection of responses to *Donum Vitae* and includes this document in an appendix. See also several articles in the *Encyclopedia of Bioethics,* ed. Reich, under "Reproductive Technologies."

113. Jean Porter, "Human Need and Natural Law," in *Infertility: A Crossroad,* ed. Wildes, 105.

114. Paul Lauritzen, *Pursuing Parenthood: Ethical Issues in Assisted Reproduction* (Bloomington: Indiana University Press, 1993), 89–97.

115. Peters, *For the Love of Children,* 33.

116. Ibid., 180.

117. Thomas H. Murray, "What Are Families For? Getting to an Ethics of Reproductive Technology," in *Reproductive Technologies,* ed. Shannon, 115.

118. Maura A. Ryan, *Ethics and Economics of Assisted Reproduction: The Cost of Longing* (Washington, DC: Georgetown University Press, 2001).

119. Ibid., 71.

120. Ibid., 78.

121. Ibid., 132.

122. Ibid., 82.

123. Blake, "Infertile Couples," 163.

124. Ibid., 159.

125. Ibid., 163.

126. Elisabeth Brinkmann, "Embracing the Deficient Body: Alternative Responses to Infertility" (Ann Arbor, MI: UMI Dissertation Services, 2001), 159.

127. Sigrid Graumann and Christof Mandry, "The Ethics of Medical Genetics: An Annotated Bibliography," in Junker-Kenny and Cahill, eds., *The Ethics of Genetic Engineering* (London: SCM and Orbis, 1998), 112–20. See also Lori B. Andrews, "Prenatal Screening and the Culture of Motherhood," *Hastings Law Journal* 47, no. 4 (1996): 967–1096.

128. Interdisciplinary representation of European authors is offered in Elisabeth Hildt and Sigrid Graumann, eds., *Genetics in Human Reproduction* (Aldershot, UK: Ashgate, 1999); Hille Haker and Deryck Beyleveld, eds., *The Ethics of Genetics in Human Procreation* (Aldershot, UK: Ashgate, 2000); Maureen Junker-Kenny, *Designing Life? Genetics, Procreation and Ethics* (Aldershot, UK: Ashgate, 1999). Some of these authors, including Hille Haker, Sigrid Graumann, and Elisabeth Hildt, are or have been students or colleagues of the German theologian and international bioethicist Dietmar Mieth, of the University of Tübingen. Maureen Junker-Kenny is a theologian at Trinity College, Dublin.

129. Regine Kollek, "Technicalization of Human Procreation and Social Living Conditions," in *The Ethics of Genetics in Human Procreation,* ed. Haker and Beyleveld, 140.

130. Kollek, "Technicalization of Human Procreation," 143, 157.

131. President's Council on Bioethics, *Reproduction and Responsibility: The Regulation of New Birth Technologies* (Washington, DC: President's Council on Bioethics, 2004), also available at www.bioethics.gov

132. Erik Parens and Lori P. Knowles, "Reprogenetics and Public Policy: Reflections and Recommendations," *Hastings Center Report* 33, no. 4 (2003): S1–S24.

133. For a discussion, see Kathy Hudson, "Something Old and Something New," *Hastings Center Report* 34, no. 4 (2004): 14–15.

134. President's Council, *Reproduction and Responsibility,* 5.

135. Parens and Knowles, "Reprogenetics," S3.

136. Ibid., S6–S7.

137. Ibid., S7.

138. Ibid., S8.

139. Ibid., S9.

140. Ibid., S12–S14.

141. Ibid., S15–S17.

142. See Dorothy Wertz, "Reproductive Technologies: Sex Selection," in *Encyclopedia of Bioethics,* ed. Reich, vol. 4, rev. ed., 2212–16.

143. For a cautious approach to sex selection that raises questions for both sides, but does not condemn it, see Bonnie Steinbock, "Sex Selection—Not Obviously Wrong," *Hastings Center Report* 32, no. 1 (2002): 23–28.

144. Dorothy C. Wertz, "International Perspectives on Ethics and Human Genetics," *Suffolk University Law Review* 27, no. 4 (1993). See also Jonathan M. Berkowitz and Jack W. Snyder, "Racism and Sexism in Medically Assisted Conception," *Bioethics* 12, no. 1 (1998): 25–44.

145. Dena S. Davis, *Genetic Dilemmas: Reproductive Technology, Parental Choices, and Children's Futures* (New York: Routledge, 2001), 160.

146. Wertz, "Reproductive Technologies," 1435.

147. Stephen G. Post, *More Lasting Unions: Christianity, the Family and Society* (Grand Rapids, MI: Eerdmans, 2000), 119–50.

148. John Paul II, *On the Family (Familiaris Consortio)*, December 15, 1981 (Washington, DC: United States Catholic Conference, 1982), no. 41.

149. John Paul II, "Address to the Meeting of Adoptive Families Organized by the Missionaries of Charity," September 5, 2000, retrieved from www.vatican.va/holy_father/john_paul_ii/speeches/2000

150. Ibid.

151. Ibid.

152. Ryan, *Cost of Longing*, 56–60. See also Christine Gudorf, "Parenthood, Mutual Love, and Sacrifice," in *Women's Consciousness, Women's Conscience: A Reader in Feminist Ethics*, ed. Barbara Hilkert Andolsen, Christine E. Gudorf, and Mary D. Pellauer (San Francisco: Harper & Row, 1987), 175–91.

153. Post, *More Lasting Unions*, 119.

154. For a much more extensive discussion of the ethics of adoption and of the role of religious institutions in adoption, see Lisa Sowle Cahill, "Adoption: A Roman Catholic Perspective," in *The Morality of Adoption: Social-Psychological, Theological, and Legal Perspectives*, ed. Timothy P. Jackson (Grand Rapids, MI: Eerdmans, forthcoming). Important religiously affiliated agencies encouraging and practicing adoption are Catholic Charities (www.catholiccharitiesinfo.org/faqs/services.htm) and Holt International Children's Services (www.holtintl.org).

Chapter 7

1. UNESCO, *Universal Declaration on the Human Genome and Human Rights*, UNESCO Document 27 V/45, adopted by the Thirty-First General Assembly of UNESCO, Paris, November 11, 1997. The *Declaration* is available in the *Journal of Medicine and Philosophy* 23, no. 3 (1998). See Articles 1 and 12.

2. For extensive coverage, see *New York Times*, June 27, 2000, www.nytimes.org

3. See Fabienne Peter and Timothy Evans, "Ethical Dimensions of Health Equity," in *Challenging Inequities in Health: From Ethics to Action*, ed. Timothy Evans, Margaret Whitehead, Finn Diderichsen, Abbas Bhuiya, and Meg Wirth, eds. (Oxford: Oxford University Press, 2001), 25–33.

4. Paul H. Silverman, "Commerce and Genetic Diagnostics," special supplement, *Hastings Center Report* 25, no. 3 (1995): S15.

5. Marcia Angell, *The Truth about Drug Companies: How They Deceive Us and What to Do about It* (New York: Random House, 2004), 91–92.

6. Ibid., 11.

7. Ibid., 200.

8. Ibid., 102.

9. Sheldon Krimsky, *Science in the Private Interest: Has the Lure of Profits Corrupted Biomedical Research?* (Lanham, MD: Rowman & Littlefield, 2003), 9.

10. Ibid., 178–79.

11. World Health Organization Advisory Committee on Health Research, *Genomics and World Health: Summary* (Geneva: World Health Organization, 2002), 17, retrieved June 2005 from www3.who.int/whosis/genomics/genomics_report.cfm

12. Ibid., 12–16.

13. See Timothy F. Murphy and Marc A. Lappe, eds., *Justice and the Human Genome Project* (Berkeley: University of California Press, 1994); Ted Peters, ed., *Genetics: Issues of Social Justice* (Cleveland, OH: Pilgrim Press, 1998); and Buchanan et al., *From Chance to Choice.*

14. Francis S. Collins and Victor A. McKusick, "Implications of the Human Genome Project for Medical Science," *Journal of the American Medical Association* 285 (2001): 540–44.

15. NBAC, *Ethical and Policy Issues in International Research: Clinical Trials in Developing Countries,* April 30, 2001, retrieved June 2005 from the website of the President's Council on Bioethics, www.bioethics.gov/reports/past_commissions/index.html

16. HUGO Ethics Committee, "Statement on Benefit-Sharing," April 9, 2000, retrieved June 2004 from www.gene.ucl.ac.uk/hugo/benefit.html

17. Marcio Fabri, "Power, Ethics, and the Poor," in *The Ethics of Genetic Engineering,* ed. Junker-Kenny and Cahill, eds., 74.

18. For basic information on patenting, see Human Genome Program, U.S. Department of Energy Office of Science, "Genetics and Patenting" (2000), retrieved June 27, 2005, from www.ornl.gov/sci/techresources/Human_Genome/elsi/patents.shtml; and Susan Cartier Poland, "Genes, Patents, and Bioethics—Will History Repeat Itself?" *Kennedy Institute of Ethics Journal* 10, no. 3 (2000)" 265–81.

19. WTO Press Release, "Decision Removes Final Patent Obstacle to Cheap Drug Imports," August 30, 2003, retrieved June 2005 from www.wto.org/english/news_e/pres03_e/pr350_e.htm

20. Audrey Chapman, "Religious Perspectives on Human Germ-Line Modifications," in *Beyond Cloning: Religion and the Remaking of Humanity,* ed. Ron Cole-Turner (Harrisburg, PA: Trinity Press International, 2001), 70.

21. CHA, *Genetics, Science, and the Church: A Synopsis of Catholic Church Teachings on Science and Genetics* (St. Louis, MO: Catholic Health Association, 2004), 13.

22. John Paul II, "Health Development Based on Equity, Solidarity, and Charity," November 1997, retrieved June 2005 from the CHA website, www.chausa.org/misssvcs/JPII.ASP, at www.healthpastoral.org/wordofpope/jpii05_en.htm

23. Townes, *Breaking the Fine Rain of Death.*

24. Ibid., 62–68.

25. Ibid., 151.

26. Susanne M. DeCrane, *Aquinas, Feminism and the Common Good* (Washington, DC: Georgetown University Press, 2004), 150. On the incidence of breast cancer in black women, and the social factors that contribute, see also Susan Brooks Thistlethwaite, "The Chemistry of Community," in *Adam, Eve, and the Genome: The Human Genome Project and Theology,* ed. Susan Brooks Thistlethwaite (Minneapolis: Fortress Press, 2003), 165–67.

27. Lee H. Butler Jr., "Dreaming the Soul: African American Skepticism Encounters the Human Genome Project," in *Adam, Eve and the Genome,* ed. Thistlethwaite, 130.

28. Laurie Zoloth, "Reasonable Magic and the Nature of Alchemy: Jewish Reflections on Human Embryonic Stem Cell Research," *Kennedy Institute of Ethics Journal* 12, no. 1 (2002): 88.

29. Sondra Wheeler, "Talking Like Believers: Christians and Jews in the Embryonic Stem Cell Debate," in *God and the Embryo*, ed. Waters and Cole-Turner, 153.

30. M. Therese Lysaught, ""What Would You Do If . . . ? Human Embryonic Stem Cell Research and the Defense of the Innocent," in *Stem Cell Research: New Frontiers in Science and Ethics*, ed. Nancy E. Snow (Notre Dame, IN: University of Notre Dame Press, 2003), 167–93.

31. Andrea Vicini, "The Ethics of Genetic Technology: Knowledge, the Common Good, and Healing: The Case of the Human Genome Project" (Ph.D. diss., Boston College, 2000).

32. Brent Waters, "Does the Embryo Have a Moral Status?" in *God and the Embryo*, ed. Waters and Cole-Turner, 73.

33. See Hefner, "Evolution of the Created Co-Creator," 211–33.

34. Maureen Junker-Kenny, "Embryos in vitro, Personhood, and Rights," in *Designing Life? Genetics, Procreation, and Ethics*, ed. Maureen Junker-Kenny (Aldershot, UK: Ashgate, 1999), 152. See also John Hardt, "Bioethics and Moral Anthropology: The Case of Genetic Enhancement" (Ph.D. diss., Boston College, 2005), which includes an extended critique of the co-creator metaphor.

35. Bart Hansen and Paul Schotsmans, "Stem Cell Research: A Theological Interpretation," *Ephemerides Theologicae Lovanienses* 80, no. 4 (2004): 364–71.

36. Chapman, *Unprecedented Choices: Religious Ethics at the Frontiers of Genetic Science* (Minneapolis: Forress Press, 1999), 256.

37. For representative statements by religious bodies, see Waters and Cole-Turner, eds., *God and the Embryo*, Appendices A–H, 163–205.

38. For a legal and policy overview of events following the president's decision, see Cynthia B Cohen, "Stem Cell Research in the U.S. after the President's Speech of August 2001," *Kennedy Institute of Ethics Journal* 14, no. 1 (2004): 97–98.

39. The President's Council on Bioethics, "Human Cloning and Human Dignity: An Ethical Inquiry," in *God and the Embryo*, ed. Waters and Cole-Turner, 206–21.

40. For a range of theological and denominational viewpoints, see Waters and Cole-Turner, eds., *God and the Embryo*; Suzanne Holland, Karen Lebacqz, and Laurie Zoloth, eds., *The Human Embryonic Stem Cell Debate: Science, Ethics and Public Policy* (Cambridge, MA: MIT Press, 2001); and Snow, ed., *Stem Cell Research*.

41. President's Council, "Human Cloning," 215.

42. Ibid., 216.

43. Eric Cohen, "Of Embryos and Empire," *The New Atlantis* 2 (summer 2003): 10.

44. Ibid., 11.

45. John M. Broder and Andrew Pollack, "Californians to Vote on Spending $3 Billion on Stem Cell Research," *New York Times*, September 20, 2004, A1, A19.

46. Daniel Callahan, "Promises, Promises: Is Embryonic Stem-Cell Research Sound Public Policy?" *Commonweal*, January 14, 2005, 12–13.

47. See *Genetic Crossroads*, the e-mail newsletter of the Center for Genetics and Society, September 23, 2004. For information, go to www.genetics-and-society.org/newsletter

48. National Academies, Committee on Guidelines for Human Embryonic Stem Cell Research, National Research Council, *Guidelines for Human Embryonic Stem Cell Research*

(Washington, DC: National Academies Press, 2005). This report is also available on the website of the National Academies, www.national-academies.org/, through the "publications" link (at http://books.nap.edu/catalog/11278.html

49. Snow, ed., *Stem Cell Research.*

50. Karen Lebacqz, "Stem Cell Ethics: Lessons from the Context," in *Stem Cell Research,* ed. Snow, 85–99.

51. Edward J. Furton, "Levels of Moral Complicity in the Act of Human Embryo Destruction," and Richard M. Doerflinger, "The Ethics and Policy of Embryonic Stem Cell Research: A Catholic Perspective," in *Stem Cell Research,* ed. Snow, 100–120 and 143–66 ff.

52. FitzGerald, "Human Embryonic Stem Cell Research," 23–36.; John Langan, "Stem Cell Research and Religious Freedom," in *Stem Cell Research,* ed. Snow, 37–46; Lisa Sowle Cahill, "Stem Cells and Social Ethics: Some Catholic Contributions," in *Stem Cell Research,* ed. Snow, 121–42; and Lysaught, "What Would You Do If."

53. Holland et al., eds., *Human Embryonic Stem Cell Debate.*

54. Ibid., "Introduction," xxii.

55. Laurie Zoloth, *Health Care and the Ethics of Encounter: A Jewish Discussion of Social Justice* (Chapel Hill: University of North Carolina Press, 1999); Karen Lebacqz, "Fair Shares: Is the Genome Project Just?" (82–110) and "Genetic Privacy: No Deal for the Poor" (239–54); and Laurie Zoloth-Dorfman, "Mapping the Normal Human Self: The Jew and the Mark of Otherness" (180–204), all in Peters, ed. *Genetics.*

56. Zoloth-Dorfman, "Mapping the Normal Human Self," 203.

57. Margaret R. McLean, "Stem Cells: Shaping the Future in Public Policy," *Human Embryonic Stem Cell Debate,* ed. Holland et al., 205.

58. Suzanne Holland, "Beyond the Embryo: A Feminist Appraisal of the Embryonic Stem Cell Debate," in *Human Embryonic Stem Cell Debate,* ed. Holland et al., 83.

59. Paul Lauritzen, "Neither Person nor Property: Embryo Research and the Status of the Early Embryo," *America,* March 26, 2001, 21.

60. According to Reuters news agency, the United Nations General Assembly's legal committee approved the declaration on February 18, though hardly unanimously. The vote passed by 71 to 35, with 43 abstentions. The proposal was put forward by Honduras, backed by the United States, and resisted by stem cell research interests. A series of amendments by Belgium to make the declaration more open to stem cell research was defeated. The nonbinding measure was to go to the full 191-nation assembly. "UN Panel Seeks Bans on Cloning," *The Washington Post,* February 19, 2005, A2. On March 8, the UN General Assembly approved the declaration, by a vote of 84 to 34, with 37 abstentions. See www.un.org/NEWS/Press/docs/2005/qa10333.doc.htm

61. Mark S. Frankel and Audrey R. Chapman, *Human Inheritable Genetic Modifications* (Washington, DC: American Association for the Advancement of Science, 2000). See also Mark S. Frankel, "Inheritable Genetic Modification and a Brave New World: Did Huxley Have It Wrong?" *Hastings Center Report* 33, no. 2 (2003): 31–36.

62. Rosario Isasi, in 2004 a postdoctoral fellow at the University of Montreal School of Law Genetics and Society Project, is pursuing international research on the law and ethics of the use of genetic enhancements in sports.

63. See Eric T. Juengst, Robert Binstock, Maxwell Mehlman, Stephen G. Post, and Peter Whitehouse, "Biogerontology, 'Anti-aging Medicine,' and the Challenges of Human

Enhancement," and David Gems, "Is More Life Always Better?" in *Hastings Center Report* 33, no. 4 (2003): 21–30, 30–39.

64. Juengst et al., "Biogerontology," 23.

65. Frankel, "Inheritable Genetic Modification," 32.

66. See Jan C. Heller, "Using Human Dignity to Constrain Genetic Research and Development: When It Works and When It Does Not," in *Genetics and Ethics: An Interdisciplinary Study,* ed. Gerard Magill (Saint Louis, MO: Saint Louis University Press, 2004), 116–25.

67. Frankel, "Inheritable Genetic Modification," 36.

68. Chapman, *Unprecedented Choices,* 123.

69. Pope John Paul II, address to the Delegation of the Jubilee 2000 Debt Campaign, September 23, 1999. Also quoted in Pontifical Council for Justice and Peace, 1999, op. cit. As cited in CIDSE (International Cooperation for Development and Solidarity), "Biopatenting and the Threat to Food Security," 2000, retrieved from www.cidse.org/pubs/tg1pppt1.htm

70. Chapman, *Unprecedented Choices,* 127.

71. The Joint Appeal is discussed extensively by Audrey Chapman in *Unprecedented Choices,* 125–31 and 156–65, and in "Religious Perspectives on Biotechnology," 120–26.

72. As cited by Chapman, *Unprecedented Choices,* 125.

73. Ibid., 131.

74. *Directives,* nos. 31, 50, 54.

75. CHA, *Harnessing the Promise of Genomics: Resources for Catholic Health Care Ministry* (St. Louis, MO: Catholic Health Association, 2004); also available at www.chausa.org/resources

76. CHA, *Harnessing the Promise,* vii.

77. Philip J. Boyle, "Genetics and Pastoral Counseling," *Second Opinion* (April 2004): 4–53. A much earlier work by Karen Lebacqz also poses questions about "normality," attitudes toward children, the need to interpret complicated genetic information, and the inevitability of illness, disappointment, and suffering, as well as of healing. Lebacqz, ed., *Genetics, Ethics, and Parenthood.* Issues regarding access and justice were not highly visible in discussions of genetics two decades ago.

78. Dennis Brodeur, "The Challenges of Advances in Genetic Medicine for the Biomedical and Organizational Ethics of Health Care Delivery," in Magill, *Genetics and Ethics,* ed. Magill, 164–75.

79. For an overview of the topic and of theological responses, see James J. Walter, "The Bioengineering of Planet Earth: Some Scientific, Moral and Theological Considerations," in *New Genetic Medicine,* ed. Shannon and Walter, 161–72.

80. CIDSE (International Cooperation for Development and Solidarity), *Biopatenting and the Threat to Food Security,* 2000, retrieved from www.cidse.org/pubs

81. A letter of invitation to me as a panelist came from Winston G. Carroo, of the Agricultural Missions, New York, NY. Another key planner was Robert Gronski, of the National Catholic Rural Life Conference in Des Moines IA.

82. Globalizing the Principles Network, "Principles for Corporate Responsibility: Bench Marks for Measuring Business Performances," 2003, retrieved from www.benchmarks.org

83. Conference 9 of the FAO Electronic Forum on Biotechnology. See www.fao.org/biotech

84. Andrew Pollack, "Panel Sees No Unique Risk from Genetic Engineering," *New York Times,* July 28, 2004, retrieved from www.nytimes.org. The title of the study, released July 27, 2004, is "Safety of Genetically Engineered Foods: Approaches to Assessing Unintended Health Effects."

85. The sponsors were the Pontifical Academy of Sciences and the U.S. Embassy to the Holy See; the conference was held on September 24, 2004.

86. Catholic News Service, "US Lobbies Vatican on GM Food and World Hunger," retrieved from www.cathnews/409/146.php; a source was John L. Allen, "World Hunger and Biotechnology Debated," *National Catholic Reporter,* September 24, 2004.

87. Caritas Internationalis and CIDSE, "GMOs and Hunger," September 24, 2004, see their websites at www.cidse.org and www.caritas.org

88. Ibid., 2.

89. WHO, *World Health Report 2003—Shaping the Future,* retrieved from www.who.int/mediacentre/releases/2003/pr93/en.

90. Abdallah S. Daar, Halla Thorsteinsdottir, Douglas K. Martin, Alyna C. Smith, Shauna Nast, and Peter A. Singer, "Top Ten Biotechnologies for Improving Health in Developing Countries," *Nature Genetics* 32 (2002): 229–32.

91. Tikki Pang, "Equal Partnership to Ensure That Developing Countries Benefit from Genomics," *Nature Genetics* 33 (2003): 18.

92. Ibid., 18.

93. Michael Kremer, "On How to Improve World Health," *Daedalus* (summer 2004): 120. Kremer is an economist at Harvard and the cofounder of the Bureau for Research and Economic Analysis of Development (BREAD). See also Michael Kremer and Rachel Glennerster, *Strong Medicine: Designing Pharmaceutical Markets to Treat Neglected Diseases* (forthcoming).

94. www.accessmed-msf.org/

95. Kremer, "Improve World Health," 122.

96. Ibid.

97. John Steinbruner and Nancy Gallagher, "Constructive Transformation: An Alternative Vision of Global Security," *Daedalus* (summer 2004): 88.

98. Ibid., 92. The report cited is Committee on Research Standards and Practices to Prevent the Destructive Application of Biotechnology, *Biotechnology Research in the Age of Terrorism: Confronting the Dual Use Dilemma* (Washington, DC: National Academies Press, 2004).

Final Reflections

1. Schillebeeckx, *Schillebeeckx Reader,*86.

2. Schreiter, *New Catholicity,* 99.

3. M. Cathleen Kaveny, "Genetics and the Future of American Law and Policy," in *The Ethics of Genetic Engineering,* ed. Junker-Kenny and Cahill, 70.

4. See Campbell, "Meaningful Resistance: Religion and Biotechnology," 1–29.

5. The phrase "network of criss-crossing communities" is a phrase of David Hollenbach, used to describe the operation of global government in seeking the common good today. *Common Good and Christian Ethics,* 229. "Web of transformation" is the phrase of Gary Gunderson. *Boundary Leaders,* 127, discussed in chapter 2.

INDEX

Ship To:

Kristina Bryce
42 kettle court
Newburgh, NY 125501285 USA

Ship From:

TEXTBOOKSNOW-ABEBOOKS
8950 W PALMER ST
RIVER GROVE, IL 60171

Return Information (cut and attach to the outside of return shipment)

TEXTBOOKSNOW-ABEBOOKS **Order #: 83930414**
8950 W PALMER ST
RIVER GROVE, IL 60171

(Attn: Returns) **DE80858**

Date: 12/20/2010 **Order #:** 83930414

SKU	Qty	Condition	Title	Price	Total
5201935U	1	Used	Theological Bioethics 9781589010758 Refund Eligible Through= 1/22/2011	$ 16.17	$ 16.17

Sub Total	$	16.17
Shipping & Handling	$	3.00
Sales Tax	$	0.00
Order Total	**$**	**19.17**

Order #: 83930414

Refund Policy: All items must be returned within 30 days of receipt. Pack your book securely, so it will arrive back to us in its original condition. To avoid delays, please use the return section and label provided with your original packing slip to identify your return. Be sure to include a return reason. For your protection, we suggest using a traceable, insured shipping service (UPS or Insured Parcel Post). We are not responsible for lost or damaged returns. Item(s) returned must be received in the original condition as sold and including all additional materials such as CDs, workbooks, etc. We will initiate a refund of your purchase price including applicable taxes within 5 business days of receipt. Shipping charges will not be refunded unless we have committed an error with your order. If there is an error with your order or the item is not received in the condition as purchased, please contact us immediately for return assistance.

Reason for Refund/Return:
Condition Incorrect Item Received Incorrect Item Ordered Dropped Class Purchased Elsewhere Other

Contact Us: For customer service, email us at customerservice@textbooksNow.com.